Evaluation of Sensibility and Re-Education of Sensation in the Hand

Evaluation of Sensibility and Re-Education of Sensation in the Hand

A. LEE DELLON, M.D.

Assistant Professor, Plastic Surgery
The Johns Hopkins University School of Medicine
Attending Hand Surgeon
Union Memorial Hospital
Baltimore, Maryland

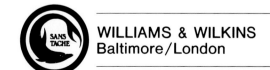

WILLIAMS & WILKINS
Baltimore/London

Made in the United States of America

Library of Congress Cataloging in Publication

Dellon, A Lee.
  Evaluation of sensibility and re-education of sensation in the hand.

  Bibliography.
  Includes index.
  1. Hand—Surgery—Complications and sequelae. 2. Nerves, Peripheral—Surgery—Complications and sequelae. 3. Hand—Innervation. 4. Sensory discrimination—Testing. 5. Exercise-therapy. I. Title. [DNLM: 1. Sensation. 2. Hand—Innervation. 3. Surgery, Plastic. 4. Peripheral nerves—Surgery. WE830 D358e]
RD559.D44   617′.57501   80-20638
ISBN 0-683-02427-2

Composed and printed at the
Waverly Press, Inc.
Mt. Royal and Guilford Aves.
Baltimore, MD 21202, U.S.A.

FOREWORD

RAYMOND M. CURTIS, M.D.

This book more than fulfills its author's purpose by providing a bridge that connects the Hand Surgeon to Neuroscientist, each of these to the Hand Therapist, and all to the patient with an injured peripheral nerve. The book is scholarly and authorative, yet written in a way that easily translates the complex material. The content is comprehensive, and arranged to be of maximal educational benefit. Each statement is referenced, and the reference appears both at the end of the chapter and at the end of the book in a separate bibliography, which will ease future recall.

To place this book in historical perspective we must realize that since Sterling Bunnell's classic monograph in 1944, the vast majority of subsequent texts have dealt with either specific surgical techniques or anatomic studies related to the hand. The trend is toward published symposia or multi-authored texts. Even the emphasis on rehabilitation has excluded the sensory aspects. Thus, Lee Dellon's contribution is unique, and we are indeed indebted to him for this tremendous undertaking. His broad background in basic science and research, his search of the past for clues to the future, his more than a decade of meticulous evaluation of patients with impaired peripheral sensibility have culminated in this single-authored book. The book is reminiscent of Bunnell, not only in specific areas, for example, use of comparative anatomy to discuss the evolution of the sensory end organ as Bunnell did for the upper limb, but also in original contributions. Dr. Dellon demonstrated in primates the fate of sensory corpuscles after denervation and following nerve repair. Dr. Dellon is responsible for urging that our evaluation techniques for sensibility have a neurophysiologic basis. He demonstrated the pattern of sensory recovery following nerve repair, initiated the use of vibratory stimuli administered by tuning forks for peripheral nerve problems, added the terms "moving-touch" and "constant-touch" to our vocabulary, and conceived the moving two-point discrimination test. Equally important he developed and refined sensory rehabilitation to be consistent with this evaluation scheme, incorporating specific sensory exercises at the appropriate time in the recovery process. These exercises emphasize finger movement and object recognition. This Sensory Re-education has produced unparalleled results.

Outstanding is the model of the sensory endings in the fingertip, which is found in Chapter 2. The Section on Evaluation of Sensibility critically reviews the relevance of every previously described clinical test. The separate existence of a vibratory sense is disproved. Finally, the author's own evaluation scheme is described in detail for each potential clinical setting. The Section on Re-education of Sensation begins with the most comprehensive review of end-results of nerve repairs, in which essentially every published report is collated and reduced to a common reporting format. The historical and technical aspects of Sensory Re-education will be welcomed by a world in which this concept increasingly is being accepted, and already producing improved results.

The volume clearly has been a labor of love of many years for Lee. He has recognized that knowledge develops from the thousands who precede, and to these he shows his gratitude. We are under a heavy debt to him. His volume takes its place as one of the outstanding contributions to medicine and biology.

Baltimore   1980

FOREWORD

ERIK MOBERG

Once the world knew only two centers of culture, one in Europe and the other in China. Only distorted rumors connected the two, arriving over endless camel trails. Neither center influenced the other. In order for Marco Polo to see in person these two different worlds and initiate communication, he needed a young unbiased brain together with an ability for fearless traveling.

In important parts of basic neuroscience and clinical nerve work the situation has been similar. On the one hand, neurophysiology is developing a micro-"electrology" capable of tracing even single nerve impulses. In animal experiments computerized studies are revealing much of great interest. On the other hand, the clinical observations of modern hand surgery have added a wealth of new knowledge concerning hand function, impossible to obtain in the animal laboratory. Patients provide the examples to distinguish the different qualities of sensory function and between afferents to the conscious and unconscious level. This is the basis for all rehabilitation. Yet between these two fields the contacts are almost missing. There is even a barrier in their terminology.

The young author of this book is the first one to connect these two antipodes, each so important to the other. Dr. Dellon's enormous enterprise, to travel through and scrutinize modern physiology and other basic sciences and to summarize and combine these with modern hand surgery reminds one of the ancient explorer.

Sterling Bunnell in his "Surgery of the Hand," in spite of the language barriers, reviewed almost all of the important literature. Similarly, as should be the rule in scientific work, Dr. Dellon has included important work from different times and languages. The references are not only mentioned, they are, when necessary, translated, read, and digested. (It is a pleasure to find even the rarely quoted but important work of Stopford from the 1920's included.) And so the information in this book will no doubt remain for a long time the source by which less penetrating authors will escape.

Sensory Rehabilitation, which has been neglected for so long a time from our follow-up work, has now been elevated to an established position through the intense personal efforts of Dr. Dellon. A thorough description of the when and how is given as a necessary guide for this critically needed therapy.

And so this book is unique in the flood of hand surgery literature of today. No doubt it will give rise to conflicting opinions and controversy, which is the basis of all progress. After reviewing the established facts, the author guides the reader to many remaining unsolved questions. This book will find readers from many fields.

It has been a rare privilege to follow Dr. Dellon's work from his early beginning to this outstanding presentation.

Gotteborg   1980

PREFACE

The purpose of this book is to bridge the potential, if not actual, gap between those involved with the neurosciences and those involved with the care of the peripheral nerve. The bridge is a personal one; its construction begun 12 years ago, attempting to seek a firmer basis for understanding and, hopefully, correcting problems encountered in the operating room and the surgical follow-up clinics. It's a bridge whose final span will continually be under construction.

Research into the mechanisms of sensibility, the neural process which transduces external stimuli, has lagged enormously behind research into motor function. Yet, without sensation, the central, conscious perception or appreciation of those peripherally generated neural impulses, the hand is virtually immobile. Without sensation, visual control must be added to guide hand action. Since the mid-1960's, neurophysiologists and anatomists have brought microdissection, single-unit nerve recording, and electron microscopy to bear upon the sensory component of the mixed nerve. These insights have provided a more valid basis for understanding the sensory receptor population in the fingertip, for evaluating sensibility following nerve injury and repair, and for rehabilitating the hand.

However, as the basic scientist and the clinician evolve into ever more highly specialized areas, separation and loss of communication result in failure to utilize each other's vital contributions. It is, unfortunately, rare for either the clinician to read the basic science literature or the basic scientist to examine a patient. Surely fruitful areas for further exploration would arise from the latter, and answers to perplexing problems derive from the former.

It is hoped that the correlated view presented in this book will reach the medical student's lecture halls in microanatomy and classrooms in physical diagnosis. It is hoped that this bridge aids the peripheral nerve surgeons (be they hand, orthopedic, plastic, or neurosurgeons) in evaluating the hand with a nerve injury, in understanding the meaning of that evaluation, and in choosing and completing the indicated therapy, sensory re-education. It is hoped that neuroscientists reading this book will take pride in finding application of their "basic" contributions and be challenged to enter the clinical arena. Finally, it is hoped that this book provides more than a bridge, rather, a bond between the surgeon and the hand therapist, providing rational techniques to allow the patient to fulfill the maximum potential for sensory recovery in the shortest possible time.

The origin of our present misconceptions of sensory receptor morphology and physiology is explored in Chapter 1. These misconceptions are corrected in Chapter 2 with a contemporary model of the glabrous skin and in Chapter 3 with a distillation and interpretation of contemporary neurophysiology. The usually neglected sensory end organs are focused upon in Chapter 4, after denervation and in Chapter 5 after reinnervation. Evolution of my technique for evaluating sensibility comprises Chapters 6 through 9, which present a historical review of sensory testing, critically review alternative approaches to sensory testing, and culminate in Chapter 10, my personal approach to evaluating sensibility. Chapter 11 reviews the end result of nerve repair since 1940 and provides the data base for an historic control. The development, technique, and results of sensory re-education conclude the book in Chapter 12.

The text is designed for maximum educational benefit. Each Chapter has its own bibliography arranged numerically as the reference arises in the text. A combined bibliography, arranged alphabetically, precedes the index. The index is comprehensive, including both subjects and authors cited in the text. The referenced works have each been read, unless the reference is specifically attributed to another author's citation or quote. This required, in many cases, language translation. At the conclusion of most chapters is a section on clinical implications, transferring theory into practice. Where appropriate, new avenues for research are suggested. Where the work referred to is my own, the text is written in the first person. Some of this material, as noted in the bibliography, is "hot-off-the-press," and as such is not yet available in the published "scientific literature." In these instances, sufficient data has been included to justify the conclusions. Thus, this text represents a highly personal approach to its subject material. It is, however, an approach which I believe incorporates the basic science and clinical knowledge of today into a unified philosophy and application.

ACKNOWLEDGMENTS

The single greatest factor permitting my dream of this book to become a reality has been the love and understanding of my wife, Marge, and my boys, Evan and Glenn. The book represents an irreplaceable and precious commodity, time spent away from them. And certainly in the last 6 months of this book's preparation, even when I was with them, I was away. For their realization that the fulfillment of this dream was so important to me, and for their providing the peace of mind required for its fulfillment, I can only say, "Thank you" and "I love you."

The preparation of the book required assistance. I was truly fortunate to be able to work with two talented medical illustrators. Sue Seif did all the book's illustrations except Chapter 2. The illustrations for Chapter 2 are by Mark Lefkowitz and are an outgrowth of his thesis project. I had the privilege to be the scientific advisor to both Sue and Mark for their Master's Theses and have been delighted with the work they've produced for this text. I know their future illustrations will enhance the medical community beyond the foreseeable future.

The photographic contributions to this book are from three sources. Robert M. McClung and Margo N. Smyrnioudis, from the Department of Audiovisual Services, the Union Memorial Hospital, did the studio-staged photography for Chapters 6, 9, and 12. Raymond (Peter) E. Lund, RBP, FBPA, Director of Pathology Photography and Instructor in Pathology at the Johns Hopkins Hospital, and his staff, did the photomicroscopy for Chapters 5 and 12, co-ordinated the special timing required to reproduce figures from journal texts which were kindly loaned from the Welch Library, and reproduced my patient slides into prints. Bryce Munger, M.D., Chairman of the Department of Anatomy of the Milton S. Hershey Medical Center, did the electron microscopy for the book, including the previously unpublished light micrographs of the Merkel cell-neurite complexes in Chapter 2. My deepest thanks to you all.

Special thanks to Walter Ehrlich, M.D., Associate Professor of Environmental Physiology in the Johns Hopkins School of Hygiene and Public Health. He combines both the literary skill of a linguist and the scholarly patience of a medical scientist. He was thus able to translate for us the works of Weber, von Frey, Valentin, and others. His is a unique contribution.

The final draft of this text was edited by my most severe (literary) critic, my wife. Marge wielded the red pen like a scalpel. And for these kind yet merciless cuts, I again can only offer my thanks.

Finally, a thank you to Susan Vitale, Senior Editor, to George Stamathis, Production Coordinator, and to the production staff at Williams & Wilkins, my publisher. The completed book reflects their skill and experience, and I am deeply grateful for their efforts and professionalism.

CONTENTS

Section 1

Back to Basics

Section 2

Evaluation of Sensibility

Section 3

Re-Education of Sensation

SECTION 1

Back to Basics

Chapter 1

CLASSICS

INTRODUCTION
ANATOMY
PHYSIOLOGY

At the outset do not be worried about this big question— Truth. It is a very simple matter if each one of you starts with the desire to get as much as possible. No human being is constituted to know the truth, the whole truth, and nothing but the truth and even the best of men must be content with fragments, with partial glimpses, never the full fruition ... what is the student but a lover courting a fickle mistress who ever eludes his grasp? ... The hardest conviction to get into the mind of a beginner is that the education upon which he is engaged is not a college course, not a medical course, but a life course.

Sir William Osler [1]

The student, new to his chosen field of endeavor, eagerly reads and memorizes the introductory material. It is in a textbook. It is taught by a Professor. It is marked right or wrong on an exam. The student assumes that what he is learning is true. Yes, the student should constantly question. But when the field of study is anatomy or physiology, human or comparative, or all of these, the totality of material to master is so huge there is no time to question its truth. There is not even time to master it all! The student usually is working to his capacity just to survive! During the late 19th century and early 20th century, a few professors of great reputation dominated scientific thinking in these areas. Many of their teachings have been handed down to us, not only unchanged but unchallenged.

An example of material transmitted to us in this manner is the following scheme of the modalities of cutaneous sensation and their corresponding receptor systems[2]:

Touch and pressure	Free nerve endings, particularly those in relation to hairs, Meissner's corpuscles and Pacinian corpuscles
Warmth	End organs of Ruffini
Cold	Krause's end bulbs or corpuscles
Pain	Free nerve endings

The modalities of deep sensation and their corresponding receptor systems are:

Pressure	Pacinian corpuscles
Pain	Free nerve endings
Proprioception	Free nerve endings, Pacinian corpuscles, muscle spindles and Golgi end organs

I began studying anatomy and physiology in 1966. This scheme is from a textbook published in 1978.[2] With the exception of pain being subserved by the free nerve end-

3

ings, this scheme is entirely wrong! The associations are wrong and the Merkel disc is omitted. It is the purpose of this chapter to explain the evolution of this scheme.

ANATOMY

The misconceptions began with the anatomy of cutaneous sensibility. Anatomy in the 19th century was a descriptive science. In 1836, Pacini redescribed the corpuscle Vater had described in 1741.[3] This corpuscle was the first to be discovered because it was the largest, being visible by gross dissection and without magnification. In 1853, Wagner, using a hand lens and maceration technique, described the corpuscle which Meissner, 1 year later, described in more detail.[4] As microscopes became available, gross anatomic description gave way to histology. There followed an outpouring of descriptive material on sensory endings, in many tissues and in many species. This investigative work was not standardized. Every new method of tissue preparation (dilute acid, dilute alkali), and every new histochemical stain brought new descriptions.

At the turn of the century the following techniques were in use: Merkel's osmic acid, Golgi's silver chromate, Ehrlich's methylene blue, Ranvier's gold chloride, Cajal's silver nitrate, and Bielschowsky's ammoniacal silver.[5] But what was truth and what was artifact? The height of this sensory ending proliferation was reached in Botezat's classification of 1912. He listed 36 separate endings in glabrous (nonhairy) skin in addition to those in the hairy skin (Table 1.1).[6]

For me, "the way out" of this seemingly hopeless maze was provided by Winkelmann.[5] Utilizing meticulous silver staining technique, he restudied the hairy and glabrous skin of many mammals. His histology was documented photographically. His book summarized a decade of this work and reviewed thoroughly the previous literature (404 references). In brief, the only sensory end organs he confirmed in glabrous skin were the Pacinian corpuscle, the Meissner corpuscle and the Merkel cell-neurite complex. These end organs, their innervation pattern, and relationship to the organization of the skin, are illustrated in Chapter 2.

What about the Krause end bulb (for cold) and the Ruffini end organ (for heat)? These holdovers from antiquity cannot be confirmed in glabrous skin with the modern techniques.

As reviewed by Winkelmann,[5] Krause's end bulb has gone by several other names: genital corpuscle (as Krause described it in the glans penis), endkopseln (as Krause described in the elephant!), Dogiel's body, and the mucocutaneous end organ. Krause's end bulbs don't occur in normal glabrous skin. The mucocutaneous end organ is the configuration imposed upon the axons by the physical confines of transitional skin. Thus in areas without hair follicles or rete ridges, the mucocutaneous end organ may be found. The Ruffini Body, as reviewed by Winkelmann,[5] does not occur in glabrous skin. Most of what Ruffini described as the most common receptors in the skin were rolled nerve trunks, i.e., artifacts. The criteria for end-organ existence, outlined by Winkelmann,[5] are: (1) repetitive observation of the structure, and (2) continuity between known nerve structure and end organ. These criteria can be fulfilled by studying serial thick sections of tissue gently handled and carefully stained. My own work has confirmed these tenets.[7] Except for Krause and Ruffini, no one has seen their end organs in glabrous skin, and it is time that modern teaching and writing reflected this.

PHYSIOLOGY

As the magnifying glass and gross anatomy were the forerunners of electron microscopy and molecular biology, so may the comparative sensory studies and physiology be considered the forerunners of single unit nerve recordings, psychophysical correlates, and neurophysiology. Johannes Muller is often cited for "the law of specific nerve energies," 1828, which stated that "for each sensation there is a specific receptor, a specific nerve pathway, and a specific central locus of appreciation."[5] In the context of cutaneous sensibility, this sounds quite "specific," yet our review of the writings of Muller suggests a

Table 1.1
Mechanisms of the Naked Skin and of the Hairy Skin[a]

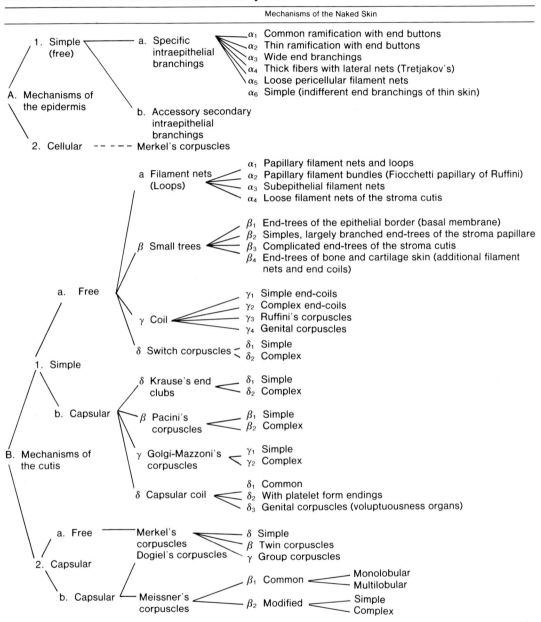

Mechanisms of the Naked Skin

A. Mechanisms of the epidermis
1. Simple (free)
  a. Specific intraepithelial branchings
    α_1 Common ramification with end buttons
    α_2 Thin ramification with end buttons
    α_3 Wide end branchings
    α_4 Thick fibers with lateral nets (Tretjakov's)
    α_5 Loose pericellular filament nets
    α_6 Simple (indifferent end branchings of thin skin)
  b. Accessory secondary intraepithelial branchings
2. Cellular ----- Merkel's corpuscles

B. Mechanisms of the cutis
1. Simple
  a. Free
    a Filament nets (Loops)
      α_1 Papillary filament nets and loops
      α_2 Papillary filament bundles (Fiocchetti papillary of Ruffini)
      α_3 Subepithelial filament nets
      α_4 Loose filament nets of the stroma cutis
    β Small trees
      β_1 End-trees of the epithelial border (basal membrane)
      β_2 Simples, largely branched end-trees of the stroma papillare
      β_3 Complicated end-trees of the stroma cutis
      β_4 End-trees of bone and cartilage skin (additional filament nets and end coils)
    γ Coil
      γ_1 Simple end-coils
      γ_2 Complex end-coils
      γ_3 Ruffini's corpuscles
      γ_4 Genital corpuscles
    δ Switch corpuscles
      δ_1 Simple
      δ_2 Complex
  b. Capsular
    δ Krause's end clubs
      δ_1 Simple
      δ_2 Complex
    β Pacini's corpuscles
      β_1 Simple
      β_2 Complex
    γ Golgi-Mazzoni's corpuscles
      γ_1 Simple
      γ_2 Complex
    δ Capsular coil
      δ_1 Common
      δ_2 With platelet form endings
      δ_3 Genital corpuscles (voluptuousness organs)
2. Capsular
  a. Free
    Merkel's corpuscles
    Dogiel's corpuscles
      δ Simple
      β Twin corpuscles
      γ Group corpuscles
  b. Capsular
    Meissner's corpuscles
      β_1 Common
        Monolobular
        Multilobular
      β_2 Modified
        Simple
        Complex

more general concept. In his book he did propose a theory of specific energy but for senses such as sight, hearing, pressure, friction, galvanism and sensation. He did not discuss cutaneous sensory submodalities.[8]

Direct experiments followed. In 1882, Magnus Blix,[9] investigating the sensory submodalities of heat, cold, and touch, described sensory spots on the skin. In view of the proliferation of sensory end organs being

Table 1.1—continued

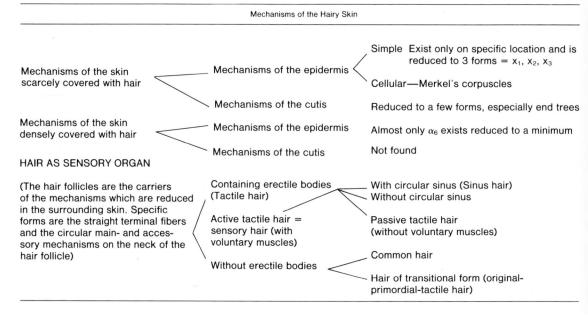

Mechanisms of the Hairy Skin

described during the last quarter of the 19th century, it was only a matter of time until the structure/function correlation began.

The correlations still being taught to our generation were formulated in detail in 1896 by Max von Frey[10] (Fig. 1.1). He was a careful observer and his investigations and writings continued into the first quarter of the 20th century. But his classic correlations were the product of arm chair theorizing.

von Frey did punctate stimulation of the skin. For example, his 1894 publication[11] "concerned the threshold and conditions of threshold in mechanical stimulation"! He found that pressure points ("Druckpunkte") have different thresholds in different parts of the body. He found a continuum between pressure points and pain points ("Schmerzpunkte"), and described punctate sensibility as a mosaic. To von Frey, touch meant pressure and he never spoke of touch as being movement, only as pressure. In studying the hairy skin, he observed that there was a place where the angle of the hair is acute to the skin, and here pressure is felt when the hair is touched. He thus preceded Pinkus by 7 years in describing the "Haar-scheibe"! He concluded his theorizing in this paper by saying that "where there is no hair,

one might think of the Meissner corpuscle as the organ of pressure sense." He believed that free nerve endings were for pain.

von Frey's deductions were made on the basis of comparing "known" receptor morphology with observed sensory capacity plus intuition. For example, he knew the cornea could perceive pain, but not cold or pressure, and that the cornea contained free nerve endings. Thus, free nerve endings subserved pain! He knew the conjunctiva had Krause's end bulbs and could perceive cold. Thus Krause's end bulbs subserved cold. He extrapolated from this to the hypothesis that the cold spots in the finger ("Kaltpunkte") contained Krause's end bulbs. Without such clear reasoning, he assigned the Rufini body to the warm spot ("Warmpunkte").[12] Up to this point he did not mention the Pacinian corpuscle or the Merkel disc.

In what truly amounted to a monograph,[10] von Frey detailed his investigational techniques, tools (Fig. 1.2), results, and theories. It is in this paper that we see the development of his "sensory hairs" (Fig. 1.3). They followed as a more ready means of testing pressure (touch to him) than his complex graphing apparatus (Fig. 1.4). von Frey discussed in more detail his assignment of pressure receptor (by which he meant touch/pressure) to the Meissner corpuscle. He wrote that the *Vater* corpuscles (he never called it the Pacinian corpuscle) were too few and too deep to be cutaneous pressure receptors, whereas the Meissner corpuscles were numerous and superficial. He emphasized again that the Meissner corpuscle was the hair follicle of the glabrous skin. With regard to the Merkel discs, von Frey wrote that "the proposition that Merkel's discs in humans are found in skin where there are not Meissners, speaks against their function as 'sensory' organs,

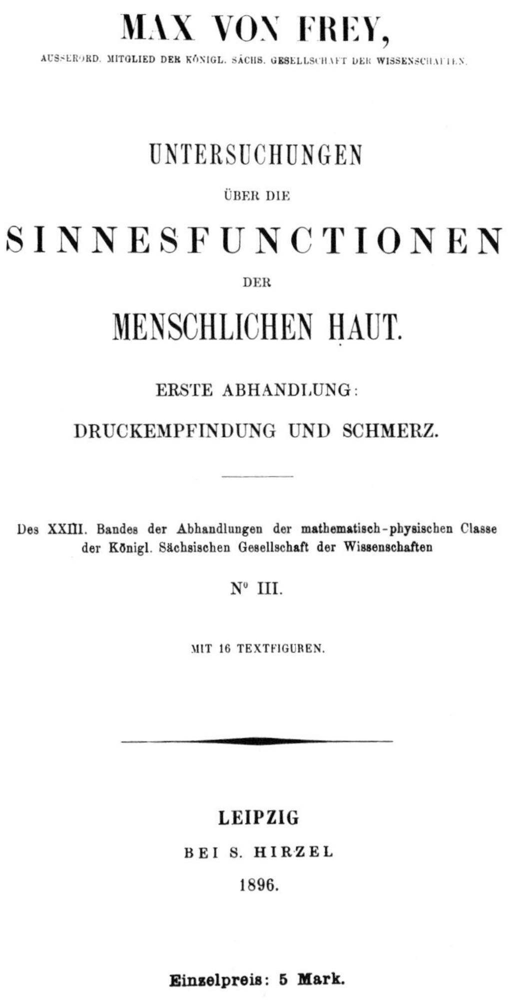

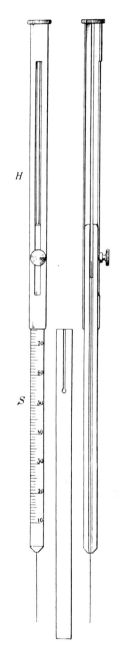

MAX VON FREY,

AUSSERORD. MITGLIED DER KÖNIGL. SÄCHS. GESELLSCHAFT DER WISSENSCHAFTEN.

UNTERSUCHUNGEN

ÜBER DIE

SINNESFUNCTIONEN

DER

MENSCHLICHEN HAUT.

ERSTE ABHANDLUNG:

DRUCKEMPFINDUNG UND SCHMERZ.

Des XXIII. Bandes der Abhandlungen der mathematisch-physischen Classe der Königl. Sächsischen Gesellschaft der Wissenschaften

N° III.

MIT 16 TEXTFIGUREN.

LEIPZIG

BEI S. HIRZEL

1896.

Einzelpreis: 5 Mark.

Figure 1.1. Frontpiece from von Frey's 1896 paper in which he correlates sensory perceptions with sensory end organs.[10]

Figure 1.2. von Frey's aesthesiometer for testing pain.[10]

because the sensory function here is always covered by hair."

To study cutaneous pressure thresholds, von Frey developed a graded series of sensory hairs. These were 40 to 100 μm. in diameter

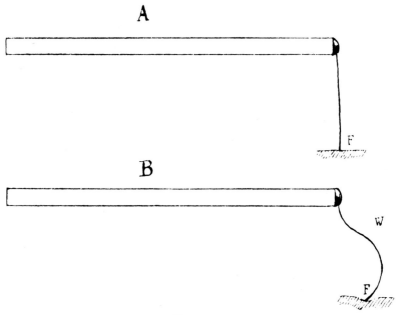

Figure 1.3.   von Frey's sensory hairs.[10] These were made by fixing a hair to a candle-stick. The cutaneous pressure threshold was the force required to bend the thinnest hair that produced a perception.

and made from human straight hair. When these hairs were bent upon application, the force required was taken as the threshold. von Frey recommended a series of hairs, first a child's, then a woman's, then a man's, and finally a horse hair. Pig's bristle was too strong, he found, and caused the sensation of pain. In time von Frey came to call the thickest sensory hairs "pain hairs." He sent a set of these to Henry Head for use in Head's classic studies.[13] An example of von Frey's use of his sensory hairs to map sensory spots is shown in Figure 1.5. Later, von Frey was to attach his sensory hairs to a tuning fork, electromagnetically driven, to evaluate punctate vibratory sensibility.[14]

The next approach of physiologists foreshadowed the psychophysical studies of today. Head,[15] Trotter and Davies,[16] and Boring,[17] each reported elective division of one of their own cutaneous nerves. They then carefully recorded the observations on their own loss and sensory recovery. The most notable controversy to come from this approach was Head's concept of protopathic and epicritic sensation. In essence, he viewed

these as representing two physiologically distinct sets of nerve fibers, receptors, and central mechanisms. The first dealt with early returning, unpleasant sensations and the second, with later returning, discriminative functions. Head did not attempt detailed structure/function correlations. His theory, however, conflicted with von Frey's and a spirited debate in the "letters to the editors" columns enlivened the journals of that day.[18]

Two diverse trends now entered the picture: Neurohistology, as evidenced by the Woolard-Weddel school, and Neurophysiology, as evidenced by the Adrian school. Woolard, and later his pupil, Weddel, correlated sensory and histologic findings, primarily by using methylene blue staining techniques. By employing thick sections and photographic documentation, they were able to record the histologic findings in a way the rest of the world could also examine. They found that a touch spot actually contained many overlapping fibers, that the measure of discriminating two points was related to the extent of this overlap, that pain sensibility was related to free nerve endings[19] and that

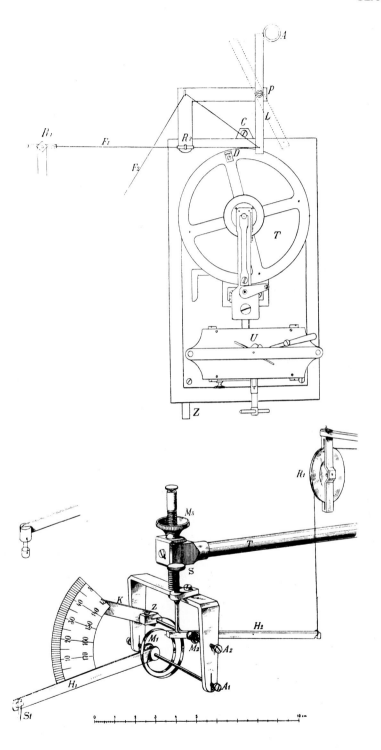

Figure 1.4. von Frey's diagrams of his pressure-recording apparatus.[10]

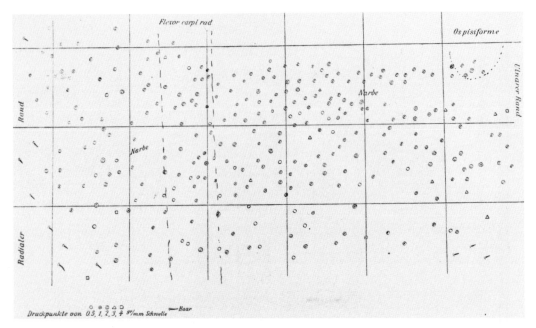

Figure 1.5.   Example of the sensory maps of von Frey.[10] This map, of the volar wrist skin, demonstrated the punctate pattern of the pressure spots.

"a single stimulus at the periphery is presented to the spinal cord as a complex spatial and temporal pattern of impulses."[20] Ultimately, they were to reject the concept of punctate sensibility in favor of a more unitarian hypothesis. They proposed two categories of endings. In hairy skin, these were the dermal nerve network and hair follicles. In glabrous skin, these were the dermal nerve networks and the nonspecific encapsulated end organs.[21]

Other reviewers of the field at that time arrived at different conclusions, however. In particular, Walsche[22] concluded that each sensory submodality was served by a fiber/receptor system that was complete from periphery to the central nervous system. Walsche based his reasoning on the pioneering electrophysiologic recording of Lord Adrian in the Physiological Laboratory, Cambridge, England.

Adrian[23] developed a technique for "single unit" fiber recording while stimulating the fiber's peripheral receptor field. He began with a nerve-muscle model in the frog, progressed to a Pacinian corpuscle—cat mesentery model, and then settled on the Pacinian

corpuscles in the plantar aspect of the hind second toe of the cat. In this final model, Adrian recorded from the internal plantar nerve.[23] In his 1926 paper, he wrote: "The end organs sensitive to pressure are not known with certainty, but they are generally supposed to be the touch corpuscles in the skin and the Pacinian and other types." Adrian applied pressure by a glass rod to the footpad by increasing the weight from 5 to 100 gm upon the pad. Continuous nerve impulses were recorded which adapted slowly to the stimulus and whose frequencies varied with stimulus intensity. In 1929, a report of further studies with this model[24] indicated that "pressure gives an immediate discharge of impulses from the (Pacinian corpuscle)." This work is the basis for the correlation "pressure-Pacinian corpuscle" which appeared in texts for the next half century.

The neurophysiology of the Pacinian corpuscle was re-examined with a more sophisticated electrophysical technique by Lowenstein and Rothkamp,[25] Lowenstein,[26, 27] and Lowenstein and Mendelson[28] at Columbia during the late 1950's and early 1960's. Lowenstein used the cat mesentery model and stimulated the corpuscle directly by "compressing it with fine rods and piezo-electric crystals." Although he clearly wrote "in a rapidly adapting receptor, such as the Pacinian corpuscle . . . ," the fact that his stimulus was one of pressure, that he did not suggest a clinical correlation in terms of sensation for the corpuscle, and that he emphasized generator potentials rather than conducted action potentials, I believe combined to perpetuate the pressure-Pacinian myth.

How can we understand the conflict between Adrian's slowly adapting Pacinian and Lowenstein's rapidly adapting one? In reply to my question, Michael Merzenich, who trained with Vernon B. Mountcastle at Johns Hopkins and is now in the Department of Physiology, School of Medicine, University of California, San Francisco, wrote:[29]

(Adrian) "erroneously described Pacinian corpuscles as pressure receptors, on the basis of what they regarded as direct evidence derived from isolated corpuscles. Vibrations introduced inadvertently with their stimulation led to continuous responses in isolated corpuscles; they then believed the receptor responded to continuous pressure, when in fact they were responding to their accidental continuous stimulation. This fact is hard to believe until you see a Pacinian corpuscle in operation! Then you believe how such a mistake could be made. Surprisingly (this) mistake was repeated shortly thereafter by Gammon and Bronk."[30]

As Winkelmann's work with morphology had led me out of the sensory receptor swamp, so too did the work of Mountcastle with neurophysiology lead me out of the sensory fiber swamp. Mountcastle had tabulated (see Table 1.2) the relationship of mechanoreceptor properties, as defined by single-unit recordings in monkey hands, with human perceptions. He correlated Merkel discs with slowly-adapting fibers, Meissner corpuscles with superficial, low-frequency vibration (flutter), and Pacinian corpuscles with deep, high-frequency vibration. The language of that table is pure neurophysiology and not intended for clinical application. The concept of the chart, relating sensation of a fiber/receptor system based on the fiber's property of adaptation, is the foundation of my approach to evaluating sensibility (see Chapter 10). (The specific neurophysiologic aspects of adaptation are described in Chapter 3.) However, Mountcastle still included proprioception as being related primarily to joint receptors (see discussion in Chapter 9). Although Mountcastle's table (Table 1.2) did not contain reference to dermal Krause's end bulbs and Ruffini endings, these endings are still included in his drawing of the skin and on a table on sensory endings.[32] For the first time, though, free nerve endings are correlated with perception of temperature,[33] and no sensory submodality

Table 1.2
First-Order Afferents Feeding Lemniscal System Via Dorsal Columns[a]

Source	Type	Mechanoreceptor Submode
Hairy skin	Quickly-adapting fibers sensitive to hair movement (movement detectors)	Touch-pressure (and flutter)
	Slowly-adapting fibers innervating touch pads (Iggo)	Touch-pressure
Glabrous skin	Quickly-adapting fibers innervating dermal ridges (probably Meissner's corpuscles) (movement detectors)	Touch-pressure (and flutter)
	Slowly-adapting fibers innervating dermal ridges (probably Merkel's discs)	Touch-pressure
Dermis and deep tissues	Fibers ending in Pacinian corpuscles (detectors of high frequency transients)	Vibratory sensibility
	Slowly-adapting fibers ending in fascia and periosteum (Ruffini-like)	Touch-pressure
	Fibers ending in joint capsules and joint ligaments (Ruffini-like)	Position-sense kinesthesia

[a] Adapted from V. B. Mountcastle and I. Darian-Smith.[31]

is attributed to the supposed dermal endings of Krause and Ruffini.

My own work attempted to base the evaluation of sensibility on a firm, neurophysiologic basis. In 1968, I began the use of 30 and 256 cps tuning fork testing to evaluate the low and high frequency, quickly-adapting fiber group. Movement detection was attributed to these fibers, although a vibratory stimulus was used to test them and the perception they mediated was termed moving-touch. Direct pressure of the examiner's fingertip, or the classic Weber two-point discrimination test was used to evaluate the slowly-adapting fiber group. Constant-touch and pressure were attributed to these fibers and their receptor presumed to be the Merkel disc. It was emphasized that the Pacinian corpuscle was not a pressure receptor.[34] Although there was no direct evidence to assign the Meissner's corpuscle and Merkel disc to these fiber groups, I felt, as Mountcastle[31] had, that by morphologic analogy these were the best assignments. This approach broke the touch-pressure categorization of all touch submodalities into moving and constant-touch, with moving-touch being further subdivided based on the tuning curves of the quickly-adapting fibers.[35]

This approach, and these correlations, were presented to the Johns Hopkins Medical Society on February 3, 1969. The tests were conducted on a series of patients in whom the pattern of sensory recovery following nerve injury had been mapped. On July 30, 1969, the manuscript was rejected by the *Johns Hopkins Medical Journal* with the comment: "There are no data which might support the opinion of the authors and therefore no real contribution is made in terms of proving or disproving any concepts."[36]

Whenever possible, thereafter, I took the opportunity to point out the correlation between Meissner's, Pacinian's and Merkel discs, fiber adaptation properties, and the sensory submodalities attributed to them[37-42] (see Table 1.3). It is gratifying, therefore, to note that in the most recent tabulation of "sensibility and receptor organs" to appear in a clinical text, George Omer has correctly correlated pressure perception with the Merkel disc, vibration with the Pacinian corpus-

Table 1.3
Correlation between Merkel, Meissner's, and Pacinian Endings, Fiber Adaptation Properties, and Sensory Submodalities[a]

Fiber Property	Sensory Perception	Sensory Receptor
Slowly-adapting	Constant-touch pressure	Merkel cell—neurite complex
Quickly-adapting	Moving-touch flutter	Meissner corpuscle
Quickly-adapting	Moving-touch vibration	Pacinian corpuscle

[a] See expansion of this scheme in Table 3.4 and 10.1.

cle, and temperature perception with free nerve endings.[43]

A recent trend is worth noting. At the beginning of the 20th century, increasing numbers of neurohistologists described increasing numbers of sensory receptors. Today we believe that there are three that can be demonstrated reproducibly. Today, near the beginning of the 21st century, increasing numbers of neuroscientists are describing increasing neurophysiologic classes (if not numbers) of nerve fiber populations. One recent categorization is based on Mountcastle's properties of adaptation, but subdivides the quickly-adapting fibers into three major groups (Pacinian afferents, hair follicle receptors, field receptors) and the slowly-adapting fibers into two major groups (SA I and SA II).[44] The current leader in "hair splitting" is the classification of cutaneous mechanoreceptors into 11 groups.[45] While this last report provides a useful algorithm for the neurophysiologist in the experimental setting, I believe that my approach, based upon Mountcastle's work, still provides the basis of a meaningful clinical examination, and the best current synthesis from antiquity and artifact.

References

1. Osler W: The student life, in Franklin AW (ed): *A Way of Life and Selected Writings of Sir William Osler.* New York: Dover, 1958, pp 172–173.
2. Sunderland S: *Nerves and Nerve Injuries,* ed 2. Edinburgh: Churchill-Livingstone, 1978, p 344.
3. Pacini F: *Nuovo Giornalle Letherali,* 1836, p 109. Cited by Winkelmann RK: *Nerve Endings in Normal and Pathologic Skin.* Springfield: Charles C Thomas, 1960.

4. Meissner G: *Beiträge sur Kenntnis der Anatomie and Physiologie der Haut.* Leipzig: Leopold Voss, 1853, p 47, and Untersuchungen uber den Tostsuin. Z Rat Med 7:92–119, 1859. Cited by Winkelmann RK: *Nerve Endings in Normal and Pathologic Skin.* Springfield: Charles C Thomas, 1960.

5. Winkelmann RK: *Nerve Endings in Normal and Pathologic Skin.* Springfield: Charles C Thomas, 1960.

6. Botezat E: Die Apparate des Gefühlssinnes der nackten und behaarten Saügetieshaut, mit Berucksechtegung des Menschen. Anat Anz 42:278–318, 1912.

7. Jabaley ME, Dellon AL: Evaluation of sensibility by microhistological studies, in Omer G, Spinner M (eds): *Management of Peripheral Nerve Problems.* Philadelphia: WB Saunders, 1980, Ch 23, 62.

8. Muller J: *Uber die phantastischen Gesichtserscheinungen.* Koblenz: J Holscher, 1826.

9. Blix M: Experimenteia bidrag till lösning of fragan om hudnervernas specifiko energi. Ups Lakarefor Forhandlingar 43:427–441, 1882.

10. von Frey M: Untersuchungen über die Sinnesfunktionen der menschlichen Haut. Abh Sächs Ges (Akad) Wiss 40:175–266, 1896.

11. von Frey M: Beitrage zur Physiologie des Schmerzsinns, II. Ber Sachs Ges Wiss 46:283–296, 1894.

12. von Frey M: Beitrage zur Physokogie zur Sinnesphysiologie der Haut, III. Ber Sachs Ges Wiss 47:166–184, 1895.

13. Rivers WHR, Head H: A human experiment in nerve division. Brain 31:323–450, 1908.

14. von Frey M: Physiologische Versuche über das Vibrationsgefuhl. Z Biol 65:417–427, 1915.

15. Head H: The afferent nervous system from a new aspect. Brain 28:99–115, 1905.

16. Trotter WB, Davies HM: The peculiarities of sensibility found in cutaneous areas supplied by regenerating nerves. J Psychol Neurol 20:102–131, 1913.

17. Boring EG: Cutaneous sensation after nerve divisions. Q J Exp Physiol 10:1–95, 1916.

18. Munger B: Personal communication, March 22, 1980.

19. Woolard HH, Weddel G, Harpman JA: Observations on the neurohistologic basis of cutaneous pain. J Anat 74:413–419, 1940.

20. Weddell G, Sinclair DC, Feindel WH: Anatomical basis for alterations in quality of pain sensibility. J Neurophysiol 11:99–109, 1948.

21. Weddell G, Palmer E, Palli W: Nerve endings in mammalian skin. Biol Rev 30:159–195, 1955.

22. Walsche FMR: The anatomy and physiology of cutaneous sensibility: A critical review. Brain 65:45–112, 1942.

23. Adrian ED, Zotterman Y: The impulses produced by sensory nerve endings. Part 3. Impulses set up by touch and pressure. J Neurophysiol 61:464–483, 1926.

24. Adrian ED, Umrath K: The impulse discharge from the Pacinian corpuscle. J Physiol 78:139–154, 1929.

25. Lowenstein WR, Rothkamp R: The sites for mechano-electrical conversion in a Pacinian corpuscle. J Gen Physiol 41:1245–1265, 1958.

26. Lowenstein WR: Biological transducers. Sci Am 203:99–108, 1960.

27. Lowenstein WR: On the "specificity" of a sensory receptor. J Neurophysiol 24:150–158, 1961.

28. Lowenstein WR, Mendelson M: Components of receptor adaptation in a Pacinian corpuscle. J Physiol 177:377–397, 1965.

29. Merzenich MM: Personal communication, October 6, 1976.

30. Gammon GS, Bronk DW: The discharge of impulses from Pacinian corpuscles in the mesentery and its relation to vascular change. Am J Physiol 114:77–84, 1935.

31. Mountcastle VB, Darian-Smith I: Neural mechanisms in somesthesic, in Mountcastle VB (ed): *Medical Physiology*, ed 12. Saint Louis: CV Mosby, 1968, Ch 62.

32. Mountcastle VB: Physiology of sensory receptors: Introduction to sensory processes, in Mountcastle VB (ed): *Medical Physiology*, ed 12. Saint Louis: CV Mosby, 1968, Ch 61.

33. Mountcastle VB: Pain and temperature sensibilities, in Mountcastle VB (ed): *Medical Physiology*, ed 12. Saint Louis: CV Mosby, 1968, Ch 63.

34. Dellon AL, Curtis RM, Edgerton MT: Evaluating recovery of sensation in the hand following nerve injury. Johns Hopkins Med J 130:235–243, 1972.

35. Mountcastle VB, Talbot WH, Darian-Smith I, et al: A neural base for the sense of flutter-vibration. Science 155:597–600, 1967.

36. Personal communication, Editor, Johns Hopkins Med J, July 30, 1969.

37. Dellon AL, Curtis RM, Edgerton MT: Re-education of sensation in the hand following nerve injury. Plast Reconstr Surg 53:297–305, 1974.

38. Dellon AL: Changes in primate Pacinian corpuscles after volar pad excision and skin grafting (Letter to the Editor). Plast Reconstr Surg 58:614–617, 1976.

39. Dellon AL: Two-point discrimination and the Meissner corpuscle (Letter to the Editor). Plast Reconstr Surg 60:270–271, 1977.

40. Dellon AL: The moving two-point discrimination test: Clinical evaluation of the quickly adapting fiber-receptor system. J Hand Surg 3:474–481, 1978.

41. Dellon AL: The paper clip: Light hardware for evaluation of hand sensibility. Contemp Orthop 1:39–44, 1979.

42. Dellon AL: The plastic ridge device and moving two-point discrimination (Letter to the Editor). J Hand Surg 5:92–93, 1980.

43. Omer GE: Sensibility testing, in Omer GE, Spinner M (eds): *Management of Peripheral Nerve Problems.* Philadelphia: WB Saunders, 1980, Ch 1.

44. Iggo A: Cutaneous and subcutaneous sense organs. Br Med Bull 33:97–102, 1977.

45. Horch KWM, Tuckett RP, Burgess PR: A key to the classification of cutaneous mechanoreceptors. J Invest Dermatol 69:75–82, 1977.

Chapter 2

NEW MORPHOLOGY

INTRODUCTION
EVOLUTION OF CORPUSCLES
VATER-PACINIAN CORPUSCLE
MEISSNER CORPUSCLE
MERKEL ''CORPUSCLE''
MODEL OF THE DISTAL GLABROUS
    SKIN

While it is as yet uncertain whether the sensitive fibres end externally in loopes or in absolutely free ends, it is generally held that a vast number are externally related in some way to the little bodies known as the corpuscles of Meissner, of Vater or Pacini ... the structure of these corpuscles does not differ so essentially as to induce the belief that they must have different physiological functions, were it not for their varying anatomical relations to tissues.

S. Weir Mitchell, *1872*[1]

It seems likely that further human experiments, in which attention is particularly directed to the end-organs, may extend our knowledge of sensation considerably, and shed light upon the problems related to the receptors themselves.

J. S. B. Stopford, *1930*[2]

INTRODUCTION

The purpose of this chapter is to present the sensory end organs of glabrous skin in their primate environment. This is done in a medical illustration that encompasses the most contemporary light and electron microscopic observations on the nature of these sensory "corpuscles," their relationship to the dermal nerves, and the basic organization of the cutis.

Aware in 1978 that all extant text illustrations of the glabrous skin were deficient in some critical aspect, and aware that the monograph I was planning must contain the most accurate and detailed illustration of the apparatus of peripheral sensibility, I approached Ranice W. Crosby. She is the Director of the Department of Art as Applied to Medicine and Associate Professor at the Johns Hopkins School of Medicine. I proposed a thesis project for one of her students that would culminate in the production of a three-dimensional model of the glabrous skin, a synthesis of current histological and neurophysiological thought. Mark Lefkowitz accepted this challenge and prepared the color plates in this chapter from the model that was prepared as his Master's thesis in 1979.[3] The original model, itself, has been donated to the Raymond M. Curtis Hand Center at the Union Memorial Hospital in Baltimore, Maryland, and has been displayed there since August 1, 1980.

It is consistent with the theme of this monograph that as recently as 1967 a review on the "comparative anatomy and physiology of the skin" excluded the area of mechanoreceptors in glabrous skin.[4] However, within a decade, reviews of light and electron microscopy of these previously ignored sensory receptors had appeared.[5-8] Accordingly, only sufficient reference will be included in the following text to support the inclusion or exclusion of material encompassed in the medical illustrations.

The sensory end organs do not stand alone! Our understanding of their supporting structure comes primarily from the work of Cauna,[9] who worked with silver impregnation techniques and later Weddel,[10] with methylene blue vital dyes. The pattern that emerges consistently is of subcutaneous digital nerves branching beneath the glabrous skin, rising to form a subdermal plexus of fasciculi, and branching again to form the subpapillary plexus or nerve network. These networks contain both myelinated and nonmyelinated nerves. From the subpapillary plexus, myelinated (group A, beta) fibers emerge to innervate specific sensory end organs. The Pacinian corpuscle is innervated at the subdermal level. The Meissner corpuscle and Merkel "corpuscle" are in specific relationship to the dermal-epidermal junction. Beneath the papillary ridge, or fingerprint, is an elongated epidermal peg, the intermediate ridge. This is bordered by a dermal papillae

on each side, each of which, in turn, is bordered by a shorter epidermal peg, the limiting ridge. Within a dermal papilla, between a limiting ridge and an intermediate ridge, is a Meissner corpuscle. At intervals along the longitudinal length or undersurface of the intermediate ridge, a sweat duct pierces the basal layer of germinal epidermis. At these junctures along the intermediate ridge lie the Merkel cell-neurite complex, the so-called Merkel corpuscle. The limiting ridges, bound down to the periosteum by collagen bundles, thus describe a mechanical transducer that transmits a touch stimuli efficiently to the sensory end organs. Along the length of the papillary ridge, these functional units are separated by septae which effectively divide the glabrous skin into small segments, each of which is maximally innervated by a single myelinated nerve for each type of sensory end organ within that segment. Yet overlap of nerve fibers below the septae provide the mechanism for the partially shifted peripheral receptive fields that permit tactile gnosis (see Chapter 3 and Figs. 2.2 and 2.3).

I believe that Miller et al.[11] are correct in concluding that peripheral cutaneous sensory receptors can be divided into three groups: free nerve endings with unexpanded tips, endings with expanded tips, like the Merkel cell-neurite complex, and encapsulated endings, like the Pacinian and Meissner corpuscle. In glabrous skin, extensive modern staining of primate material has failed to demonstrate Krause's end bulbs or Ruffini endings.[12, 13] The end bulbs seen by Krause in mucous membranes have been confirmed,[12] and these, probably with Winkelman's mucocutaneous end organ, represent an attempt by quickly-adapting fibers to form end organs in skin which is devoid of hair follicles or dermal papillae. That is, the mucocutaneous end organ is the transitional ending of the quickly-adapting fiber between Meissner corpuscles in glabrous skin and the innervated hair follicle in hairy skin. As the Merkel cell-neurite complex represents the expanded tip ending in glabrous skin, so the Ruffini spray endings represent the end organ of the slowly-adapting fibers in nonglabrous skin. These Ruffini spray endings have been observed on hair follicles in hairy skin[14] and primate hairy facial skin.[15] This scheme is carried out in tissues other than skin, too. In joints, for example, the slowly-adapting fibers are represented by Ruffini spray endings (expanded bulb endings), and the quickly-adapting fibers are represented by Pacinian corpuscles (encapsulated endings)[16] (see Table 2.1).

EVOLUTION OF CORPUSCLES

In the evolution of the species homo sapiens, the development of the cerebral cortex is a dominant feature. A significant portion of the cerebral cortex is the parietal lobe, which contains a broad area, critical to sensation. It would appear logical that the peripheral mechanisms of cutaneous sensibility that are the input to this central computing area also should be highly evolved. I am unaware of any treatise on the evolution of the cutaneous sensory end organs, but I believe insight can be gained from correlating previous comparative anatomy reports, the classification of the animal kingdom, geologic time, and observations on patients following nerve repair.

In Table 2.2, a greatly shortened classification of the animal kingdom is correlated with geologic time periods for a few critical animal species, using standard reference works.[17, 18] The geologic periods are listed in Table 2.3 for chronologic comparison.[19]

The earliest peripheral cutaneous sensory mechanisms were simple nerve networks as in the invertebrates. These evolved into nerve networks plus free nerve endings in the earliest vertebrates.[20] Such early vertebrates, like the lamprey eel, developed in the Jurassic Period, about 150 million years ago. The Cretaceous Period was at the end of the Mesozoic Era, and was the time of the dying out of the great reptiles, and the origin of the smaller mammals and birds. Deciduous trees and grass were developing, and in this setting ducks and geese, opossum and moles appeared. For these animals, a sensitive nose was essential. In the case of the birds, the forelimbs were wings, and their hard beak, for example, had to serve to detect seeds or larvae in marshland. The beak developed, therefore, as an organ of touch.[21] In the mole, the limbs were digging tools, the eyes were blind, and so, again, the snout developed into a touch organ.

As the need for tactile discrimination was added to the need for simple protective sensibility, peripheral sensory structures differentiated. The best studied birds are ducks and geese,[12, 20-25] and they have two well-defined sensory end organs in their bills. The Herbst (1848) corpuscle is a Pacinian-like corpuscle, and the Grandry (1869) corpuscle is a Merkel cell-neurite-like corpuscle. The contrasts and similarities are best described by Munger,[22, 23] and these represent in evolutionary terms the development of a specific encapsulated end organ for the quickly-adapting fibers (Herbst) and an expanded tip ending associated with an epithelial cell for

Table 2.1
General Pattern of Nerve Endings

Nerve Ending	Skin			Joint
	Glabrous	Transitional	Hairy	
Free nerve	Present	Present	Present	Present
Expanded tip	Merkel cell-neurite complex	None known	Pilo-Ruffini complex Haar-scheibe	Ruffini spray endings
Encapsulated	Pacinian corpuscle Meissner corpuscle	Krause end-bulb Mucocutaneous end organ	Hair follicle	Pacinian corpuscle

Table 2.2
Animal Kingdom

Classification			Geologic Period
Phylum	Protozoa		
	Mollusca		
	Arthropoda		
	Chordata		
Subphylum		Vertebrata	
Class		Marsipobranchii (lampreys)	Jurassic
		Pisces	
		Amphibia	
		Reptilia	
		Aves	
Subclass		Anseres (duck, goose)	Cretaceous
		Passeres (songbirds)	Eocene
		Mammalia	
		Theria	
Order		Marsupialica (opossum)	Cretaceous
		Eutheria	
		Insectivora (mole)	Cretaceous
		Rodentia (mouse)	Eocene
		Carnivora (raccoon)	Eocene
		Primates	Eocene
Suborder		Prosimiae (lemur)	
		Simiae (monkey)	
		(baboon)	
		(gorilla)	
		(man)	

Table 2.3
Geologic Time

Era	Period	Epoch	Years Ago
Cenozoic	Quaternary	Recent	Present
	Tertiary	Pleistocene	
		Pliocene	
		Miocene	
		Oligocene	
		Eocene	55,000,000–35,000,000
		Paleocene	70,000,000–55,000,000
Mesozoic	Cretaceous		135,000,000–70,000,000
	Jurassic		180,000,000–135,000,000
	Triassic		225,000,000–180,000,000

the slowly-adapting fibers (Grandry). An end organ analogous to the Meissner corpuscle is not present in these species. Among mammals from this Cretaceous Period, the mole, and especially the opossum, have been studied. The mole's snout has a sensory apparatus described by Eimer (1871) and elaborated upon by Boecke[12] and Munger.[26] This organ of Eimer has small encapsulated nerve terminals at its base as well as expanded nerve endings in relation to epithelial cells at its base. The opossum snout has both Pacinian corpuscles and Merkel cell-neurite complexes.[22] Thus, the mammals of this period that were requiring increasingly finer tactile discrimination also developed sensory receptors along the pattern described for the bird's bill. But no sensory end organ analogous to the Meissner corpuscle has been observed in the mammals that developed more than 70 million years ago.

As evolution implies transition, I believe we should not be surprised to find a transitional form of sensory corpuscle develop prior to the Meissner corpuscle. The transitional corpuscle has been named variously over the last century. It is Krause's end bulb, Krause's genital corpuscle, Winkelmann's mammalian end organ or mucocutaneous end organ, etc.[12] In essence, in response to a need for finer discrimination of moving stimuli, small corpuscles composed of a few lamellar cells around a nerve terminal developed in the deep to superficial dermis, such as have been noted in the opossum, beneath the hairless snout skin,[27] and in many mammalian species in the glans penis and clitoris,[12] and by Krause in the conjunctiva and lip.[12] The opossum, although evolving in the Cretaceous Period, did not evolve until the Eocene Period or later in many parts of the world, and thus represents a good species for this transitional end organ.[28] The raccoon, developing more recently in the Eocene, was first noted to have these small encapsulated corpuscles by Zollmann and Winkelmann[29] in 1962. Munger and Pubols[27] documented these simple corpuscles extensively and demonstrated them to be quickly-adapting receptors. The raccoon has five flexible toes on each foot, no clavicles, and generally diminished vision and hearing.[28] They are excellent tree climbers and are extremely dextrous with their forepaws. The simple corpuscles in the raccoon lie just at the base of the dermal papillae adjacent to the Merkel-Rete papillae.

The Meissner corpuscle represents, I believe, the most recent sensory corpuscle to evolve. The earliest species in which I am aware that a Meissner corpuscle has been described is the mouse.[30] In the mouse, small lamellated corpuscles, some with multiple innervation, are located within the dermal papillae. Meissner corpuscles, to be described in greater detail below, have been identified in every primate studied.[12]

Thus, in the most recently evolved mammals, the primates, there are three sensory end organs that serve as the mechanoreceptors to transduce touch stimuli. The organization of these receptors with respect to the skin and their nerve fibers is the subject of the rest of this chapter. But, for emphasis here with respect to evolution, I believe the Meissner fiber/receptor system not only provides the basis for the highest degree of tactile discrimination, tactile gnosis, but also provides a high degree of "overkill." By overkill, I mean a high ratio of nerve fibers to receptor. The degree of peripheral receptive field overlap possible in this fiber/receptor system has great survival value. Following a nerve repair,

when a significant number of axons fail to regenerate to the fingertip, the Pacinian system with few fibers to start and a 1:1 fiber to receptor ratio has a small chance to recover, while the Merkel cell-neurite system, with more fibers to start with but with less than a 1:1 fiber to receptor ratio, has the least chance to recover. The Meissner system, with the greatest number of fibers to start with, and a greater than 1:1 fiber to receptor ratio, has the best chance to reinnervate the necessary peripheral innervation density to permit recovery of functional sensation (see Fig. 7.5). Recognition of the Meissner corpuscle as the most recent corpuscle to evolve gives further emphasis to the use of the moving two-point discrimination test (Chapter 8) to evalute sensibility and the object recognition tasks involved in sensory re-education (Chapter 12).

VATER-PACINIAN CORPUSCLE

The facts regarding the historical priority for naming this end organ are best outlined by Lee.[31] Vater was the first to describe the presence of this structure, which he termed "papillae nervae." Almost a century later, Pacini redescribed these structures, adding the description of the concentric lamellae separated by fluid. He believed these were part of the lymphatic system. In 1844, Henle and Kolliker were the first to relate the corpuscle to a nerve fiber, thereby describing the first nerve ending.

The entire subject of the Pacinian corpuscle is reviewed by Winkelmann[12] (but is inaccurate regarding its role as a pressure detector, see Chapter 3). Cauna and Mannan[32] have reported its embryologic development, and ultrastructural reports are numerous.[33-35]

To be emphasized here is that the Pacinian corpuscle is a deep dermal and subcutaneous sensory receptor, 1 to 4 mm long and 0.5 to 1 mm wide, innervated by a single myelinated nerve. Estimates of the number of corpuscles present vary from 200 per thumb, 600 per hand, 120 per centimeter of volar pulp. The corpuscle develops between the 3rd and 5th month of fetal life, which is earlier than the Meissner corpuscle. The axon enters the corpuscle, loses its myelin sheath, and enters the inner core. The inner core contains a granular material that stains for nonspecific cholinesterase. The axon terminal tip contains numerous mitochondria. The axon is surrounded by 40 to 60 concentric lamellae. The inner few lamellae are split by a fissure, while the outer lamellar cells are contiguous with the epineurium of the nerve fiber.

The Pacinian corpuscle may be found in clusters, but in such cases each is usually innervated by its own nerve fiber. The Pacinian corpuscle may be occasionally bilobed, and in such a situation, a cross-section would give a picture similar to the so-called Golgi-Mazzoni body (1878).[12] The arteriovenous glomerular apparatus is found often near a Pacinian corpuscle.

In this book, light microscopy of the Pacinian corpuscle is illustrated with the Masson trichrome stain (Fig. 5.19), hematoxylin and eosin (Fig. 12.25), and with silver stain (Fig. 5.19).

MEISSNER CORPUSCLE

The Meissner corpuscle was described originally in a paper co-authored by Wagner and Meissner in 1852, with the description of the corpuscle further elaborated by Meissner in two subsequent papers in 1852 and 1856.[36] This corpuscle has been identified repeatedly by many current investigators, and descriptions are available in excellent light microscopic studies by Cauna[36, 37] with frozen section and silver staining techniques, by Weddell[38] with methylene blue, by Ridley[39] in human normal and pathologic states, and ultrastructural studies.[40–42]

Under light microscopy, the Meissner corpuscle appears as an encapsulated, oval end organ within the dermal papilla. There may be bilobed corpuscles, but most commonly a single lobed corpuscle is present. The lobulations may be two to four, each appearing full and plump. Within each lobulation, there appears to be a stacked series of flattened discs which, in fact, represent the lamellar cells. The nuclei which appear usually at the edge or side of the "capsule" are lamellar cell nuclei. With Masson trichrome stain, the pink-staining tissue within the corpuscle is axoplasm and the blue-staining fibers are the connective tissue that comprises structural framework for the lobular architecture.[43] With silver and methylene blue techniques, each corpuscle is demonstrated to have multiple innervation, ranging from two to nine separate nerve fibers. Two to three fibers enter at the base of the corpuscle, others rising in the dermal papilla to enter the corpuscle from its sides or top. The fibers lose their myelin sheath as they enter the corpuscle, and the lamellar cells may represent either perineurial (Schwann) cells or modified epithelial cells, or both.

The Meissner corpuscles are related to the papillary ridge and more specifically to the intermediary ridge. They vary in frequency from one every other or every third ridge at the digital pulp, to a frequency of every fifth or sixth in the palm. Rudimentary Meissner-like corpuscles are located in the distal dorsal (still glabrous) finger skin. Meissner corpuscles arise about the 7th month of fetal life and diminish in frequency with advanced age.[36, 39, 44]

Within the Meissner corpuscle, the terminal nerve filaments end as either multiple fine enlargements, bulbs, or loops, or as fine networks by light microscopy. By electron microscopy, each terminal nerve filament contains numerous mitochondina and is ensheathed by a lamellar cell process. No desmosomes have been noted. Between lamellar cell processes is a fine, interlamellar ground substance. There is no true capsule and this interlamellar substance is in communication or is contiguous with the extracellular space of the dermal papilla.

The multiple fiber innervation of the Meissner corpuscle allows for overlap of the peripheral receptive fields of individual fibers in a manner not possible with the Pacinian corpuscle or the Merkel cell-neurite complex.

The innervated hair follicle of hairy skin is most certainly the morphologic and neurophysiologic analog of the Meissner corpuscle in glabrous skin.

In this book Meissner corpuscles are illustrated in trichrome (Figs. 4.3 and 5.3), silver (Figs. 4.4, 5.4, 5.16, 5.17, and 12.25), and nonspecific cholinesterase (Fig. 4.2) stains from light microscopy and from electron micrographs (Figs. 4.5, 5.5, 5.6, and 10.5).

MERKEL "CORPUSCLE"

In 1875, Merkel[45] wrote a very thorough paper, in which he described Tastzellen (touch cells) and Tastkorperchen (touch corpuscles) in geese, ducks, pigs, cows, sheep, and man. That Merkel was thorough is evident, not only from his exhaustive comparative anatomy studies, but also from his referral to the Pacinian corpuscle as the Vater corpuscle, and to the Meissner corpuscle as the Wagner corpuscle.[45] Merkel described nerve terminals ending in relationship to clear cells in the basal layer of epidermis of rete pegs in human fingertips. He called the clear cells "touch cells" and the combination of epithelial cell and nerve terminal a "corpuscle." He never implied an encapsulated end organ for his corpuscle. He believed it to be an end organ for touch.

Merkel's osmium preparations may well have been demonstrating melanocytes, but other investigators of his era made similar observations, such as Ranvier, using gold chloride (1877) and Retzius using silver (1894).[12] Nevertheless, the Merkel "corpuscle" never seemed to make it into the orthodoxy of anatomy. von Frey never included it in his scheme of sensory-histology correlations (see Chapter 1). He didn't need another "touch corpuscle." For von Frey, touch was pressure and he already had Pacinian and Meissner corpuscles for his correlations! Subsequent (and present day) textbooks simply excluded the Merkel corpuscle. As recently as 1955, the Merkel corpuscle was said to be an artifact.[46] Winkelmann[12] states that Cauna "did not find them," referring to Merkel's corpuscle; however, Figure 18 in Cauna's 1954 paper[9] is clearly a Merkel corpuscle, although Cauna identified it only as a nerve network beneath the intermediate ridge. In 1960, Winkelmann consistently demonstrated what he termed "hederiform," or ivy-like nerve terminals ending along the intermediate epidermal ridge in relation to clear cells in the basal layer of glabrous skin. However, Winkelmann believed the Merkel corpuscle was similar to a Meissner corpuscle, listed it as a subclass under the Meissner corpuscle, suggested it should stain for cholinesterase activity since the Meissner does

(but in fact the Merkel doesn't), suggested it subserved touch and, in particular, motion.

Thus, although after a generation of neglect the Merkel corpuscle was rediscovered, there was still a long way to go. There have been few published photomicrographs of the Merkel corpuscle in man, and to this end I have included Figure 2.1, kindly contributed by Bryce L. Munger, M.D., Chairman of the Department and Professor of Anatomy at the Milton S. Hershey Medical School. It is appropriate that these illustrations come from him since in 1965 he published the first electron micrographs of the Merkel cell and its secretory granules, and coined the term that is most appropriate, and which I have adopted in this book, the Merkel cell-neurite complex.[26]

Munger described the Merkel cell-neurite complex in glabrous opossum snout in 1965. That same year, Mann and Straille described a structure in the cat with clear cells and nerve terminals associated with a tylotrich (thickened, nonpellage body) hair and an intimately associated epidermal pad.[47] This complex was slowly-adapting. Previously, Iggo and Muir[48] had demonstrated the cat touch dome to be a receptor related to a slowly-adapting fiber. This touch dome, although unassociated with a hair, is located on the hairy cat paw and was morphologically analogous to the Haarscheibe (hair disc) described by Pinkus in 1904 on the hairy skin of man.[49] The Haarscheibe of man and the tylotrich follicle and touch pad of cats, although in hairy skin, had in common with Munger's glabrous opossum snout receptor the association of a clear epithelial cell and an expanded bulb nerve termination.

There can no longer be any question of the existence of a Merkel cell-neurite complex that is the receptor part of the slowly-adapting fiber/receptor system. It has been described on the human trunk (1966),[55] the rat back as well as hairy skin of rabbits, mice, and guinea pigs (1967),[51] hairy skin of monkey forearm and hand (1969),[52] and the glabrous fingertips of the raccoon (1971).[53] There have been many confirmatory reports.[54-60] The description to follow is based upon these studies.

The Merkel cell is a large cell located in

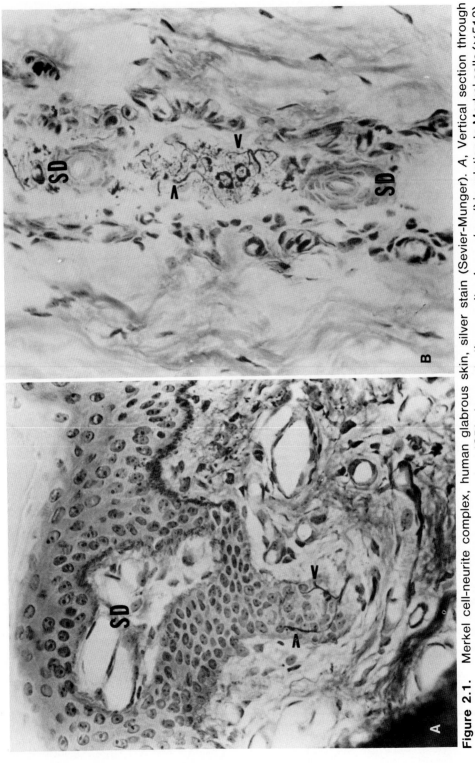

Figure 2.1. Merkel cell-neurite complex, human glabrous skin, silver stain (Sevier-Munger). *A,* Vertical section through intermediate epidermal ridge at level of sweat duct (*SD*), demonstrating neurites (*arrowhead*) in relation to Merkel cells (×512). *B,* Horizontal section through base of intermediate ridge to demonstrate relationship of neurites (*arrowhead*) to sweat ducts (*SD*) (×380).

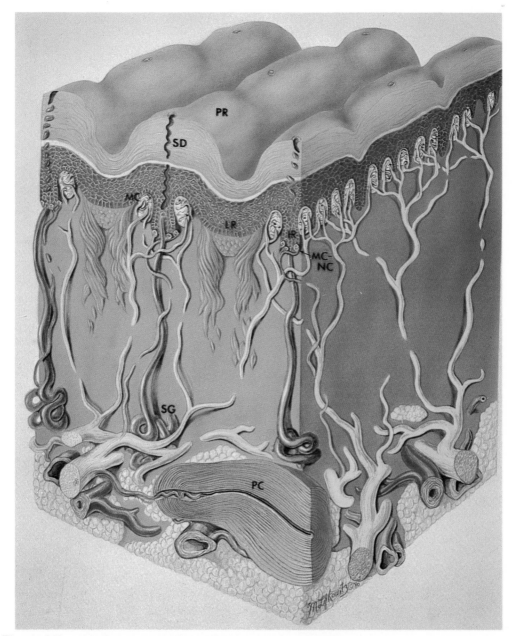

Figure 2.2.   Model of distal glabrous human skin: MC, Meissner corpuscle; MD, Merkel cell-neurite complex; PC, Pacinian corpuscle; LR, limiting ridge; IR, intermediate ridge; PR, papillary ridge; SG, sweat gland; SD, sweat duct. Note multiple innervation for Meissner corpuscles, single innervation for Pacinian corpuscle and Merkel cell-neurite complex. Note overlapping peripheral receptive fields.

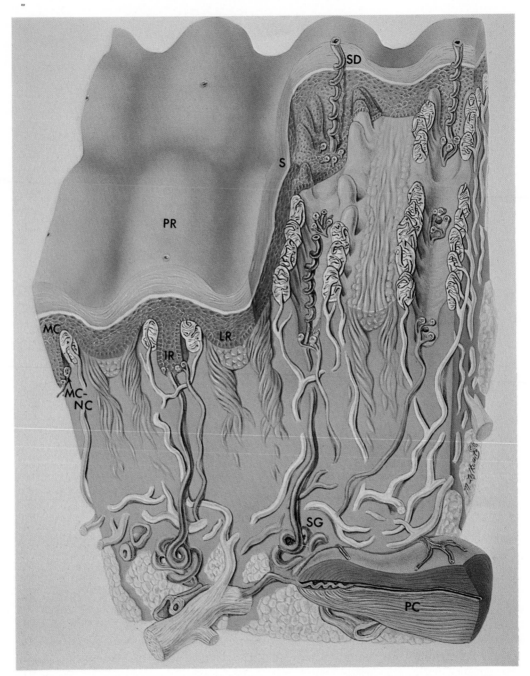

Figure 2.3. Model of distal glabrous human skin. Abbreviations are same as in Figure 2.2.

the basal layer of the epidermis. In hairy skin, it is either in groups below an elevated pad (Haarscheibe) or associated with a hair (tylotrich or vibrissae), while in the glabrous digital skin it lies in groups of four about the entrance of the sweat duct into the intermediate ridge (Fig. 2.1). A single myelinated nerve innervates a Haarscheibe in humans, a tylotrich hair in cats, and a group of Merkel cells about the sweat duct in the glabrous skin. In cats, a single nerve fiber may innervate four to seven touch domes on the hindleg. The Merkel cells of the Haarscheiben and tylotrich are associated intimately with hairs, those of the touch dome and glabrous skin are not. The Merkel cell has a nucleus with irregular borders and contains electron-dense cytoplasmic granules polarized toward the side adjacent to the nerve terminal. The granule's histochemical content remains unknown. In man, desmosome-like communications have been identified, between the Merkel cell and neurite. The origin of the Merkel cell, neural crest versus nonneural epithelium, remains debated. The Merkel cell is intimately associated with the neurite, which has lost its myelin and ends in expanded bulbs in a disc-like array around or about the Merkel cell.

Although Adrian and Zottermann[61] suggested that the Pacinian corpuscle was the pressure receptor, the work of Werner and Mountcastle[62] demonstrated that only a slowly-adapting fiber/receptor system was responsive to vertical skin displacement in a linear fashion. The Merkel cell-neurite complex, then, must be the pressure receptor (see Chapter 3).

In this book, in addition to Figure 2.1, the Merkel cell-neurite complex is illustrated in hematoxylin and eosin (Figs. 4.7 and 5.7) and in silver (Figs. 5.16 and 12.25) stain for light microscopy and for electron microscopy (Figs. 10.6 and 10.7).

MODEL OF THE DISTAL GLABROUS SKIN

Figures 2.2 and 2.3 are medical illustrations prepared to illustrate the histology of the distal glabrous skin of the primate, based upon the references and material developed above, and Lefkowitz's thesis.[3]

References

1. Mitchell SW: *Injuries of Nerves and Their Consequences*, 1872. American Academy of Neurology Reprint Series, p 19, New York: Dover, 1965.
2. Stopford JSB: *Sensation and the Sensory Pathway*. London: Longsmans, Green, 1930, Ch XI.
3. Lefkowitz M: *A Model of the Glabrous Skin of the Fingertip*, Master's thesis. Johns Hopkins University, Baltimore, 1979.
4. Montagna W: Comparative anatomy and physiology of the skin. Arch Dermatol 96:357–363, 1967.
5. Iggo A: Cutaneous receptors, in Hubbard JF (ed): *The Peripheral Nervous System*. New York: Plenum Press, 1974, Ch 12, pp 374–404.
6. Breathnach AS: Electron microscopy of cutaneous nerves and receptors. J Invest Dermatol 69:8–26, 1977.
7. Horch KW, Tuckett RP, Burgess PR: A key to the classification of cutaneous mechanoreceptors. J Invest Dermatol 69:75–82, 1977.
8. Iggo A: Cutaneous and subcutaneous sense organs. Br Med Bull 33:97–102, 1977.
9. Cauna N: Nature and functions of the papillary ridges of the digital skin. Anat Rec 119:449–468, 1954.
10. Weddell G: Nerve endings in mammalian skin. Biol Rev 30:159–195, 1955.
11. Miller MR, Ralston HJ, Kasahara M: The pattern of cutaneous innervation of the human hand. Am J Anat 102:183–201, 1958.
12. Winkelmann RK: *Nerve Endings in Normal and Pathologic Skin*. Springfield, Ill: Charles C Thomas, 1960.
13. Dellon AL: Personal observations, unpublished.
14. Halata, Z: Spezifische innervation, Ch 6, in Orfanos CE (ed): *Haar und Haarkrankheiten*. Stuttgart: Gustav Fischer Verlag, 1979.
15. Biemesderfer D, Munger BL, Binck J, et al: The Pilo-Ruffini complex: A non-sinus hair and associated slowly-adapting mechanoreceptor in primate facial skin. Brain Res 142:197–222, 1978.
16. Halata Z: The ultrastructure of the sensory nerve endings in the articular capsule of the knee joint of the domestic cat (Ruffini corpuscles and Pacinian corpuscles). J Anat 124:717–729, 1977.
17. Blackwelder RD: *Classification of the Animal Kingdom*. Carbondale, Ill: Southern Illinois Univ Press, 1963.
18. Rothschild NMV: *A Classification of Living Animals*. New York: John Wiley & Sons, 1961.
19. Webster N: *The Living Webster Encyclopedic Dictionary*. Chicago: English Language Inst of America, 1975.
20. Kappers CVA, Huber GC, Crosby EC: *The Comparative Anatomy of the Nervous System of Vertebrates, including Man*. New York: Hafner, 1960.
21. Marshall AJ: *Biology and Comparative Physiology of Birds*. New York: Academic Press, 1960.
22. Munger BL: The comparative ultrastructure of slowly and rapidly adapting mechanoreceptors, in Dubner R, Kawamuro Y (eds): *Oral-Facial Sensory and Motor Mechanisms*. New York: Appelton-Century-Crofts, 1971, Ch 6.

23. Munger BL: Patterns of organization of peripheral sensory receptors, in Lowenstein WR (ed): *Handbook of Sensory Physiology*. Berlin: Springer-Verlag, 1971, Ch 17.

24. Saxod R: Developmental origin of the Herbst cutaneous sensory corpuscle: Experimental analysis using cellular markers. Dev Biol 32:167–178, 1973.

25. Gottschaldt KM, Lausmann S: Mechanoreceptors and their properties in the beak skin of geese (Anser anser). Brain Res 65:510–515, 1974.

26. Munger BL: The intraepidermal innervation of the snout skin of the opossum. J Cell Biol 26:79–97, 1965.

27. Munger BL, Pubols LM: The sensorineural organization of the digital skin of the raccoon. Brain Behav Evol 5:367–393, 1972.

28. Anderson S, Jones JK: *Recent Mammals of the World: A Synopsis of Families.* New York: Ronald Press, 1967.

29. Zollmann PE, Winkelmann RK: The sensory innervation of the common North American racoon (Procyon lotor). J Compt Neurol 119:149–157, 1962.

30. Ide C: The fine structure of the digital corpuscle of the mouse toe pad, with special reference to nerve fibers. Am J Anat 147:329–356, 1976.

31. Lee F: A study of the Pacinian corpuscle. J Comp Neurol 64:497–522, 1936.

32. Cauna N, Mannan G: Development and postnatal change of digital Pacinian corpuscles (corpuscular lamellosa) in the human hand. J Anat 93:271–286, 1959.

33. Pease DC, Quilliam TA: Electron microscopy of the Pacinian corpuscle. J Biophys Biochem Cytol 3:331–342, 1957.

34. Nishi K, Oura C, Paillie W: Fine structure of Pacinian corpuscles in the mesentery of the cat. J Cell Biol 43:539–552, 1969.

35. Spencer PS, Schaumberg HH: An ultrastructural study of the inner core of the Pacinian corpuscle. J Neurocytol 2:217–235, 1973.

36. Cauna N: Nerve supply and nerve endings in Meissner's corpuscles. Am J Anat 99:315–350, 1956.

37. Cauna N: Structure of digital touch corpuscles. Acta Anat (Basel) 32:1–23, 1958.

38. Weddell G: Multiple innervation of sensory spots in skin. J Anat 75:441–446, 1941.

39. Ridley A: Silver staining of nerve endings in human digital glabrous skin. J Anat 104:41–48, 1969.

40. Cauna N, Ross LL: The fine structure of Meissner's touch corpuscles of human fingers. J Cell Biol 8:467–482, 1960.

41. Breathnach AS: *An Atlas of the Ultrastructure of Human Skin.* London: JA Churchill, 1971.

42. Hashimoto K: Fine structure of the Meissner corpuscle of human palmar skin. J Invest Dermatol 60:20–28, 1973.

43. Dellon AL, Witebsky FG, Terrill RE: The denervated Meissner corpuscle: A sequential histologic study after nerve division in the Rhesus monkey. Plast Reconstr Surg 56:182–193, 1975.

44. Dickens WN, Winkelmann RK, Mulder DW: Cholinesterase demonstration of dermal nerve endings in patients with impaired sensation. Neurology (Minneap) 13:91–100, 1963.

45. Merkel F: Tastzellen und Tastkorperchen bei den Hausthieren und beim Menschen. Arch Mikrosk Anat 11:636–652, 1875.

46. Weddell G, Palmer E, Palie W: Nerve endings in mammalian skin. Biol Rev 30:159–195, 1955.

47. Mann SJ, Straille WE: Tylotrich (hair) follicle: Association with a slowly adapting tactile receptor in the cat. Science 147:1043–1045, 1965.

48. Iggo A, Muir AR: A cutaneous sense organ in the hairy skin of cats. J Anat 97:151, 1963.

49. Pinkus F: Ueber Hautsinnesorgars neben den menshlichen Haar (Haarscheiben) und ihre verglesisehend anatomische Bedentung. Arch Mikrosk Anat EntwMech 65:124–179, 1904.

50. Kawamura T, Nishiyama S, Ikeda S, et al: The human haarscheibe, its structure and function. J Invest Dermatol 42:87–90, 1966.

51. Smith KR: The structure and function of the Haarscheibe. J Comp Neurol 131:459–474, 1967.

52. Iggo A, Muir AR: The structure and function of a slowly-adapting touch corpuscle in hair skin. J Physiol 200:763–796, 1969.

53. Munger BL, Pubols LM, Pubols BH: The Merkel rete papilla—a slowly adapting sensory receptor in mammalian glabrous skin. Brain Res 29:47–61, 1971.

54. Smith HR: The ultrastructure of the human haarscheibe and Merkel cell. J Invest Dermatol 54:150–159, 1970.

55. Kasprzak H, Tapper DN, Craig PH: Functional development of the tactile pad receptor system. Exp Neurol 26:439–446, 1970.

56. Kawamura T: Fine structure of the dendritic cells and Merkel cells in the epidermis of various mammals. Jpn J Dermatol 81:343–351, 1971.

57. Winkelmann RK, Breathnach AS: The Merkel cell. J Invest Dermatol 60:2–15, 1973.

58. English KB: Cell types in cutaneous type 1 mechanoreceptors (Haarscheiben) and their alterations with injury. Am J Anat 1:105–126, 1974.

59. Munger BL: Neural-epithelial interactions in sensory receptors. J Invest Dermatol 69:27–40, 1977.

60. English KB: Morphogenesis of Haarscheiben in rats. J Invest Dermatol 69:58–67, 1977.

61. Adrian ED, Zottermann Y: The impulses produced by sensory nerve endings: The responses of a single nerve organ. J Physiol (Lond) 61:151–171, 1926.

62. Werner G, Mountcastle VB: Neural activity in mechanoreceptive cutaneous afferents: Stimulus-response relations, Weber functions, and information transmission. J Neurophysiol 28:359–397, 1965.

Chapter 3

NEUROPHYSIOLOGIC BASIS OF SENSATION

INTRODUCTION
PERIPHERAL SENSIBILITY
CENTRAL ORGANIZATION

The study of the sense is a point of convergence, where, in the future, the science of physiology, psychology and physics will come together.

E. H. Weber, *1835*[1]

There is one field of enquiry in which neither animal experiment nor access to a large number of patients is of much use; the study of disturbances of sensibility, more particularly, cutaneous sensibility. It is no accident that the renowned investigations of Head, Trotter and Davis, Boring, Woolard and Weddell were done in times of peace. It is a leisurely occupation. Animal experiments . . . have helped a little; but man alone . . . can describe the manifold sensations experienced after an injury to a nerve or during regeneration. Moreover, the injuries themselves must be deliberately inflicted, with great precision, and the subject has to be a fully informed member of the experimental team . . . It may be said that this is rather the province of the physiologist and the anatomist. In methodology this is true enough, but the problem is intensely practical . . . What is so astonishing is that in spite of the devoted efforts of many workers the riddle of sensibility is still not yet solved.

H. J. Seddon, *1972*[2]

INTRODUCTION

Ernst Heinrich Weber was expressing, perhaps, optimism as he looked ahead to the challenge provided by the study of peripheral sensibility. Sir Herbert Seddon, almost a century and a half later, was expressing, perhaps, frustration. His monograph reviews a lifetime of work, recording his own observations on more than 2,200 nerve injuries. Sir Sidney Sunderland's massive book on the peripheral nerve[3] and Barnes Woodhall's review[4] of more than 3,600 peripheral nerve injuries already had been published. The British, Australian, and United States experiences had been carefully documented. Seddon wrote these words in his Preface about 6 years before his death. He looked back over the past 3 decades of clinical experience and realized that the surgeon still did not have statistical evidence from a controlled series to know whether primary or secondary nerve repair gave better results, whether nerve grafting was superior to either or neither. He realized further that published reports on the end results of nerve repair continued in the absence of a standardized scheme for evaluating functional sensation in the hand. Seddon would have had cause for optimism, however, had he been aware of the work coming forth from Vernon B. Mountcastle's neurophysiology lab at Johns Hopkins. Seddon's book contains more than 450 references in its bibliography, but none to the basic mechanisms of sensibility elucidated by Mountcastle. Mountcastle's textbook of neurophysiology is a good starting place, for in just two chapters[4] are reviewed the elements that permitted me to develop a clinical approach to evaluating peripheral sensibility that would have pleased Sir Herbert.

I have had the privilege of visiting Doctor Mountcastle's laboratory. There are the special plexiglass chairs, stereotactic devices, behavorial reward devices, and mechanical testing devices for the monkey subjects. These were arrayed before a phalanx of computers, oscilloscopes, stimulating and recording devices. But the hardware only hints at the guiding genius, of his "view from within." On October 28, 1974, Doctor Mountcastle presented the Dean's Lecture to the Johns Hopkins University School of Medicine.[6] This provides an overview of the activities of Mountcastle's laboratory and spans almost 2 decades of work.

PERIPHERAL SENSIBILITY

The sensory part of the peripheral nervous system may be thought of as being comprised of sensory units. Each unit includes a neuron, located in the dorsal spinal ganglion, its central termination with the central nervous system, its peripheral afferent fibers, and its most distal termination. This distal termination may be called the sensory ending and may be a "free" ending, a nerve network, or an ending in relationship to a nonneural structure. These nonneural structures may be hair follicles or a form of "encapsulated end organ." The encapsulated end organs, as described in Chapter 2, are Merkel cell-neurite complexes, Meissner corpuscles, and Pacinian corpuscles. Those receptors found in joints, fascia, and muscle spindles will not be considered here.

Each afferent nerve fiber is related to a defined peripheral receptive field. A stimulus of proper quality and intensity will evoke a neural impulse (response) from this axon from anywhere within its receptive field. The threshold (stimulus required to generate impulse) is lowest in the center of the field. Adjacent peripheral receptive fields partially overlap. Thus, a stimulus to a point on the skin evokes a profile of neural impulses from the overlapping afferent fibers (Fig. 3.1). The number of nerve fibers present in a given area of skin is referred to as the peripheral innervation density and is related to the volume of cerebral cortex representing that area. Thus, for example, the hand, and in particular the fingertips, have among the highest innervation density of any place on the body surface and are represented by one of the largest areas on the sensory cortex.[5]

The peripheral nerve is classified conveniently by its fiber size and whether or not it is myelinated.[7] For our purposes, the classification may be simplified to the group A, myelinated fibers, and the group C, unmyelinated fibers. The C fibers are small, being just 1 to 2 μm. Group A is subdivided by fiber size into A-delta, 2 to 5 μm.; A-beta, 10 to 15 μm.; and A-alpha, 15 to 20 μm. The A-alpha are motor fibers. Erlanger and Gasser correlated the A-beta fibers with touch, the A-delta with sticking pain and temperature, and the C fibers with burning pain. The A-delta and C fiber groups will not be discussed further, but detailed accounts of their neurophysiology are available.[8-10]

The group A-beta fibers, therefore, are those heavily myelinated fibers subserving the sense of touch. Mountcastle found these

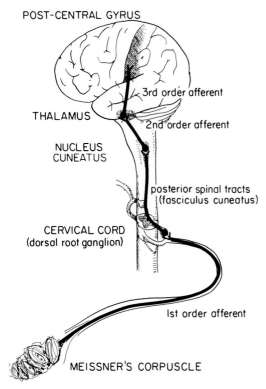

POST-CENTRAL GYRUS

3rd order afferent

THALAMUS

2nd order afferent

NUCLEUS
CUNEATUS

posterior spinal tracts
(fasciculus cuneatus)

CERVICAL CORD
(dorsal root ganglion)

1st order afferent

MEISSNER'S CORPUSCLE

Figure 3.1. Each sensory unit consists of a neuron, located in the dorsal root ganglion, a central connection, and a peripheral termination. Peripherally, each fiber has a defined receptive field.

fibers could be subdivided based upon their adaptation to a constant-touch stimulus. A fiber is termed rapidly-adapting if its impulse response drops off rapidly to zero. A fiber is termed slowly-adapting if its pulse response continues throughout the stimulus duration. Only the slowly-adapting fibers increase their rate of firing, or impulse frequency, as the stimulus intensity is increased (Fig. 3.2). Thus, only a slowly-adapting fiber can convey information regarding constant-touch (Fig. 3.3) and pressure (Fig. 3.4). The Weber test, classical two-point discrimination, in which the ends of the caliper are held in constant contact with the skin, measures the innervation density of the slowly-adapting fiber/receptor population (Fig. 3.5). The quickly-adapting fiber conveys information about transients, movement. Thus, the quickly-adapting fiber/receptor system detects moving-touch (Fig. 3.6). The "moving two-point discrimination test," in which the two ends of the caliper (paper clip) are moved, measures the peripheral innervation density of the quickly-adapting fiber/receptor system (Fig. 3.7).[11]

After defining the quickly- and slowly-adapting fiber populations by their response to a constant mechanical stimulus, it remained to further test each subpopulation and attempt to relate the fiber types with their specific mechanoreceptors. The

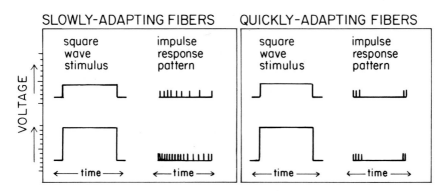

SLOWLY-ADAPTING FIBERS QUICKLY-ADAPTING FIBERS

square wave stimulus impulse response pattern square wave stimulus impulse response pattern

VOLTAGE

←— time —→ ←—time —→ ←— time —→ ←— time —→

Figure 3.2. Properties of adaptation to a constant-touch stimulus. Slowly-adapting fibers continue to discharge impulses throughout duration of stimulus and increase impulse frequency in response to increased stimulus intensity. Quickly-adapting fibers fire very briefly after stimulation and then cease. There may be an "off" response. There is no change in impulse pattern with intensity change for this stimulus.

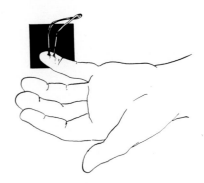

Figure 3.5. The Weber test, classical two-point discrimination, measures the innervation density of the slowly-adapting fiber/receptor system.

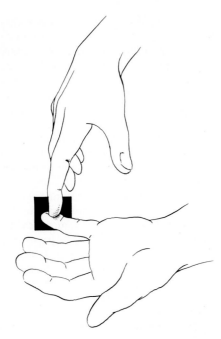

Figure 3.3. Perception of constant-touch is mediated by the slowly-adapting fiber/receptor system.

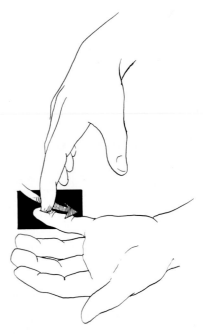

Figure 3.6. Perception of moving-touch is mediated by the quickly-adapting fiber/receptor system.

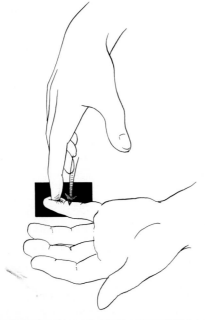

Figure 3.4. Perception of pressure is mediated by the slowly-adapting fiber/receptor system.

mechanoreceptor, an end organ, is actually a transducer. It transforms a mechanical stimulus into a conducted neural impulse. While the exact mechanism of this transducer process remains to be defined, much is known about the behavior of the individual types of mechanoreceptors. It will be seen that mechanoreceptors signal to the sensory cortex by

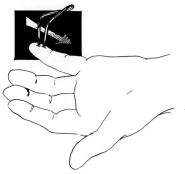

Figure 3.7. The moving two-point discrimination test measures the peripheral innervation density of the quickly-adapting fiber/receptor system.

a frequency code, that is, a temporal pattern of impulses.

Slowly-Adapting Fiber/Receptor System

The slowly-adapting fiber/receptor system was first directly studied in the touch-pad of the cat's hairy skin by Iggo.[12] Since then it has been well-defined in the cat,[13-15, 29-30] rabbit,[14] alligator,[15] opossum,[16] raccoon,[17-23] monkey,[17, 18, 28, 47] baboon,[45] and man [24-27] both in hairy[12-15, 24-30] and glabrous[16-19, 21-23, 26, 45, 47] skin.

There are two neurophysiologic properties that define slowly-adapting fiber/receptor systems. The first is that the neural impulses continue to discharge throughout the duration of the stimulus, although the frequency diminishes with duration (Fig. 3.8). The second is that there is a change in response (frequency of impulse) with stimulus intensity change (Fig. 3.9). Thus, when the mechanical probe is pushed deeper into the skin, there are more frequent neural discharges recorded from the fiber. The slowly-adaptors are the pressure sensors.

What are the receptors for the slowly-adapting mechanoreceptors of the skin? In hairy skin they are the Merkel cell-neurite complex. Pinkus[31] described these in man in 1904. Pinkus' drawings of the Haarscheibe are morphologically analogous to the touchpad of the cat. The Merkel cell-neurite complex may be intimately associated with the base of a hair follicle as described by Straille for the "tylotrich" hair[32] and Andres for the

"sinus" hair[33] in the cat. These receptors may be stimulated by direct pressure or by deflection of the associated hair. In glabrous skin, the Merkel cells are again located in the basal layer of epidermis but in certain relationship to the epidermal rete. In monkey and man they are located only at the base of the intermediate ridge about the entrance site of the sweat duct. These are the so-called type I slowly-adapting receptor.

Neurophysiologically, the slowly-adapting response fibers can be subdivided based upon other considerations. These are summarized in Table 3.1 from the Iggo's review.[34] Essentially, the type II fiber/receptor system is uncommon, appears similar to the endings described by Ruffini [it is not associated with Merkel (epithelial) cells,[35] although it has been observed at the base of a hair follicle[36]], responds to stretching of skin adjacent to its receptive field, and has a resting (nonstimulated) discharge. A type II receptor may be thought of as a Merkel cell-neurite complex without the Merkel cell! They are almost rare. Brown and Iggo found them to comprise just 3% of the slowly-adaptors in the rabbit and 9% of those in the cat's hairy skin.[14] Knibestal and Vallbo[27] found only 7% of their slowly-adapting fibers in human glabrous skin to fit into the type II category.

Do slowly-adapting cutaneous mechanoreceptors respond to stimuli other than constant-touch and pressure? Slowly-adapting fibers have been demonstrated to alter their impulse frequency to mechanical stimulus when their environmental temperature changes, but these rate changes are very much less than those generated by changes in the mechanical stimulus.[15, 35] Thus, although they do respond to changes in temperature, they do not convey the perception of temperature. Similarly, for sinusoidal mechanical stimuli, slow-adaptors showed a frequency modulation in phase with low frequency vibration, but the stimulus amplitudes were not appropriate for human perception of movement.[25, 38] In an earlier study, human Haarscheibe were directly stimulated with a 100-cps vibratory punctate stimulus. There was no sensation elicited.[37]

One additional point is worth discussing for our purposes about the slowly-adapting

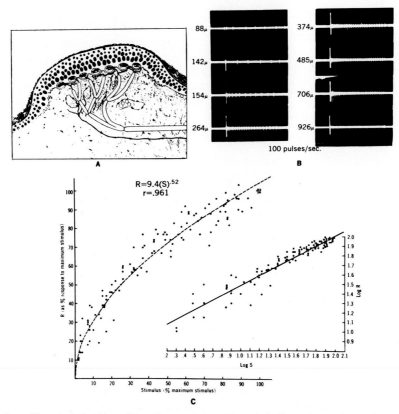

Figure 3.8. Slowly-adapting fiber/receptor system. *A,* Drawing of touch-pad found in cat hairy skin, from light and electron microscopic studies by Iggo and Muir.[13] *B,* Records of nerve impulses evoked in single fiber by mechanical stimulation of touch-pad it innervated. Skin indentation in micrometers shown to left of record. *C,* Data pooled from 10 of the studies illustrated in *B,* demonstrating power-law relationship between stimulus and response. (Adapted with permission from V. B. Mountcastle (ed): *Medical Physiology,* ed 12. Saint Louis: CV Mosby, 1968, Ch 61–62.[5])

fibers. What percent of peripheral cutaneous afferents are slowly-adapting? No one knows. To answer the question would require single-unit analysis of every fiber in a nerve. Even at the level of the digital "nerve," there are 2500 axons. We can arrive at an estimate, however. In 1966, Mountcastle[8] estimated that just 10% were slowly-adapting. This figure may have come from the work later reported by his students,[28] in which it was noted that of 505 fibers tested, there were 53 type I SA. But what should be the denominator? Should we include C fibers and A-delta fibers? A useful comparison for the clinician interested in *functional recovery* (see Chapter 6) is the percentage of slowly-adapting fibers to the total A-beta group. Several studies have recorded large numbers of single units and reported their results. Implicit in this statement is the realization of the bias in the selection of the axons that were counted. However, a brief tabulation of these (see Table 3.2) reveals that about 36% of the group of A-betas are slowly-adapting.

Quickly-Adapting Fiber/Receptor System

The quickly-adapting fiber/receptor system was the first to be investigated by microdissection. First, Lowenstein removed the

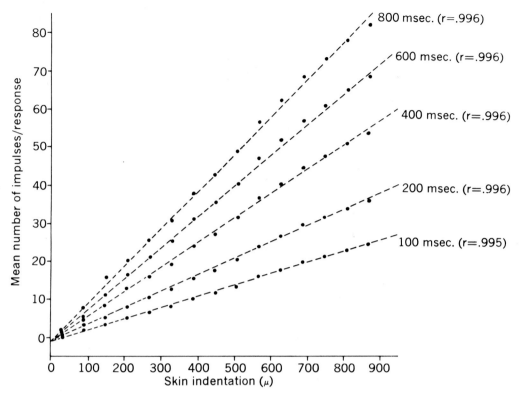

Figure 3.9.   Slowly-adapting fiber/receptor system. Single unit recordings from glabrous skin of the monkey from a 1-mm receptive field on the fingertip. Each line demonstrates the relationship between stimulus intensity (skin indentation) and impulse response. The series of lines demonstrates that this relationship holds for stimuli of varying (longer) duration. (Adapted with permission from V. B. Mountcastle (ed): *Medical Physiology*, ed 12. Saint Louis: CV Mosby, 1968, Ch 61–62.[5])

Table 3.1
Slowly-Adapting Cutaneous Mechanoreceptors[a]

	Type I	Type II
Slowly-adapting	x	x
Responds to vertical displacement	x	x
Responds to lateral skin stretch		x
Resting discharge, usual		x
Receptors per axon	1–5	1
Receptor type	Merkel	Ruffini
Usual frequency response to stimulus	High	Low
Usual discharge to maintained stimulus	Irregular	Regular

[a] Adapted from A. Iggo.[34]

onion-like capsule and demonstrated that the site of the generator potential, the unmyelinated intracorpuscular axon, was distinct from the site of the all-or-nothing potential, the first node of Ranvier.[40] It was also noted that the threshold for stimulation rose after capsulectomy. These concepts were depicted graphically in 1960 (Fig. 3.10).[41] Next, Lowenstein was one of the first to demonstrate fiber specificity by showing that:

the mechano-receptor membrane of the nerve ending of the Pacinian corpuscles is insensitive to thermal stimuli ... Although a change in temperature per se does not excite the receptor membrane it modifies markedly the mechanically excited charge transfer through the membrane ... In a

Table 3.2
Estimate of Percentage of Group A-beta That Are Slowly-Adapting Fibers

Reference No.	Animal	Skin	No. of Group A-beta Fibers	Slowly-Adapting (%)
14	Cat	Hairy	501	31
14	Rabbit	Hairy	271	32
16	Monkey	Glabrous	70	21
27	Human	Glabrous	61	75
37	Monkey	Hairy	221	34
38	Monkey	Glabrous	523	40
45	Baboon	Glabrous	21	52
Total			1,672	36

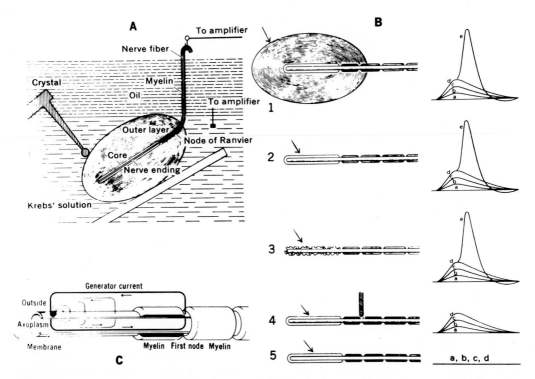

Figure 3.10. Quickly-adapting fiber/receptor system. *A,* Method of stimulating Pacinian corpuscle. Electrical impulse drives the crystal which applies force from capsule to the axon after capsule is removed. *B,* Records show increasing generator potentials (*a, b, c, d*) produced by increasing stimuli until a generator potential is produced (*e*) that reaches firing level for the axon resulting in a conducted action potential. In 4, pressure at first node of Ranvier blocks production of action potential but not generator potential. In 5, axon has degenerated after nerve section. *C,* Concept of local change in membrane permeability that results in generator potential. (Adapted with permission from V. B. Mountcastle (ed): *Medical Physiology,* ed 12. Saint Louis: CV Mosby, 1968, Ch 61–62.[5] Modified from W. R. Lowenstein: *Sci Am* 203:99–108, 1960.[41])

rapidly-adapting receptor, such as the Pacinian corpuscle, ... the exciting agent can be clearly distinguished from the modifying agent.[42]

In a further study with this model, which was the cat mesentery, an artifical capsule was made for the "decapsulated" axon. They found that they needed multilayered sheets of mesothelium (thin and elastic) with fluid between the layers to obtain good mechanical filtering.[43] They interpreted this to mean that the capsule shortens the "active" phase of a stimulus, causes rapid decay of the generator potential, and thereby limits impulse generation, i.e., the capsule is critical to rapid adaptation.[43] However, a second factor was felt to be present, too, because electrical stimulation at the first node of Ranvier still produced just a few conducted neural impulses.[43] In the summary of that paper, the statement "under these (decapsulated) conditions, the electrical response of the ending behaves as that of more slowly-adapting sensory ends:" refers to the generator potential, not the fiber's conducted response properties of adaptation. Lowenstein concluded this report with a proposed model for "high pass mechanical filter":

The primary elements of this mechanical filter are the lamellae, their inter-connexions and the fluid. The former two provide the structural stiffness and the elasticity, and the latter, the viscosity. The system has thus the elements of capacitative reactance (elasticity) and resistance (viscosity) ... The system behaves essentially like a dashpot with pistons (the lamellae) in series. To mechanical stimuli of slow rates of use, that is, compressions of the outer surface, such a system offers relatively little viscous resistance ... Elastic force is virtually the only force produced, and this is small and falls steeply from periphery to centre. With fast rising stimuli ... viscous resistance is high. Hence a high viscous force is developed in addition to the elastic one. The viscous force is transmitted with relatively little spatial decrement through the system ... This will give rise in the intact corpuscle to a brief pulse of pressure at the centre where the sensor is located, lasting only as long as the fast rising phase of the stimulus ... During the "off-phase of the stimulus, stimulus energy stored in the elastic elements of the system is released ... The sensory ending at the centre receives than during the "off-phase" pressure pulse similar to that of the "on-phase."[43]

Lowenstein[43] credits Gray[44, 45] with first describing the Pacinian corpuscle as having rapid properties of adaptation.

The quickly-adapting fiber/receptor system has been studied in the cat,[14] rabbit,[14] raccoon,[21, 23] monkey,[16, 27, 38, 48] baboon,[46] and human[24-27] in both hairy[14, 24-26, 37] and glabrous[16, 21, 23, 26, 27, 38, 46, 48] skin. The quickly-adapting population can be subdivided based upon the response of single fibers to peripheral vibratory stimuli.[38]

If a vibratory stimuli (an oscillating mechanical probe, electrical sine wave, or tuning fork) is applied to the peripheral receptive field of a quickly-adapting fiber, a threshold (amplitude of wave) will be found for that frequency at which the stimulus is transmitted (or perceived in an awake subject being studied percutaneously). This is the absolute threshold at which an action potential is generated. There will be higher stimulus intensity (amplitude voltage) at which stimulation of the receptive field results in a one-to-one entrainment of neural impulses in the fiber. That threshold at which the impulse frequency equals the stimulus frequency is termed the tuning point. The plot of these points for a given fiber is its tuning curve.

In a combined psychophysical experiment on humans and single-unit recording in monkeys, Mountcastle's group described the sense of flutter-vibration.[39] In brief, the quickly-adapting population of group A-beta fibers in glabrous skin contains one group most sensitive to low frequency stimuli (range of 5 to 40 cps), maximally sensitive to about 30 cps, and another group most sensitive to high frequency stimuli (range of 60 to 300 cps), maximally sensitive to about 250 cps. Thresholds were obtained in the human volunteers, and the tuning curves from the monkeys superimposed (see Fig. 3.11). In another study, the epidermis of the human volunteers was anesthetized by cocaine iontophoresis. This raised the threshold for the low-frequency responsive group of fibers (see Fig. 3.12). It was concluded from these studies that one subset of quickly-adapting fibers existed that was responsive to low-frequency stimuli, had a receptor located in the epidermis (probably the Meissner corpuscle), and was responsible for detecting

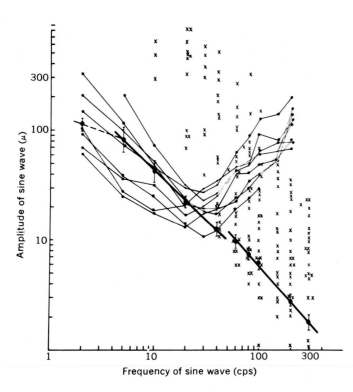

Figure 3.11. Quickly adapting fiber/receptor system. *Heavy lines* plot human threshold for perception of vibratory stimulus to index fingertip. *Lighter lines* plot threshold tuning curves for monkey median nerve fibers. *Crosses* plot tuning points for median nerve fibers that end in Pacinian corpuscles. If the crosses were joined, tuning curves would be plotted that cover the high frequency limb of the human threshold curve. (Adapted with permission from V. B. Mountcastle (ed): *Medical Physiology*, ed 12. Saint Louis: CV Mosby, 1968, Ch 61–62.[5])

transient stimuli (movement) and flutter. The second subset was responsive to high-frequency stimuli, had a receptor located below the epidermis (probably the Pacinian corpuscle), and was responsible for detecting transients (movement) and vibration. Furthermore, Pacinian afferents were more sensitive and had a larger receptive field (see Table 3.3).[39]

What is the distribution between these two subdivisions? In glabrous skin, several studies permit reanalysis of their published data to give an approximate answer. In monkeys, 16% of 310 quickly-adapting fibers were Pacinian afferents.[39] In baboons, 23% of 26 fibers were Pacinian afferents.[46] In humans, 6% of 15 fibers were Pacinian afferents.[27] It has been said that there are no Pacinian afferents in hairy skin.[37]

A characteristic set of responses to clinical stimuli is illustrated in Figure 3.13.

It remained to be learned how the quickly-adapting population of fiber/receptors signalled magnitude of response. It could not be by impulse frequency, as the slow-adaptors

do, because the rapid-adaptors' impulse frequency is related to stimulus frequency. K. O. Johnson investigated this problem in a single-unit analysis, monkey glabrous skin model, where the site of vibratory stimulus was related to its location within the receptor field. The distance of the probe from field center was related to minimum stimulus amplitude eliciting an action potential in the fiber. These data allowed the formation of spatiotemporal response profiles, essentially reconstructing the response of the population of fibers to the stimulus. Vibratory magnitude (intensity of vibratory stimulus) was found to be signalled by (1) total impulse frequency; (2) total number of active fibers; (3) total number of entrained fibers.[47]

Although it had seemed that the primate glabrous skin was too packed with sensory end organs to permit identification of the slowly-and quickly-adapting fiber's specific mechanoreceptor, recent work from Munger[48] appears to achieve this correlation. The general approach was to excise dorsal sensory ganglia, thereby diminishing the population

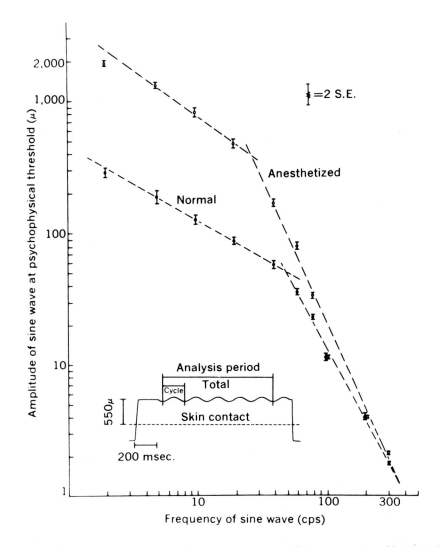

Figure 3.12.   Quickly-adapting fiber/receptor system. Measurements of human thresholds for sense of flutter-vibration tested over thenar eminence. In the anesthetized curve, cocaine was applied to skin, blocking the superficial receptors. Note that this resulted in a threshold change only over the low-frequency portion of the curve. Thus, the Meissner corpuscles are the receptors for the low-frequency responsive group. (Adapted with permission from V. B. Mountcastle (ed): *Medical Physiology*, ed 12. Saint Louis: CV Mosby, 1968, Ch 61–62.[5])

of sensory receptors. Subsequent to ganglionectomy, single-unit analysis of median nerve fibers is related to a given peripheral receptive field, which is then biopsied. The histologic, electron microscopic, and neurophysiologic correlates found an innervated Meissner corpuscle in the rapidly-adapting field, and an innervated Merkel cell-neurite complex in the slowly-adapting field.

Summaries of the information on slowly- and quickly-adapting fiber/receptor systems are given in Figure 3.14 and Table 3.4.

CENTRAL ORGANIZATION

Spinal Cord Level

In the peripheral nervous system we saw that cutaneous sensibility is organized according to submodality specific fiber/receptor systems. These fibers are the first order afferents, and their proximal connections end within the central nervous system, synapsing with the second order afferents. The neuron for the second order afferent is in the nucleus cunneatus and gracilis. Third order afferent neurons are in the ventroposterolateral nucleus of the thalamus. Here they receive input from the second order afferents and relay this centrally to the somatosensory cortex, the postcentral gyrus of the parietal lobe[49] (Fig. 3.15).

There is evidence suggesting that the submodality-specific profile of neural impulses, generated at the fingertip, reaches the thalamic level essentially unchanged. That is, fiber sorting mechanisms existing within the spinal cord continue the submodality segregation.[50-53]

Thalamic Level

The ventrobasal complex of the thalamus, and the ventroposterolateral nuclei in particular, receives the medial lemniscal pathway. The medial lemniscus carries the second order afferent fibers. Mountcastle's group[54, 55] recorded the evoked potentials in this nucleus after tactile stimulation of the skin. They found that the nucleus contains a detailed representation of the contralateral body and that its neurons (third order afferents) were highly specific as regards place (area of periphery stimulated) and sensory submodality (Fig. 3.16). The body pattern represented on the surface of the thalamus is distorted with respect to the relative surface

Table 3.3
Quickly-Adapting Cutaneous Mechanoreceptors

	Meissner	Pacinian
Quickly-adapting	x	x
Responds to oscillation	x	x
Frequency range	10–300 cps	10–300 cps
Maximum sensitivity	30 cps	250 cps
Thresholds	Higher	Lower
Receptive field	Smaller	Larger
Receptor: proven	±	+
Location	Superficial	Deep
Axon	>1	1

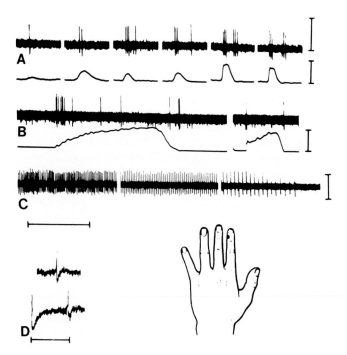

Figure 3.13. Quickly-adapting fiber/receptor example of percutaneous recording from awake human subject's response to (A) taps, (B) continuous pressure, (C) vibration, (D) mechanically (upper) and electrically (lower) induced impulse. Black spot on hand is receptive field of the recorded single fiber. Note: good response to transients (moving-touch) in A and C. Just an "on-off" type of response to constant-touch and pressure. (Adapted with permission from A. B. Vallbo and K. E. Hagbarth: *Exp Neurol* 21: 270 – 289, 1968.[26])

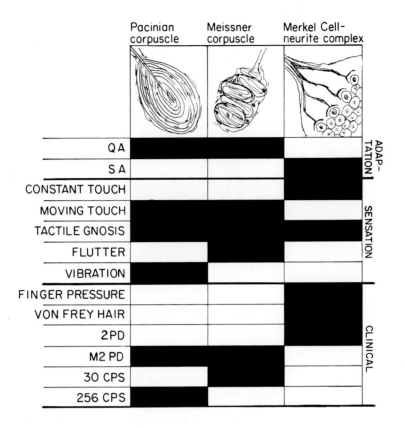

Figure 3.14.   Summary diagram of slowly- and quickly-adapting fiber/receptor systems with clinical correlates.

Table 3.4
Summary

Nerve Fiber Property	Peripheral Receptor	Sensation	Clinical Test	Neurophysiologic Correlate
Slowly-Adapting	Merkel cell-neurite complex	Constant-touch Pressure Tactile gnosis (static)	Fingertip touch von Frey hair Classic two-point discrimination	Stimulus Threshold Innervation density
Quickly-adapting	Meissner corpuscle	Moving-touch Flutter Tactile gnosis (moving)	Fingertip stroking 30-cps tuning fork Vibrometer Moving two-point discrimination	Stimulus Threshold Innervation density
Quickly-adapting	Pacinian corpuscle	Moving-touch Vibration Tactile gnosis (moving)	Fingertip stroking 256-cps tuning fork Vibrometer Moving two-point discrimination	Stimulus Threshold Innervation density

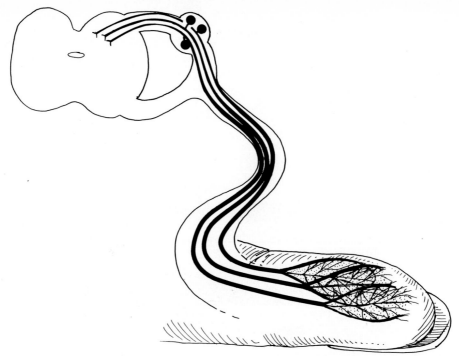

Figure 3.15. Three sets of afferent fibers transmit a submodality-specific profile of neural impulses to the somatosensory cortex. Note overlapping peripheral receptive fields.

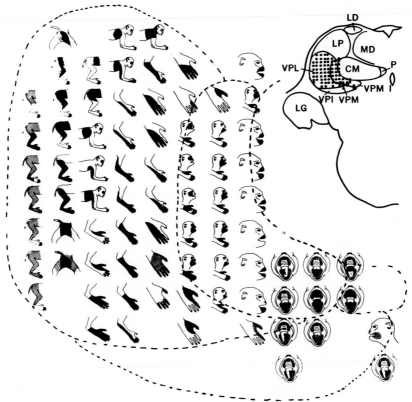

Figure 3.16. Thalamic sensory organization: Representation of cutaneous sensibility in one frontal plane of thalamus of monkey. Tactile stimulation of skin of areas marked on figurines evoked responses at points indicated. VPL, Ventroposterolateral nuclei. (Adapted from Mountcastle[54])

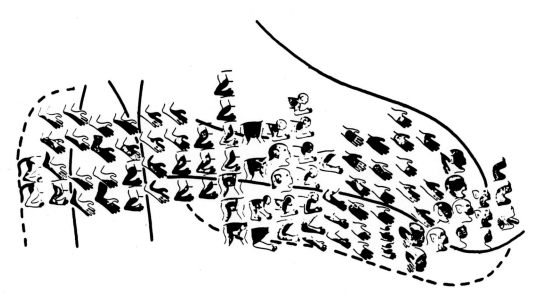

Figure 3.17. Postcentral cortex sensory organization: Representation of cutaneous sensibility rostral surface postcentral gyrus of monkey (area 1). Central sulcus is *heavy wavy line* to the right. Tactile stimulation of skin of areas marked on figurines evoked responses at points indicated. (Adapted from Woolsey.[57])

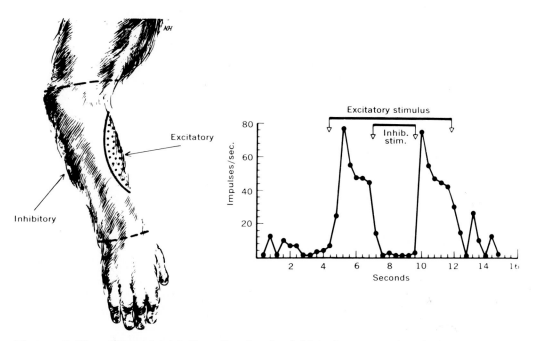

Figure 3.18. Afferent inhibition: Tracing to right is from a postcentral gyrus neuron which reacted to stimulation in the contralateral forearm excitatory zone. During this response, tactile stimulation of the zone surrounding this central excitatory zone produced inhibition of the response. (Adapted from Mountcastle and Powell.[60])

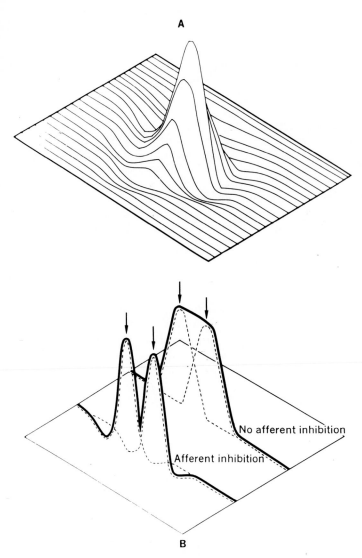

Figure 3.19. Afferent inhibition: Conceptualization of the reshaping or contouring of the profile of neural impulses by afferent inhibition. This may be the mechanism operational in two-point discrimination. (Adapted with permission from V. B. Mountcastle (ed): *Medical Physiology*, ed 12. Saint Louis: CV Mosby, 1968, Ch 61–62.[5])

areas of the periphery. The area represented by the head, hands, and feet is disproportionately large. Thus, this representation is in proportion to the peripheral innervation density, not to body geometry. From point to point on the thalamic surface, there is also a partially shifted overlap of the peripheral receptive fields.

From the thalamus, this submodality specificity is projected to somatosensory cortex.

Somatosensory Cortex

The postcentral gyrus was first mapped generally in awake humans by direct stimulation by Penfield and Rasmussen,[56] and in detail in monkeys by evoked potential by Woolsey.[57] These studies yielded the familiar, distorted homunculus in which, as we saw for the thalamus, body shape was proportionate to the peripheral innervation density, with partially shifted overlapping peripheral receptive fields (Fig. 3.17).

The surface of the postcentral gyrus can be divided by the cytoarchitecture gradient that extends from anterior (within the sulcus) area 3, to the rostral half of the gyrus surface, area 1, to the caudal half of the gyrus surface, area 2, as described by Brodmann. Area 2 contains neurons primarily activated by rotation of joints, while areas 1 and 3 contain neurons

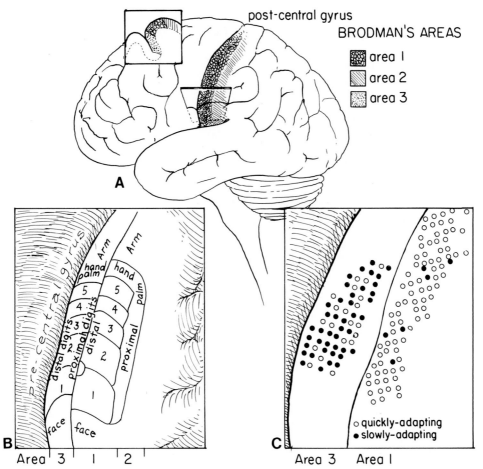

Figure 3.20. Dual representation of the hand area: *A,* The postcentral gyrus is cytoarchitecturally divided into Brodmann's areas: 3 (within sulcus), 1 (rostral half of gyrus surface) and 2. *B,* The hand area is topographically present in areas 3 and 1. *C,* Each ○ or ● represents a direct recording from a neuron, labeled after appropriate peripheral stimulations. Area 1 was found to average 95% quickly-adapting units, whereas area 3 was found to average 56% slowly-adapting units. (Adapted with permission from R. L. Paul et al.: *Brain Res* 36: 229–249, 1972.[61])

activated by skin stimulation.[5] Mountcastle's work[58, 59] demonstrated that the basic organization of postcentral gyrus neurons within each area was vertical. Utilizing a technique that penetrated the surface of the gyrus with a microelectrode, it was demonstrated that for a given penetration the neurons in that column of cortical tissue responded in the same manner to the same peripheral cutaneous stimulus. There was a columnar submodality-specific organization related to the same peripheral receptive field.

How does the postcentral gyrus organization permit two point discrimination? During the work of Mountcastle and Powell[60] on the cortex, 53 neurons of the 593 studied were not only excited by stimulation of one skin area, but were also inhibited by stimulation of another (Fig. 3.18). They found that general anesthesia could abolish this inhibitory effect, perhaps explaining why the phenomenon had been so rarely seen (the monkeys studied had received anesthesia). Afferent inhibition, in a center-surround pattern such

Table 3.5
Peripheral and Cortical Coding Mechanisms for Sense of Flutter-Vibration[a]

Psychophysical Event	Peripheral Neural Code	Central Neural Code
Identification: flutter vs vibration	Place code: which set of peripheral fibers is active	Place code: which set of cortical neurons is active
Detection of flutter	Place plus frequency code: appearance of any activity in Meissner afferents	Place plus frequency code: increment in activity in a give set of cortical neurons
Frequency discrimination	Place plus temporal order code: appearance of tuned discharges in some small number of Meissner afferents	Place plus temporal order code: cyclic entrainment of activity of a given set of cortical neurons
Subjective magnitude estimate (amplitude)	Place and spatial distribution code: linear increase in size of Meissner population activated by stimulus	Place and spatial distribution code: linear growth in size of cortical cell population in which increments in activity occur

[a] Adapted from V. B. Mountcastle.[6]

as this, shapes and limits the profile of neural impulses (as conceptualized in Fig. 3.19). Thus a broad profile may be centrally inhibited to reveal two peaks. This mechanism may be operational in two-point discrimination.[5]

Recently, careful remapping of the postcentral gyrus by Merzenich and co-workers[61] have demonstrated a duplication of the hand area within Brodmann's areas 3 and 1. This work, in the monkey species *Macaca mulatta*, was subsequently confirmed in another species, *Aotus trivirgatus*, the owl monkey[62] and recently reviewed[63] (Fig. 3.20, and also Figs. 5.11, 5.12). As first described in the macque, appropriate stimuli to peripheral receptive fields resulted in postcentral neuron responses which could be recorded as quickly- or slowly-adapting. In area 3 (within the sulcus), 56% of the responses were slowly-adaptive. In area 1 (rostral half of gyrus surface), 95% of the responses were quickly-adapting.[61] This duplication was shown to occur first at this, the highest level of sensory organization, as it was not present (by horseradish peroxidase staining) in the thalamus.[64] These authors believe this dual representation is firmly established, as they have now studied 3500 recording sites in New World Monkeys (three species) and 4400 recording sites in Old World Monkeys.[63]

A summary, adapted from Mountcastle, of the coding of peripheral sensibility is presented in Table 3.5.

References

1. Weber EH: Ueber den Tastsinn. Arch Anat Physiol 1:152–159, 1835.
2. Seddon HJ: *Surgical Disorders of the Peripheral Nerves.* Baltimore: Williams and Wilkins, 1972, p viii.
3. Sunderland S: *Nerves and Nerve Injuries.* Edinburgh: Churchill-Livingstone, 1978.
4. Woodhall B, Beebe GW: *Peripheral Nerve Regeneration.* Washington, DC: US Gov Print Office, 1956.
5. Mountcastle VB (ed): *Medical Physiology,* ed 12. Saint Louis: CV Mosby, 1968, Ch 61–62.
6. Mountcastle VB: The view from within: Pathways to the study of perception. Johns Hopkins Med J 136: 109–131, 1975.
7. Erlanger J, Gasser HS: *Electrical Signs of Nervous Activity.* Philadelphia: Univ Penn Press, 1937.
8. Mountcastle VB: Pain and temperature sensibilities, in Mountcastle VB (ed): *Medical Physiology,* ed 12. Saint Louis: CV Mosby, 1968, Ch 63.
9. LaMotte RH, Campbell JN: Comparison of responses of warm and nociceptive C-fiber afferents in monkey with human judgments of thermal pain. J Neurophysiol 41:509–528, 1978.
10. Campbell JN, Meyer RA, La Motte RH: Sensitization of myelinated nociceptive afferents that innervate monkey hand. J Neurophysiol 42:1669–1679, 1979.
11. Dellon AL: The moving two-point discrimination test: Quantitative evaluation of the quickly-adapting fiber/receptor system. J Hand Surg 3:474–481, 1978.
12. Iggo A: New specific sensory structures in hairy skin. Acta Neuroveg 24:175–180, 1963.
13. Iggo A, Muir AR: A cutaneous sense organ in the hairy skin of cats. J Anat 97:151, 1963.
14. Brown AG, Iggo A: A quantitative study of cutaneous receptor and afferent fibers in the cat and rabbit. J Physiol 193:707–733, 1967.
15. Iggo A, Muir AR: The structure and function of a slowly-adapting touch corpuscle in hairy skin. J Physiol 200:763–796, 1969.

16. Lindblom U: Properties of touch receptors in distal glabrous skin of the monkey. J Neurophysiol 28: 966–985, 1965.

17. Werner G, Mountcastle VB: Neural activity in mechanoreceptive afferents: Stimulus response relations, Weber functions, and information transmission. J Neurophysiol 28:359–397, 1965.

18. Mountcastle VB, Talbot WH, Kornhuber HH: *The Neural Transformation of Mechanical Stimuli Delivered to the Monkey's Hand.* Ciba Foundation Symposium on Touch, Heat and Pain, de Rueck AVS, Knight J (eds). London: JA Churchill, 1966.

19. Siminoff R: Quantitative properties of slowly-adapting mechanoreceptors in alligator skin. Exp Neurol 21:290–306, 1968.

20. Munger BL: The intraepidermal innervation of the snout skin of the opossum: A light and electron microscopic study, with observations on the nature of Merkel's Tastzellen. J Cell Biol 26:79–96, 1965.

21. Pubols LM, Pubols BH Jr, Munger BL: Functional properties of mechanoreceptors in glabrous skin of the raccoon's forepaw. Exp Neurol 31:165–182, 1971.

22. Munger BL, Pubols LM, Pubols BH Jr: The Merkel rete papilla—a slowly-adapting sensory receptor in mammalian glabrous skin. Brain Res 29:47–61, 1971.

23. Munger BL, Pubols LM: The sensorineural organization of the digital skin of the raccoon. Brain Behav Evol 5:367–393, 1972.

24. Hensel H, Boman KA: Afferent impulses in cutaneous sensory nerves in human subjects. J Neurophysiol 23:564–578, 1960.

25. Konietzny F, Hensel H: Response of rapidly and slowly-adapting mechanoreceptors and vibratory sensitivity in human hairy skin. Pfluegers Arch 368: 39–44, 1977.

26. Vallbo AB, Hagbarth KE: Activity from skin mechanoreceptors recorded percutaneously in awake human subjects. Exp Neurol 21:270–289, 1968.

27. Knibestol M, Vallbo AB: Single unit analysis of mechanoreceptor activity from the human glabrous skin. Acta Physiol Scand 80:178–195, 1970.

28. Harrington T, Merzenich MM: Neural coding in the sense of touch: Human sensations of skin indentation compared with responses of slowly-adapting mechanoreceptive afferents innervating the hairy skin of monkeys. Exp Brain Res 10:251–264, 1970.

29. Horch KW, Whitehorn D, Burgess PR: Impulse generation in type I cutaneous mechanoreceptors. J Neurophysiol 37:267–281, 1974.

30. Horch KW, Burgess PR: Responses to threshold and suprathreshold stimuli by slowly-adapting cutaneous mechanoreceptors in the cat. J Comp Physiol 110:307–315, 1976.

31. Pinkus F: Uber Hautsinnesorgane neben den menschlichen Haar (Haarscheiben) und ihre vergleickenden anatomische Bedeutung. Arch Mikrosk Anat EntwMech 65:121–128, 1904.

32. Straille WE: Sensory hair follicles in mammalian skin: The tylotrich follicle. Am J Anat 106:133–148, 1960.

33. Andres KH: *The Peripheral Nervous System*, Hubbard JI (ed). New York: Plenum Press, 1974, Ch 12.

34. Iggo A: Cutaneous receptors, in Hubbard JI (ed): *The Peripheral Nervous System.* New York: Plenum Press, 1974, Ch 12, pp 347–404 (101 references).

35. Chambers MR, Andres KH, von Duering M, et al: The structure and function of the slowly-adapting type II mechanoreceptors in hairy skin. Q J Exp Physiol 57:417–445, 1972.

36. Biemesderfer D, Munger BL, Binck J, et al: The Pilo-Ruffini complex: A non-sinus hair and associated slowly-adapting mechanoreceptor in primate facial skin. Brain Res 142:197–222, 1978.

37. Merzenich MM, Harrington T: The sense of flutter-vibration evoked by stimulation of the hairy skin of primates: Comparison of human sensory capacity with the responses of mechanoreceptive afferents innervating the hairy skin of monkeys. Exp Brain Res 9:236–260, 1969.

38. Mountcastle VB: Discussion section of CIBA Foundation Symposium on *Touch, Heat and Pain.* London: JA Churchill, 1966.

39. Talbot WH, Darian-Smith I, Kornhuber HH, et al: The sense of flutter-vibration: Comparison of the human capacity with response patterns of mechanoreceptive afferents from the monkey hand. J Neurophysiol 31:301–334, 1968.

40. Lowenstein WR, Rothkamp, R: The sites for mechanoelectric conversion in a Pacinian corpuscle. J Gen Physiol 41:1245–1265, 1958.

41. Lowenstein WR: Biological transducers. Sci Am 203: 99–108, 1960.

42. Lowenstein WR: On the "specificity" of a sensory receptor. J Neurophysiol 24:150–158, 1961.

43. Lowenstein WR, Mendelson M: Components of receptor adaptation in a Pacinian corpuscle. J Physiol 177:377–397, 1965.

44. Gray JAB, Malcolm JL: The initiation of a nerve impulse by mesenteric Pacinian corpuscles. Proc R Soc Lond [Biol] 137:96, 1950.

45. Gray JAB, Mathews PBR: A comparison of the adaptation of the Pacinian corpuscle with the accommodation of its own axon. J Physiol 114:454–464, 1951.

46. Dykes RW, Terzis JK: Reinnervation of glabrous skin in baboons: Properties of cutaneous mechanoreceptors subsequent to nerve crush. J Neurophysiol 42:1461–1478, 1979.

47. Johnson KO: Reconstruction of population response to a vibratory stimulus in quickly-adapting mechanoreceptive afferent fiber population innervating glabrous skin of the monkey. J Neurophysiol 37:48–71, 1974.

48. Munger BL, Page RB, Pubols BH Jr: Identification of specific mechanosensory receptors in glabrous skin of dorsal root ganglionectomized primates. Anat Rec 93:630–631, 1979.

49. Wall P, Dubner R: Somatosensory pathways. Annu Rev Physiol 34:315–336, 1972.

50. Whitsel BL, Petrucelli LM, Sapiro G, et al: Modality representation in the lumbar and cervical fasciculus gracilis of squirrel monkeys. Brain Res 15:67–78, 1969.

51. Whitsel BL, Petrucelli LM, Ha H, et al: The resorting of spinal afferents as antecedent to the body representation in the post central gyrus. Brain Behav Evol 5:303–341, 1972.

52. Dreyer DA, Schneider RJ, Metz CB, et al: Differential contributions of spinal pathways to body representation in post-central gyrus. J Neurophysiol 37:119–145, 1945.

53. Schneider RJ, Kulics AT, Ducker TB: Proprioceptive pathways of the spinal cord. J Neurol Neurosurg Psychiatry 40:417–433, 1977.

54. Mountcastle VB, Henneman E: The representation of tactile sensibility in the thalamus of the monkey. J Comp Neurol 97:409–440, 1952.

55. Mountcastle VB, Poggio GF, Werner G: The relation of thalamic cell response to peripheral stimuli varied over an intensive continuum. J Neurophysiol 26:807–834, 1963.

56. Penfield W, Rasmussen AT: *The Cerebral Cortex of Man: A Clinical Study of Localization of Function.* New York: Macmillan, 1950.

57. Woolsey CN: Organization of somatic sensory and motor areas of cerebral cortex, in Harlow HF, Woolsey CN (eds): *Biological and Biochemical Basis of Behavior.* Madison: Univ Wisc Press, 1958.

58. Mountcastle VB: Modality and topographic properties of single neurons of cat's somatic sensory cortex. J Neurophysiol 20:408–434, 1957.

59. Powell TPS, Mountcastle VB: Some aspects of the functional organization of the cortex of the post-central gyrus of the monkey: A correlation of findings obtained in a single unit analysis with cytoarchitecture. Bull Johns Hopkins Hosp 105:133–162, 1959.

60. Mountcastle VB, Powell TPS: Neural mechanisms subserving cutaneous sensibility, with special reference to the role of afferent inhibition in sensory perception and discrimination. Bull Johns Hopkins Hosp 105:201–232, 1959.

61. Paul RL, Merzenich M, Goodman H: Representation of slowly and rapidly-adapting cutaneous mechanoreceptors of the hand in the Brodmann's areas 3 and 1 of Macaca mulatta. Brain Res 36:229–249, 1972.

62. Merzenich MM, Kaas JH, Sur M, et al: Double representation of the body surface within cytoarchitecture areas 3b and 1 in "S1" in the Owl Monkey (Aotus trivirgatus). J Comp Neurol 181:41–74, 1978.

63. Kaas JH, Nelson RJ, Sur M, et al: Multiple representations of the body within the somatosensory cortex of primates. Science 204:521–523, 1979.

64. Lin C, Merzenich MM, Sur M, et al: Connections of areas 3b and 1 of the parietal somatosensory strip with the ventroposterior nucleus in the Owl Monkey (Aotus trivirgatus). J Comp Neurol 185:355–372, 1979.

Chapter 4

SENSORY CORPUSCLES AFTER NERVE DIVISION

INTRODUCTION
EARLY SENSORY INVESTIGATIONS
PACINIAN CORPUSCLE
MEISSNER CORPUSCLE
MERKEL CELL-NEURITE COMPLEX
CLINICAL IMPLICATIONS

INTRODUCTION

In 1850, August Waller described the axonal consequences of dividing the IX and XII cranial nerves of the frog.[1] Ranson's classic light microscopic[2] and more recent electron microscopic[3, 4] investigations have described in great detail the axoplasmic, myelin, and Schwann' cell alterations that characterize the peripheral nerve fiber following complete nerve division, and which we call "Wallerian Degeneration." Virtually every minute detail of this process has been reviewed recently by Sunderland,[5] who cites 533 reference sources. Following complete transection of a nerve, both retrograde and antegrade changes occur. Retrograde changes include not only a variable degree of axoplasmic disintegration and absorption, followed by axonal remnant swelling, but also central neuronal chromatolysis, followed by cell death (or recovery). The proximal axonal swelling represents the build up, through axoplasmic flow, of materials required for the axoplasm sprouts to regenerate and corresponds with a central nuclear polarity during chromosynthesis or recovery. The severity of the retrograde changes is directly proportional to the severity of the injury (avulsion causes more chro-

matolysis than laceration) and inversely proportional to the distance between the neuron and the site of injury (shoulder level causes more chromatolysis than forearm level). The antegrade changes comprise axonal swelling, axonal breakup, myelin degeneration, Schwann-cell dedifferentiation into macrophage-like cells, phagocytosis of degenerated axoplasm and myelin, and subsequent partial collapse of the endoneurial tube. The most distal antegrade change, the counterpart of the central component of retrograde change, is not discussed. *The fate of sensory corpuscles following nerve division is not mentioned.*

Sensory function is more difficult to assess at every level of investigation than motor function. For this reason, investigation of every phase of neuromuscular activity has preceded similar work in sensory function. Until the last 2 decades sensory function has been relatively ignored. Sunderland[6] devotes five full chapters (with at least 550 references) to the effect of denervation upon muscle without a single reference to the effect of denervation upon sensory corpuscles!

A brief account of change in the motor system following denervation is offered for comparison with the sensory material to follow. After complete nerve division, progressive gross muscle atrophy occurs, although histologically the remaining fibers retain striations and relatively normal subsarcolemmal nuclei. Atrophy is due to myofibrillar fragmentation and subsequent loss. Motor end-plates degenerate. There is a relative increase in the connective tissue component which may give the appearance of "fibrosis." Motor fiber bulk may be reduced by 80%. The pathophysiologic, biochemical, and ultrastructural changes occurring in denervation muscles are beyond the scope of this text.

EARLY SENSORY INVESTIGATION

Two basic approaches have been used to investigate the fate of denervated sensory corpuscles: (1) The nerve is injured (crushed, ligated, or transected) and previously innervated tissue examined at some point later in time. (2) The tissue containing the sensory end organs is excised and transplanted, and this transplanted tissue is then examined at some point later in time.

The series of experiments carried out in the laboratory of J. Boeke, in Utrecht, Netherlands in the 1920's and 1930's remains classic.[7, 8] A succession of co-workers, including Klein, Dykstra, Heringa, and Van Straten, were present with Boeke during this time.[9] Their early work involved the mole's snout: this specialized sensory end organ (the organ of Eimer) contains expanded bulb nerve endings adjacent to epidermal papillae. The organ of Eimer was observed to "degenerate" following trigeminal nerve transection. A similar study in the duck demonstrates that the bill's corpuscular endings, Grandry corpuscles (a neurofibrillar disc morphologically analogous to a Merkel cell-neurite complex) and Herbst corpuscles (Pacinian-like corpuscles) degenerated following division of the V cranial nerve. Also in the duck, bill skin was excised and transplanted onto the foot with subsequent degeneration of these corpuscles (Fig. 4.1).

The sensory end organ most intensely studied with respect to nerve sectioning experiments has been the taste bud. Guth[10, 11] (then at the National Institutes of Health, and now at the University of Maryland's Department of Anatomy) pursued Waller's experimental design. Using a rat model, the IX cranial nerve was divided and the circumvallate papillae studied; they were found to degenerate and desquamate. Recent electron microscopy has confirmed these observations.[12, 13]

In the skin graft type of study, small corpuscular sensory endings were observed to degenerate completely in pig snout transplanted to the pig's back[14] and in rabbit scrotal skin transplanted to the rabbit's ear.[15]

Although these studies suggest that denervated sensory corpuscles degenerate, recent authorities imply that sensory end organs persist, at least to the extent that the regenerating axon "re-establishes" continuity with the end organ.[16, 17] Seddon cites an example of "Pacinian and Meissner Corpuscles found in man nine months after nerve injury," documented by Lyons and Woodhall in 1949. Careful review, however, reveals a histologic section from a fingertip biopsy from the amputated arm of a soldier injured 9 months earlier. The soldier had sustained a high velocity missile injury to the axilla with laceration of the subclavian artery and brachial plexus. In the biopsy, one Pacinian and one Meissner corpuscle were found: they were described as being "aneuric and fibrotic." Though "persisting" following "nerve injury," I believe these corpuscles had degenerated.

Winkelman's observation of Meissner corpuscles in the toe of one dog 18 months following sciatic nerve division[19] is often quoted as demonstrating that sensory corpuscles persist following nerve division. Winkelman used a nonspecific cholinesterase stain to identify these corpuscles. Using silver stain, however, he noted that the corpuscle was "denervated." The cholinesterase histochemical technique has been utilized to study biopsy material from fingertips of patients with neuropathy.[20] Qualitative changes were observed in these disease states. The interpretation of these studies is difficult. They essentially demonstrate an aneuritic corpuscular remnant that contains an active enzyme. Application of a cholinesterase inhibitor to the skin fails to alter the clinical response to sensory testing,[21] and therefore positive non-

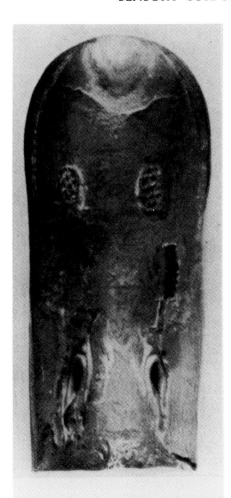

Figure 4.1. Photograph of duck's bill, with two sites of successfully transplanted scaly skin from the duck's foot. No Herbst or Grandry corpuscles regenerated *de novo* in these grafts. (Reproduced with permission from J. Boeke: *The Problems of Nervous Anatomy.* London Oxford University Press, 1940.[9])

FIG. 8. Photograph of duck's bill containing two pieces of transplanted 'scaly' skin of the foot. After Dijkstra, 1933.

specific cholinesterase staining does not have functional significance clinically. The positive staining material appears to be localized between the axoplasm and the Schwann-cell,[22] or, by analogy, between the axon tip and the lamellar cell process in the Meissner corpuscle. No comments were made in the study of the neuropathies as to whether the numerically diminished corpuscles that remained were of normal size or atrophic! I feel that this staining technique cannot be utilized to demonstrate anything more than the location of a Meissner corpuscle, and inferences regarding corpuscles' integrity or function are not justified.[23] My own investigations with this technique also demonstrate presence of positive-staining Meissner corpuscles in denervated primate fingertips, but careful comparison with controls suggests that the overall shape of the Meissner corpuscle is distorted and smaller[24] (Fig. 4.2). I believe these observations suggest that even though Meissner corpuscle remnants are nonspecific cholinesterase-positive in staining characteristics, these end organs are degenerating following denervation.

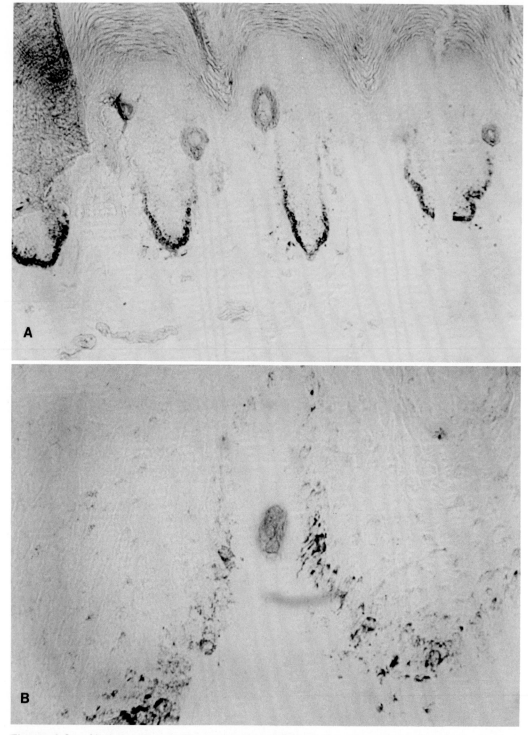

Figure 4.2. Nonspecific cholinesterase staining of the Meissner corpuscle. Control sections: *A* at ×25 and *B* at ×100. At 4 months after denervation (*C*, ×100) the corpuscle still stains well but has altered morphology.

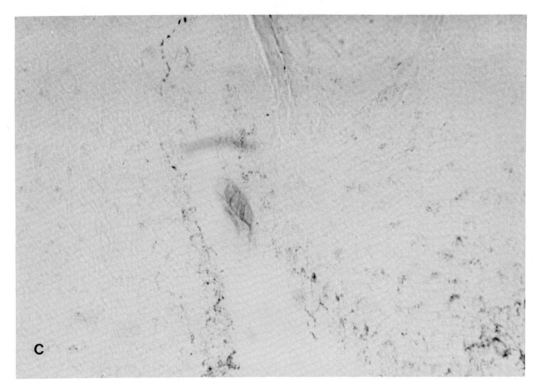

Figure 4.2.   (*C*)

PACINIAN CORPUSCLE

It was natural for detailed sensory investigations to begin with the Pacinian corpuscle. As discussed in Chapter 1, this corpuscle was the first sensory end organ discovered because it is macroscopic. It is ubiquitous in mammals and quite abundant in the mesentery of the cat. Ferdinand C. Lee,[25] in a remarkable series of experiments from the Hunterian Surgical Laboratory (begun by William Stewart Halstead) at Johns Hopkins, demonstrated degeneration *in* the Pacinian corpuscle. These were reported in 1936. He divided the myelinated fiber to the corpuscle in the cat mesentery and observed, histologically, degeneration of the axon and its completion within 2 weeks. His surgery was performed under an early (Greenough) operating microscope. His short-term observation showed no change in the lamellar corpuscle. Lee also studied the physiology of the corpuscle and the effect of "regeneration" following partial excision of the corpuscle (it rounded over and contracted, not really "regenerated").

In 1949 Glees et al.[26] made long-term observations on the effect of denervation upon the Pacinian corpuscle itself. They excised Pacinian corpuscles from cat mesentery and implanted them into cat cerebrum and thigh muscle. Up to 400 days later there were no signs of degeneration of the lamellar corpuscular structure. There were also no signs of reinnervation either by cerebral axons or those "cutaneous" axons adjacent to the thigh muscle.

Lowenstein's neurophysiologic studies of this receptor, discussed in detail in Chapter 3, led to a series of experiments on the effect of denervation upon the Pacinian corpuscle. Attempting to learn the relationship of the different components of this fiber/receptor system to neural conduction, Lowenstein[27] crushed and divided the myelinated axon to the corpuscle. The axon ending degenerated and the corpuscle's laminated capsule remained unchanged. In attempting "nerve union" studies, corpuscles, themselves, were still present in failed "nerve unions" 7 weeks after nerve division.

The effect of denervation upon Pacinian corpuscles has been investigated in subhuman primates.[28, 29] After nerve division, the axon terminal within the corpuscles was completely absent within 3 to 4 weeks. Specific descriptions of later corpuscle changes were not given, although noninnervated corpuscles could be "identified" at 40 weeks postdenervation. Histochemical studies demonstrated loss of acetylcholinesterase staining in the Pacinian corpuscle by 8 weeks postdenervation, while nonspecific cholinesterase staining showed no difference from controls.

Ultrastructural evaluation of the immediate events following denervation has been reported in the cat, sciatic nerve, hind footpad model.[30] These findings confirmed those discussed above and added that the lamellar cell processes were responsible for the phagocytosis of the unmyelinated portion of the axon within the Pacinian corpuscle's inner core, analogous to the Schwann cell phagocytosis of the myelinated portion of the axon. This suggested that the lamellar cells were modified Schwann cells.

The single reported observation, of which I am aware, in man is that described earlier[18] following brachial plexus trauma. At 9 months postinjury, fingertip biopsy demonstrated a single "aneuritic and fibrotic" Pacinian corpuscle.

It may be concluded that Wallerian degeneration occurs following division of the sensory nerve fibers to a Pacinian corpuscle. The end organ's tightly wound lamellae, probably over a great length of time, undergoes progressive degeneration. This latter process is slow and its time course remains to be defined. The relationship between the activity of the enzymes of the cholinesterase system upon neurotropism or capsular integrity remains unknown.

MEISSNER CORPUSCLE

Although the observations by Winkelman[19] of the effects of denervation upon Meissner corpuscles (utilizing *non-specific* cholinesterase staining techniques) has been interpreted as demonstrating persistence of these corpuscles) further work has altered these interpretations. In a series of precise morphologic and histochemical investigations, Silver, Versaci, and Montagna studied control and "pathologic" biopsy material from patients' fingertips.[31, 32] These patients had various median and ulnar nerve injuries from 2½ to 12 months prior to biopsy. The staining reaction to acetylcholinesterase became greatly reduced following denervation and that to butyrocholinesterase also became reduced. Nonspecific cholinesterase staining was not employed. Furthermore, serial sections of corpuscles were measured in terms of capsular height, length, and width, and volumes estimated. In two patients, 10 months and 12 months postdenervation, Meissner corpuscle volume was reduced by 53% versus control! For example, one of these patients demonstrated Meissner corpuscle degeneration from an estimated volume of 98 cu μm to one of 47 cu μm, a change statistically significant at the p less than 0.001 level.

The effect of nerve crush and division in subhuman primates was studied at 3 to 4 weeks, 6 weeks and 8 weeks postinjury utilizing acetylcholinesterase and nonspecific cholinesterase and silver techniques.[27] By 3 to 4 weeks, all corpuscles were aneuritic, acetylcholinesterase staining was diminished, and nonspecific cholinesterase staining unchanged. By 8 weeks, the acetylcholinesterase staining characteristics were returning in the crushed nerve specimens, while in the nerve division specimens the acetylcholinesterase reaction was absent and the nonspecific cholinesterase reaction was normal.

These earlier studies demonstrated that at 3 to 4 weeks the Meissner corpuscle had undergone Wallerian degeneration and that at 8 weeks postdenervation alterations in histochemical staining occurred. In at least two isolated observations, the capsular structure degenerated by 10 months.

We investigated the effects of prolonged denervation upon the Meissner corpuscle in the Rhesus monkey, utilizing a sequential light and electron microscopic technique that permitted controlled observations.[24] In these studies, an Azzopardi silver and Masson trichrome staining technique was used to study 72-hour, 2-week, 4-month, 7-month, and 9-month postdenervation fingertip biopsies. In each monkey, the median, ulnar, and radial sensory nerves were excised for a length of 1 cm at the wrist level to totally deafferent the volar pads and eliminate anomalous innervation. At 72 hours postdenervation, the Meissner corpuscle had lost the pink-staining material usually present between the lamellae, and the lobular architecture was less prominent. Silver staining showed the axon terminals were fragmenting. At 2 weeks, lobular subdivisions were less evident, the lamellae appeared to be "collapsing," and no axon terminal remained. There was little further change in 4 months. By 7 months, the corpuscles were shrinking in size. By 9 months, they were markedly shrunken (Fig. 4.3 and 4.4).

Ultrastructural changes paralleled and confirmed the light microscopic observations.[24]* The electron microscopy at 48 hours showed that terminals were degenerating and being phagocytized by lamellar cell processes. At 4 months postdenervation, axon terminals were absent, lamellar cell processes had become blunt, and there was a relative increase in interlamellar substance (Fig. 4.5). The observation of lamellar cell phagocytosis of the axon terminals is analogous to the Schwann cell phagocytosis of the axon in classical Wallerian degeneration,[33] of the Dark Cell phagocytosis of the axon filaments in the rat fungiform taste bud,[12] and of those reported above in the Pacinian corpuscle.[30]

We conclude that the denervated Meissner corpuscle undergoes progressive degeneration, beginning first with its axon terminal, then with enzyme systems within the lamellar cell (e.g., acetylcholinesterase) and then with atrophy of the lamellar cell complex itself.

MERKEL CELL-NEURITE COMPLEX

During studies following discovery of the "Touch Corpuscle" in the cat, Brown and Iggo[34] observed that crushing the saphenous nerve caused the tactile cells and the nerve fibers to degenerate and the dome to flatten. Palmer[35] extended these observations to the opossum. In an abstract, he reported dividing the infraorbital nerve and observing snout Merkel cells and the axon terminals to be

degenerated completely by 72 hours after nerve section. Kasprzak et al.[36] in 1970 confirmed Brown and Iggo's earlier observations on the cat's footpad.

An apparent species difference in the trophic dependence of the Merkel cell on the presence of the axon was noted by Smith.[37] In the rat, division of the cutaneous nerve caused degeneration of the axon terminals beneath the tylotrich hair, but up to 90 days later the Merkel cells remained intact. Kasprzak et al.[36] confirmed these observations in the rat.

Burgess et al in 1974[38] divided the femoral cutaneous nerve of the cat and observed its effect upon the previously identified touch dome population. This site was depilated, the domes tatooed, the domes counted under magnification, and the site photographed. The site was re-examined at intervals up to 1 year after the crush and denervation. Electrophysiologic recording was done from the nerve with simultaneous stimulation of the touch domes in the receptive fields before and after nerve crush and division. At 16 days following nerve division, the neural component of the dome was completely degenerated. By 35 days following nerve division, the entire dome had disappeared (Figs. 4.6 and 4.7).

Recently, Munger and Ide[39] have studied degeneration of the Merkel cell-neurite complex in the raccoon at the ultrastructural level. They have confirmed the neural degeneration and observed a decrease in the Merkel cell, as well as decreased numbers of the synaptic vesicles in the Merkel cell. (see Fig. 10.7).

It may be concluded that the Merkel cell-neurite complex also undergoes progressive degeneration postdenervation.

CLINICAL IMPLICATIONS

Length of Delay Before Nerve Repair

What is the effect of delaying a nerve repair for a period of time after nerve division? In general, there is little effect for a "short delay" and a decrease in quality of recovery of function for delays greater than 4 months. But "good" recovery has been reported even after delays of 2 years.[40] One report stated that "in marked contrast to the analysis of motor recovery, it is extremely

---

* Electron microscopy was generously done by Bryce Munger, M.D., Chairman of the Department of Anatomy at Milton S. Hershey Medical Center, Hershey, Pennsylvania.

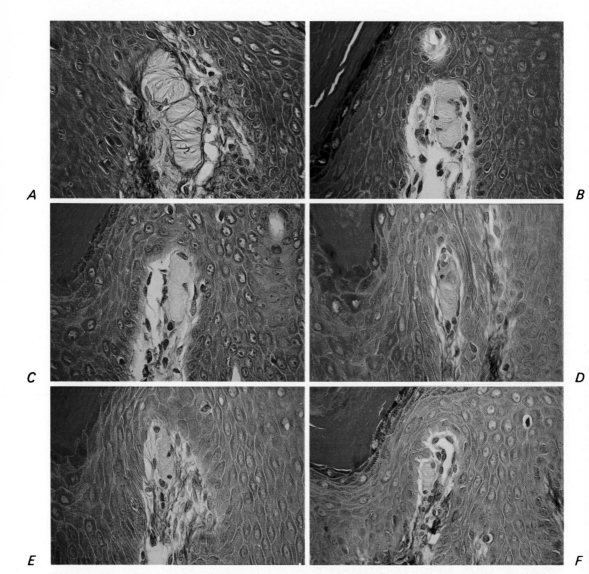

Figure 4.3. Progressive changes in the Meissner corpuscle after denervation. *A*, Representative normal Meissner corpuscle from a control fingertip; all the other photographs are of denervated Meissner corpuscle. *B*, At 72 hours after denervation, showing early loss of lobular subdivisions and of pink-staining material. *C*, At 2 weeks, there is complete loss of the lobular subdivision and lamellar collapse appears, with progressive diminution in the size of Meissner corpuscle at 4 months (*D*) and at 7 months (*E*). By 9 months (*F*), a markedly shrunken Meissner corpuscle is seen adjacent to the capillary in the dermal papilla (Masson trichrome, ×160). (Reproduced with permission from A. L. Dellon et al. *Plast Reconstr Surg* 56:182–193, 1975.[24])

significant that the analysis here yielded no evidence that time from injury to suture influenced (sensory) recovery in any way."[41] A critical review of those studies suggesting that a long delay has no effect, however, reveals that these studies are based on an "arbitrary grading system,"[42] or they define delay as "greater than two weeks."[43] One study which suggests that delay is detrimental[44] does not distinguish between sensory and motor re-

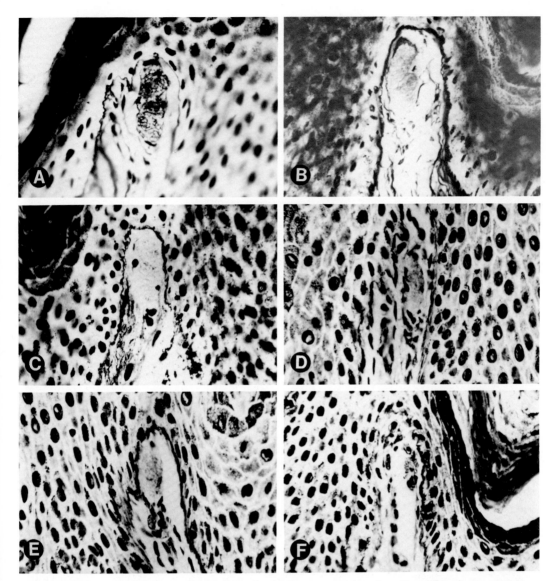

Figure 4.4.   Progressive changes in the Meissner corpuscle after denervation (*above left*). *A,* Representative normal Meissner corpuscle from a control fingertip; note the fine meshwork of nerve terminals within the corpuscle. The other photographs are of denervated Meissner corpuscles. *B,* Axonal fragments remain within Meissner corpuscle at 72 hours after denervation. *C,* At 2 weeks. *D,* At 4 months. *E,* At 7 months. *F,* At 9 months after denervation, nerve terminals are absent from the Meissner corpuscle and there is a progressive decrease in the size of the Meissner corpuscle. In the last photograph *F* the Meissner corpuscle is adjacent to a capillary (Silver stain, ×160). (Reproduced with permission from A. L. Dellon et al.: *Plast Reconstr Surg* 56:182–193, 1975.[24])

covery. This distinction is essential, of course, because the motor end-plates persist in good condition for a year and muscle atrophy does not begin for an even longer period of time.[45]

If one includes only those studies that report specifically on the sensory components of the median and ulnar nerves, and then grades the degree of functional recovery (e.g., S1 to S4),

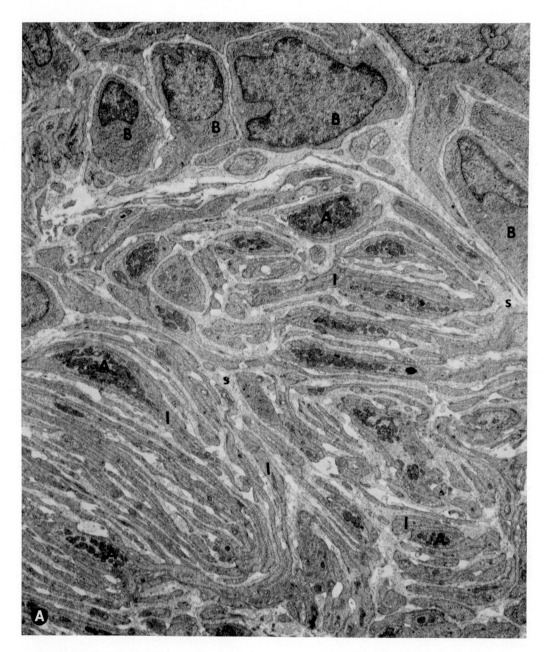

Figure 4.5.   *A,* Electron micrograph of a normal Meissner corpuscle. In a dermal papilla beneath the epidermal basal cells (B), the Meissner corpuscle contains stacks of lamellar cell processes, (*I*), which ensheath the axon terminals (*A*). The axon terminals contain numerous mitochondria. Between the processes is the interlamellar substance (*s*). (×12,450). (Reproduced with permission from A. L. Dellon et al.: *Plast Reconstr Surg* 56:182–193, 1975.[24])

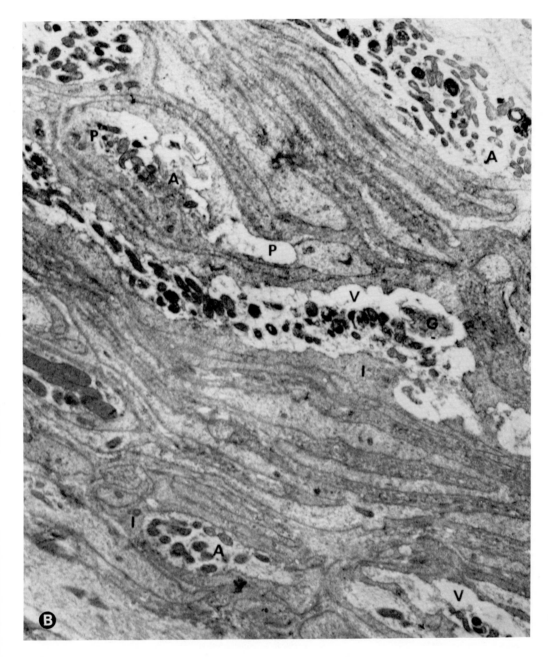

Figure 4.5.   *B,* Electron micrograph of Meissner corpuscle 48 hours after denervation. Degenerating axon terminals (*A*) are characterized by granular axoplasm (*G*) and vacuolization (*V*). Possible example of axonal phagocytosis (*P*) within a lamellar cell process (*I*) (×21,200). (Reproduced with permission from A. L. Dellon et al: *Plast Reconstr Surg* 56:182–193, 1975.[24])

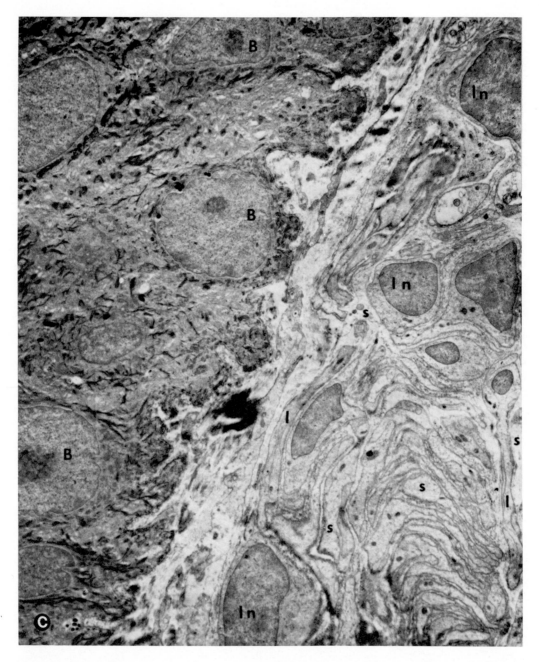

Figure 4.5. *C,* Electron micrograph of a Meissner corpuscle 4 months after denervation. Beneath the epidermal basal cells (*B*), the lamellar cell nuclei (*ln*) are crowded together in the shrunken Meissner corpuscle. No axon terminals are present. There is a relative increase in the interlamellar substance (*s*) between the collapsed and narrowed lamellar cell processes (*l*). (×12,450). (Reproduced with permission from A. L. Dellon et al: *Plast Reconstr Surg* 56:182–193, 1975.[24])

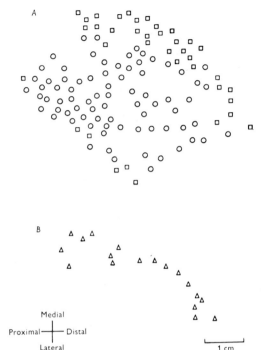

Figure 4.6. Distribution of touch domes in the cat thigh before (*A*) and after (*B*) division of the femoral cutaneous nerve. The squares and triangles are domes from overlapping, nonfemoral cutaneous nerves. (Reproduced with permission from P. R. Burgess et al: *J Physiol* 236:57–82, 1974.[38])

the results indicate a significant loss in the percentage of patients achieving a given grade of recovery and a decrease in the highest grade attained when the delay interval exceeds 4 months[46–49] (Figs. 4.8 and 4.9).

These clinical observations may be explained if one assumes that the recovery of normal sensation requires a regenerating axon to reinnervate a persisting sensory end organ. During the first 6 months of denervation, the Meissner corpuscle, for example, loses its nerve fibers and its general architecture, but it has not undergone major reduction in size and it can probably still respond fully to the reinnervating nerve. After 6 months, the progressive retraction and collapse of lamellae, the steadily diminishing corpuscular size, and the increased collagen-

ation probably render the Meissner corpuscle incapable of responding fully to a reinnervating axon's trophic influence. These structural changes probably prevent the Meissner corpuscle from ever regaining its normal threshold characteristics and, therefore, its potential for mechanoreception.

The Meissner corpuscle appears to be about midway in the rate of degeneration between the rapid deterioration (review above) of the Merkel cell-neurite complex and the relative stability of the Pacinian corpuscle. Thus, a period of delay of even 6 months will find the sensory end organ population in less than optimal condition to receive the regenerating axons.

How Long to Wait Prior to Re-exploration

Although you want to allow sufficient time to elapse to permit axonal regeneration across the repair site and distally to the fingertip, and allow for the patient's age, etc. you must remember the progressive degenerative changes occurring in the end organ population. If, for an injury at the wrist, the predicted pattern of sensory recovery (see Chapter 7) is not proceeding on schedule, we believe re-exploration, between the 4th and 6th postoperative month, is indicated. To permit a greater interval to elapse is to permit such peripheral end organ degeneration that the salvage procedure (neurolysis, nerve graft, etc.) will be handicapped severely.

Effect of Ischemia on End Organ Degeneration

This is, essentially, unknown and remains an area for future investigation. Two recent studies are pertinent. The effect of forearm arterial injuries upon recovery of sensation from concomitant nerve injury has been reviewed.[50] The conclusion was that "associated unrepaired arterial lacerations have no apparent effect on the rate or completeness of neurological recovery following repair." Presumably, this was because "following single arterial injury in the forearm, the intact artery consistently demonstrates a compensatory increased flow." However, in these cases, significant ischemia to distal sensory end organs probably doesn't occur. More

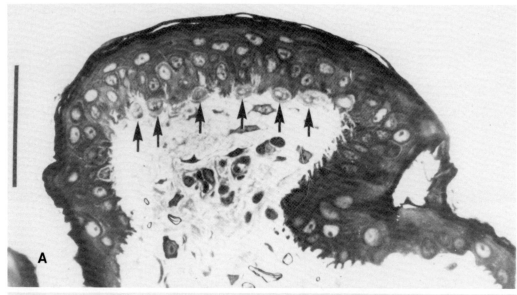

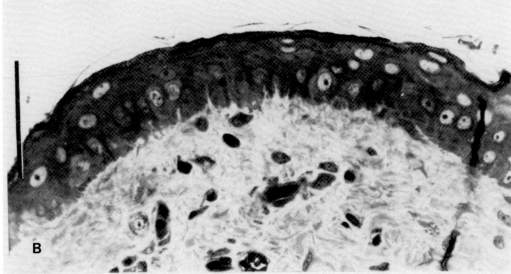

Figure 4.7. Cat touch domes before (A) and 22 days after (B) nerve division. Note complete loss of the Merkel cells (*arrows, A*) and flattening of the dome after denervation. Calibration bar (left of figures) is 50 μm. (Reproduced with permission from P. R. Burgess et al: *J Physiol* 236:57–82, 1974[38])

pertinent are the results of the Duke replantation experience.[51] Detailed evaluation of recovered sensibility was correlated with the replanted digit's pulse-volume recordings. Those patients who recovered less that 6-mm two-point discrimination all had pulse-volume recordings at least 85% of normal. Re-

sults of two-point discrimination, overall, in their series was not as good as that for digital nerve repairs in nonamputated digits.

I believe that the sensory corpuscles, being highly active metabolically, have a low tolerance to ischemia and thereby differ from the other digital components, e.g., epidermis,

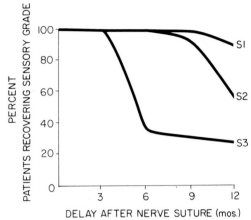

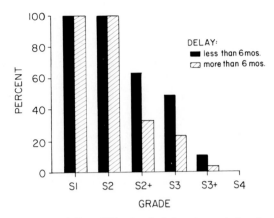

Figure 4.8. Effect of delay in nerve suture upon the degree of sensory recovery following wartime distal median nerve injuries. After delays of more than 4 months, there was a significant decrease in the percent of patients recovering to the S3 level. (Adapted from Kirklin et al.[49])

Figure 4.9. Effect of delay in repair of divided nerve upon degree of sensory recovery, for distal median nerve, wartime injuries. After delay of 6 months, there was a significant decrease in percent of patients recovering to the S2+ and S3 levels. (Adapted from Zachary.[47])

tendon, bone, in their absolute requirement for oxygen. Although a replanted digit with a cold ischemia time of 24 hours may survive, we feel that even the most meticulous nerve repair will only result in axons regenerating to ischemia-injured end organs. Following prolonged ischemia, for example, the enzyme systems of the lamellar cell processes of Meissner corpuscles are probably irreversibly damaged, rendering them either unable to be reinnervated or unable to respond to neurotropism (these may be the same thing). Ischemia is probably the cause of the "ghost" Pacinian corpuscle observed in autografted primate volar pads,[52] while lack of ischemia is the basis of the persistent neural structures observed in the distal end of the pedicle flap.[53] My own observations (see Chapter 5) on sensory corpuscles in flaps and grafts support this view (see Figs. 5.13 through 5.17).

Sensory Neurotropism

The interaction between the axon and epithelial (mesenchymal) component of the sensory corpuscle is poorly understood. To what extent is the integrity of the epidermis and dermis dependent upon neurotrophic factors? Why do fingertips undergo acral-

sclerosis after nerve division? To what extent do the corpuscular components control the course, the ultimate destination of regeneration axons? What is the role of the synaptic vesicles in the Merkel cell, and of what significance are the various cholinesterases and their varying response to denervation? These questions and more remain to be answered. An intriguing start has been made in the reviews by Harris,[54] Werner,[55] and Drachman's multiauthored monograph.[56]

References

1. Waller A: Experiments on the section of the glossopharyngeal and hypoglossal nerves of the frog, and observations of the alterations produced thereby in the structure of their primitive fibers. Philos Trans R Soc Lond 140:423–429, 1850.
2. Ranson SW: Degeneration and regeneration of nerve fibers. J Comp Neurol 22:487–546, 1912.
3. Webster HF: The relationship between Schmidt-Lantermann incisures and myelin segmentation during Wallerian degeneration. Ann NY Acad Sci 122:29–38, 1965.
4. Engel AG, Stonnington HH: Morphologic effects of denervation of muscle: A qualitative ultrastructural study, in Drachman DB (ed): *Trophic Functions of the Neuron.* New York: New York Academy of Sciences, 1974, pp 68–88.
5. Sunderland S: *Nerve and Nerve Injuries,* ed 2. Edinburgh: Churchill-Livingstone, 1978, Ch 7.

6. Sunderland S: *Nerve and Nerve Injuries*, ed 2. Edinburgh: Churchill-Livingston, 1978, Ch 17–20, 22.
7. Boeke J: On the regeneration of sensitive end-corpuscles after section of the nerve. K Acad van Wetenschoppen (Amsterdam) 25:319–323, 1922.
8. Boeke, J, Dijkstra C: De- and regeneration of sensible end-corpuscles in the duck's bill (corpuscles of Grandy and Herbst) after the cutting of the nerve, the removing of the entire skin or the transplantation of the skin in another region. K Acad van Wetenschoppen (Amsterdam) 35:1114–1119, 1932.
9. Boeke J: *The Problems of Nervous Anatomy*. London: Oxford University Press, 1940, pp 12–44.
10. Guth L: The effects of glossopharyngeal nerve transection on the circumvallate papilla of the rat. Anat Rec 128:715–731, 1957.
11. Guth L: Degeneration and regeneration of taste buds, in Beidler LM (ed): *Handbook of Sensory Physiology*, Vol. VI. Berlin: Springer-Verlag, 1971, pp 63–74.
12. Farbman AI: Fine structure of degenerating taste buds after denervation. J Embryol Exp Morphol 22:55–68, 1969.
13. Fujimoto S, Murray RG: Fine structure of degeneration and regeneration in denervated rabbit vallate taste buds. Anat Rec 168:393, 1970.
14. Fitzgerald MJT, Martin F, Paletta FX: Innervation of skin grafts. Surg Gynecol Obstet 124:808–812, 1967.
15. Orgel M, Aguayo A, Williams HB: Sensory nerve regeneration: An experimental study of skin grafts in the rabbit. J Anat 111:121–135, 1972.
16. Seddon H: *Surgical Disorders of Peripheral Nerves*. Baltimore: Williams & Wilkins Co, 1972, Ch 2,14.
17. Sunderland S: *Nerve and Nerve Injuries*, ed 2. Edinburgh: Churchill-Livingstone, 1978, Ch 31.
18. Lyons WR, Woodhall B: *Atlas of Peripheral Nerve Injury*. Philadelphia: WB Saunders, 1949, p 215.
19. Winkelmann RK: Effect of sciatic nerve section on enzymatic reactions of sensory end-organs. J Neuropathol Exp Neurol 21:655–657, 1962.
20. Ridley A: Silver staining of the innervation of Meissner corpuscles in peripheral neuropathy. Brain 91:539–552, 1968.
21. Hurley HG, Koelle GB: The effect of inhibition of nonspecific cholinesterase in perception of tactile sensation in human volar skin. J Invest Dermatol 31:243–245, 1958.
22. Orphanos CE, Mahrle G: Ultrastructural and cytochemistry of human cutaneous nerves. J Invest Dermatol 61:108–120, 1973.
23. Jabaley ME, Dellon AL: Evaluation of sensibility by microhistological studies, in Omer GE, Spinner M (eds): *Management of Peripheral Nerve Problems*. Philadelphia: WB Saunders, 1980, Ch 62.
24. Dellon AL, Witebsky FG, Terrill RE: The denervated Meissner corpuscle: A sequential histologic study after nerve division in the Rhesus monkey. Plast Reconstr Surg 56:182–193, 1975.
25. Lee FC: A study of the Pacinian corpuscle. J Comp Neurol 64:497–522, 1936.
26. Glees P, Mohiuddin A, Smith AG: Transplantation of Pacinian bodies in the brain and thigh of the cat. Acta Anat (Basel) 7:213–224, 1949.
27. Lowenstein WR, Rothkamp R: The sites for mechanoelectric conversion in a Pacinian corpuscle. J Gen Physiol 41:1245–1265, 1958.
28. Wong WC, Kanagastuntheram R: Early and late effects of median nerve injury on Meissner's and Pacinian corpuscles of the hand of the macaque (M. fascicularis). J Anat 109:135–142, 1971.
29. Krishnamurti A, Kanagasuntheram R, Vy S: Failure of reinnervation of Pacinian corpuscle after nerve crush: An electron microscopic study. Acta Neuropathol (Berl) 23:338–341, 1973.
30. Karthals JK, Wisniewski HM, Ghetti B, et al: The fate of the axon and its terminal in the Pacinian corpuscle following sciatic nerve section. J Neurophysiol 3:385–403, 1974.
31. Silver A, Versaci A, Montagna W: Studies of sweating and sensory function in cases of peripheral nerve injuries of the hand. J Invest Dermatol 40:243–258, 1963.
32. Silver A, Montagna W, Versaci A: The effect of denervation on sweat glands and Meissner corpuscles of human hands. J Invest Dermatol 42:307–324, 1964.
33. Satinsky D, Pepe FA, Liu CN: The neurilemma cell in peripheral nerve degeneration and regeneration. Exp Neurol 9:441–451, 1964.
34. Brown A, Iggo A: The structure and function of cutaneous "touch corpuscles" after nerve crush. J Physiol 165:28–29P, 1963.
35. Palmer P: Ultrastructural alterations of Merkel cells following denervation. Anat Rec 151:396–397, 1965.
36. Kasprzak H, Tapper DN, Craig PH: Functional development of the tactile pad receptor system. Exp Neurol 26:439–446, 1970.
37. Smith KR: The structure and function of the Haarscheibe. J Comp Neurol 131:459–474, 1967.
38. Burgess PR, English KB, Horch KW, et al: Patterning in the regeneration of type I cutaneous receptors. J Physiol 236:57–82, 1974.
39. Munger B: Personal communication (Munger B, Ide H, manuscript in preparation).
40. Sunderland S: *Nerve and Nerve Injuries*, ed 2. Edinburgh: Churchill-Livingstone, 1978, Ch 48.
41. Woodhall B, Beebe GW: *Peripheral Nerve Regeneration— A Follow-Up Study of 3635 World War II Injuries*, Veterans Administration Medical Monograph. Washington, DC: US Govt Print Office, 1956, p 309.
43. Thomson JL, Ritchie WP, French LO: A plan for care of peripheral nerve injuries overseas. Arch Surg 52:557–570, 1946.
43. Weckesser EC: The repair of nerves in the palm and fingers. Clin Orthop 19:200–207, 1961.
44. Hamlin E, Watkins AL: Regeneration in the ulnar, median and radial nerves. Surg Clin North Am 27:1052–1061, 1947.
45. Sunderland S: Capacity of reinnervated muscles to function efficiently after prolonged denervation. Arch Neurol Psychiatry 64:755–771, 1950.
46. Shaffer JM, Cleveland F: Delayed suture of sensory nerves of the hand. Ann Surg 131:556–563, 1950.
47. Zachary RB: Results of nerve suture, in Seddon HJ (ed): *Peripheral Nerve Injuries*. London: Her Majesties Stationery Office, 1954, pp 254–388.
48. Nicholson OR, Seddon HJ: Nerve repair in civilian

practice: Results of treatment of median and ulnar lesions. Br Med J 2:1065–1071, 1957.

49. Kirklin JW, Murphy F, Berkson J: Suture of peripheral nerves: Factors affecting prognosis. Surg Gynecol Obstet 88:719–730, 1959.

50. Gelberman RH, Blasingame TP, Feonek A, et al: Forearm arterial injuries. J Hand Surg 4:401–408, 1979.

51. Gelberman RH, Urbaniak JR, Bright DS, et al: Digital sensibility following replantation. J Hand Surg 3: 313–319, 1978.

52. Miller SH, Reisenas I: Changes in primate Pacinian corpuscles following volar pad excision and skin

grafting: A preliminary report. Plast Reconstr Surg 57:627–636, 1976.

53. Santoni-Rugiu P: Experimental study on reinnervation of free grafts and pedicle flaps. Plast Reconstr Surg 38:98–104, 1966.

54. Harris AJ: Inductive function of the nervous system. Annu Rev Physiol 36:251–305, 1974 (403 references.)

55. Werner JK: Trophic influence of nerves in the development and maintenance of sensory receptors. Am J Phys Med 53:127–142, 1974 (68 references).

56. Drachman DB (ed): Trophic Function of the Neuron. New York: New York Academy of Sciences, 1974.

Chapter 5

SENSORY CORPUSCLES AFTER NERVE REPAIR

INTRODUCTION
EARLY REINNERVATION STUDIES
PACINIAN CORPUSCLE
MEISSNER CORPUSCLE
MERKEL CELL-NEURITE COMPLEX
CROSS-REINNERVATION STUDIES
CLINICAL IMPLICATIONS

INTRODUCTION

This chapter is concerned with the most distal events by which an injured sensory nerve re-establishes contact with the external world. The process is regeneration. "Regeneration is an active invasion and displacement process in which the pushing forces of axonal streaming, increased axoplasmic pressure, and central protein synthesis are opposed by distal Schwann cell proliferation, collapsed tubules, and collagen accumulation."[1] This excellent general description focuses upon the nerve fiber, as has most previous investigation and writing in this field. Seddon,[2] for example, extended the process to the periphery but was concerned only with muscle reinnervation. Sunderland's comprehensive review of regeneration comprises 239 references on axonal regeneration,[3] 88 references on the pattern of motor recovery associated with regeneration of motor nerve fibers,[4] but just 27 references on the pattern of sensory recovery associated with regeneration of sensory nerve fibers. Of these 27 references, only five actually describe the effect of regen-

eration upon sensory corpuscles. These five references have appeared in the last decade and are included in the review to follow.

Very few studies have focused on sensory receptors. In fact, some of those referred to as demonstrating "end organ reinnervation" have not concerned sensory receptors. For example, the series of studies by Sanders and Young in the mid 1940's[6-8] is usually quoted as showing "the importance of end organ reinnervation." What these investigators actually did was to divide mixed nerves and, in some instances, pure motor nerves (e.g., to the gastrocnemius) and then to permit some nerves to regenerate and others not to regenerate. They then studied nerve *fiber* diameter in those nerves allowed to regenerate. They never evaluated sensory receptors. They concluded that although the shrunken distal Schwann tubes "restricted the diameter attained by the regenerating fibers within them,"[6] "both sensory and motor nerve fibers became larger when allowed to reach their end-organs."[8] Thus, "the most powerful influence lies not centrally but in connection with the end-organ."[8] But, these studies did not evaluate the effect of regeneration upon the sensory end organ.

One of the central areas of controversy has been whether regenerating sensory axons re-establish contact with sensory end organs, that is, reinnervate persisting sensory corpuscles, or whether regenerating sensory axons arrive at the periphery and induce the new sensory end organs, that is, develop new or *de novo* sensory corpuscles. Chapter 4 established that sensory corpuscles undergo progressive degenerative changes following denervation. The sensory corpuscles, therefore, do "persist" for a time after nerve injury, but if they remain without innervation sufficiently long, they are altered significantly. This chapter will attempt to answer the following questions: Can sensory corpuscles arise *de novo*? Can degenerating corpuscles be reinnervated? What happens if a persisting end organ is reinnervated by an axon that previously had innervated a different type of sensory end organ?

EARLY REINNERVATION STUDIES
Boeke

J. Boeke's observations on the organ of Eimer in the mole snout are quoted as demonstrating *de novo* end organ formation.[9] However, Boeke's observations were made during the mole's growth and development when the early fibers into the mole's snout (the organ of Eimer) were noted to degenerate. Following this degeneration "entirely new innervation" was found which was identical with the adult form of this organ. Thus, these observations probably cannot be extrapolated into the primate nerve repair setting.

In ducks Boeke[10,11] transected the trigeminal innervation and subsequently biopsied the duck's bill to evaluate the effect of the regenerating axons upon the Grandry (a morphologic analog to the Merkel cell-neurite complex) and Herbst (a morphologic analog to the Pacinian) corpuscles. He observed axons re-entering, thereby reinnervating, each of these corpuscles. The Grandry tactile cell, which had "shriveled" in size, regained normal size as the axon developed into the neurofibrillar disc. Developmentally, the tactile cells were of lemnoblastic (sheath cells) ori-

gin. Boeke specifically distinguishes what I call "reinnervation" from *de novo* origin as follows: "Besides a regeneration of the old existing sensory corpuscles, a great number of new corpuscles is formed."[11]

In duck bill-to-leg and leg-to-bill skin "transplant" experiments, graft biopsies at 2 months after surgery were observed to contain only degenerated corpuscles, including the Herbst corpuscles. These were smaller than normal and infiltrated by "blood capillaries apparently being organized by the surrounding connective tissue. No 'new' corpuscles developed in the leg-to-bill transplants by eleven months after surgery. In the bill-to-leg transplants, however, 'new' Grandry corpuscles developed and 'here and there' newly-formed Herbst corpuscles."[11]

In related experiments often quoted as demonstrating *de novo* origin of sensory end organs, Boeke's approach was to excise an area of skin, allow this area to heal "primarily," and to evaluate the end organs of this "regenerating skin." This approach was utilized in the duck's bill, where "newly formed Herbst and Grandry corpuscles "developed," in monkey fingertips and in the little fingertip of his assistant, Doctor von Straaten, where "new" Meissner corpuscles developed.[9,11]

Boeke's laboratory carried out imaginative and excellent work and the observations will remain classics. However, as wound healing is understood today, all the work based on "primary" healing of excised wounds is fallacious. Secondary healing by wound contracture transposed normal corpuscles from the periphery of the excised wounds into the healed central, and future biopsy site (see Fig. 5.1). Recall it was only this type of study in the duck that "new" Herbst corpuscles were observed. Problems with experimental design in sensory investigations still persist. A recent study reported "new" Pacinian corpuscles "regenerating" after nerve repair.[12] Analysis of that study[13] suggested wound contracture and transposition of normal adjacent Pacinian corpuscles as the source of the *de novo* corpuscles. Indeed, Boeke's own serial drawings of "primary healing" in the monkey's and in von Straaten's finger clearly show the wound contracture (Fig. 5.2). New skin did not form. *De novo* corpuscle formation did not occur.

Boeke's work does document that following nerve division, Grandry and Herbst corpuscles are reinnervated by regenerating axons. The study also apparently shows that *de novo* Grandry corpuscles arise in ducks during axonal regeneration.

The extrapolation of the response of sensory end organs to denervation and axon regeneration in lower vertebrates to that of higher vertebrates is probably not justified. For example, the mole is blind and "sees" primarily with its nose for food and shelter. The duck, whose forearms are wings and whose fingertips are feathers and claws, relies on its beak not only to hold its food but also to filter seeds and insects from sand, in the water and mud.[14] Although some birds, like the duck, and perhaps some mammals, like the mole, can regenerate bill or nose sensory corpuscles, increasing specialization proceeds during evolution at the expense of regenerative potential. The primates probably cannot regenerate sensory corpuscles *de novo*.

Taste Buds

Werner[15] has reviewed the literature on the taste bud as a model of sensory receptor change during embryogenesis, denervation,

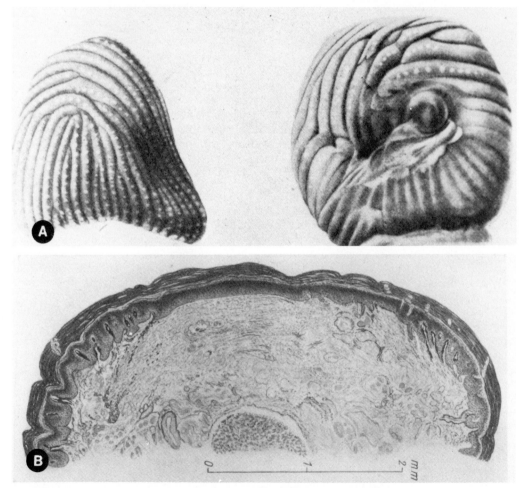

Figure 5.1.   From Boeke's study of "regenerated" skin in the monkey.[9] *A*, Note that the central, previously biopsied area, in the fingertip has not "regenerated" but healed secondarily by wound contracture. *B*, The histologic section of this area shows not new skin but scar with sensory receptors transposed centripetally, not regenerated *de novo*.

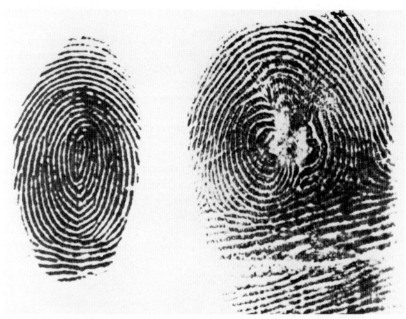

Figure 5.2.   From Boeke's study of "regenerated" skin in man.[9] Note the healed central area has done so by secondary intention. Sensory corpuscles present in the histologic section of this area are pre-existing corpuscles pulled centrally by the force of wound contracture.

and reinnervation. It is relevant that the epithelial anlage of fungiform papillae in the rat develops prior to neural ingrowth into the tongue, and that these cells have ultrastructure-size vesicles that may release a trophic substance to guide gustatory axons. Normally, taste buds are replenished on a weekly basis.[17] As reviewed in Chapter 4, taste buds degenerate completely following division of any cranial nerve carrying gustatory fibers. Repair of the divided gustatory nerve results in taste bud regeneraton.[18,19] (Additional discussion of taste bud studies is found later in this Chapter in the "Cross Innervation" section.)

Skin Grafts

The extensive literature on the reinnervation of skin grafts and flaps was the closest the researchers prior to the 1960's came to the question of sensory corpuscle reinnervation or regeneration. These studies attempted to answer two general questions: (1) By what anatomic pathway does reinnervation occur, e.g., longitudinally via pre-existing neurovascular pathways or at random through the edge or bed of the graft or flap. (2) Was the pattern of recovered sensation that of the donor or the recipient environment, e.g., would abdominal skin grafted onto the fingertip eventually recover sensation more like the abdomen or like the fingertip? A corollary of the last question was, what type of sensory corpuscle present in the graft is related to the recovered sensation? A review of these areas will lead directly to the studies on the sensory end organs themselves. Aspects of these questions have been reviewed recently by Jabaley[20] and Terzis.[21]

Several studies attempting to determine which type of soft tissue coverage recovered sensation (touch, pain, temperature) earliest concluded that detached, distant pedicle flaps recovered sensation earlier than grafts, and full thickness grafts earlier than split-thickness grafts.[22-24] Another study[25] reached the opposite conclusion. The controversy begun in the 1930's continued into the 1950's with observers on both the "flap first"[26,27] and the "flap last"[28] side of the controversy. When viewed from today's perspective, many of the differing results of these studies were due to (1) the quality of the recipient bed, (2) the time interval between injury and resurfacing and testing, (3) the testing techniques, and (4) the size and location of test area (in small test areas, perception is often through areas adjacent to the resurfaced areas). For example, in all of these studies on grafts, the donor sites were thigh and abdomen and the grafts were transferred to the trunk, face, or extremities, but not to fingertips!! Flaps were abdominal and transferred to the head and neck or hand's dorsum or palm, but not to the fingertips!! Defects were frequently those with extensive deep scarring, such as burns. Thus, resurfacing tissue contained few, if any, sensory corpuscles, and resurfaced areas were those with a normally low innervation density. These early observations, some of which are meticulous, monumental, and truly classic,[24,30] nevertheless contribute little to our understanding of sensibility in the hand or the reinnervation of sensory corpuscles.

The course which the regenerating axons followed into the graft or flap generally was agreed upon. The earliest investigators[22-25] observed that in detached pedicle flaps, sensation recovered first proximally, and proceeded distally, from the edges to the center, while in grafts the recovery was more from peripheral to central. Later studies generally concurred regarding graft innervations,[29,30] with the degree of subdermal reinnervation being related to the condition of the graft bed.[29] Reinnervating nerve axons from proximal bundles, where aligned with neurovascular bundles in the resurfacing tissue, followed them into the graft.[29,31] The greatest number of axon sprouts, however, entered the resurfacing tissue randomly, at the periphery and subdermally, and traveled randomly. They either ended as free nerve terminals, joined the cutaneous plexus of the resurfacing tissue, or, by chance, reinnervated a sensory corpuscle or hair follicle.[29,31]

The classic studies by Hutchinson, Tough and Wyburn in 1949,[32] Ponten in 1960,[30] and Mannerfelt in 1962[33] established conclusively that transplanted soft tissue recovers a sensory pattern more like its recipient bed than its donor site *if* sufficient reinnervation occurs.

The influence of Moberg[34] begins to be seen here, as Ponten's[30] studies emphasized functional recovery and recorded sensation in terms of two-point discrimination. Mannerfelt's comprehensive sensory evaluation[33] on 28 patients included not only two-point discrimination testing but the pick-up test, the coin test, and the ninhydrin test.[32] Although Ponten[30] reported examples of recovery of *tactile gnosis*, Moberg and Mannerfelt have stated that skin grafts never recover *tactile gnosis*. Skin grafts generally recover better sensation than flaps.[33] (This will be discussed further in the "Clinical Implications" section, later in this chapter.)

In the decade of the 1970's, histochemistry, electron microscopy, and sophisticated neurophysiologic recording techniques were applied to experiments similar to those done in the preceding 40 years. Ridley[35] biopsied human fingertips previously skin grafted with forearm skin in trauma patients. He observed no encapsulated endings, but did identify an occasional Merkel-like ending in relation to an epidermal ridge. He noted the apparent paradox that the patient had two-point discrimination but no Meissner corpuscles. His results have been variously interpreted. I believe they demonstrated: (1) that regenerating sensory axons do not form *de novo* encapsulated corpuscles (and therefore this observation is consistent with the results of my work on the Meissner corpuscles[36]); (2) that the observed Merkel disc may represent reinnervation of a Haarscheibe by a slowly-adapting fiber (see "Cross Innervation" section); and (3) that presence of two-point discrimination and Merkel disc *is* the appropriate correlation (see Chapter 3).

Orgel, Aguayo, and Williams[37] studied the regenerating fiber population, observing an imbalance in favor of many more small, myelinated fibers over the larger myelinated fibers. This altered ratio correlated with absent end-corpuscles in grafted rabbit skin. Terzis[21] extended these observations by noting a decreased conduction velocity in the regenerating population of axons entering the rabbit ear grafts.

Celli and Caroli,[38] in a long review, essentially have confirmed many of the observations previously presented, as has a recent publication from Japan.[39] This latter report also documents the reinnervation of hair follicles in grafted hairy skin.

In my opinion, if the resurfaced area is a fingertip, and if the resurfacing is done primarily on a nonscarred base, the perception of pain, temperature, and touch will be recovered first in the thin split-thickness graft, then in a full-thickness graft, and last in a flap. The degree of recovery of functional sensation will be related to the innervation density of sensory corpuscles in the resurfacing tissue.

A separate but related question is whether the noninjured nerves in an area adjacent to the receptive field of an injured nerve can send axon sprouts into this injured nerve's receptive field. Thus, reinnervation would occur from normal adjacent nerves rather than regenerating axons of the injured nerve. This question need not arise with the question of graft reinnervation because the nerves about the periphery of the graft have all been injured. Weddell, Guttmann, and Guttmann[40] in 1941, using a rabbit hindlimb model and whole mount, horizontal sections stained with methylene blue, concluded that there was such local extension of nerve fibers into adjacent denervated areas. Hoffman demonstrated similar findings for muscle, in the rat hindlimb. Adjacent normal axons sprouted to reinnervate a denervated motor end-plate.[41] Livingstone reported two cases in which patients' reinnervated hand areas were demonstrated by nerve block to have been reinnervated (or were these cases of anomalous innervation?) by adjacent noninjured nerves. I believe that the axons in the overlap areas of receptive fields can be either stimulated by a substance released from the degenerating axon or are released from contact inhibition by the degenerating axons and can extend into adjacent areas.

PACINIAN CORPUSCLE

In 1970, Wong and Kanagasutheram[43] made preliminary observations on the effect of crushing, sectioning, and ligating a primate (macaque) median nerve. Silver and histochemical staining techniques were done on palm biopsies using the contralateral hand as a control in a total of three animals. At 40 weeks after nerve crush, there was just an occasional Pacinian corpuscle reinnervated. I infer from the authors' lack of commentary upon long-term result of the ligation and section parts of their study, that no reinnervated Pacinian corpuscles were identified. In the crush study (one nerve, crushed at the wrist), cholinesterase staining was "nil to intense," and acetylcholinesterase staining was "nil to moderate" in Pacinian corpuscles.

In 1972, Lowenstein[44] studied the physiology of Pacinian corpuscle in the cat mesentery. In six cats the inferior mesenteric nerve was divided and "reunited" (autologous clot within a polycarbonate membrane sleeve). At 30 to 40 days after "union," just eight of the 54 tested corpuscles in the mesenteries innervated by these six nerves were mechanoreceptive.

During that same time period, Kanagasuntheram's group[45] further evaluated this difficulty in reinnervating the Pacinian corpuscle. This time they studied the ultrastructure of five corpuscles from the middle finger of a primate (slow loris) 75 days after median nerve crush in the forearm. They observed unremoved myelin debris and endoneurial fibrosis within the corpuscle's inner core, "preventing" reinnervation.

Jabaley[46] did not comment on Pacinian corpuscles in his biopsy study of human fingertips after nerve repair.

The study by Krishnamurti and Kanagasuntheram[45] may be criticized. Although they studied primates and employed excellent histochemical and ultrastructural techniques, their experimental design was poor. In their earlier study,[43] they evaluated potential reinnervation following nerve section (technique of repair unspecified) and after ligation (regeneration theoretically may not occur at all) at the wrist with a palm biopsy. They did not totally deafferent this area where a palmar cutaneous nerve, originating above the area of crush, or a musculocutaneous nerve might also be innervating the palm. In that study, the time chosen for postinjury evaluation, 40 weeks, was appropriate for the injury-test site separation of a few centimeters. The time chosen in their next study,[45] however, was too short; the injury and test site were now widely separated (forearm-to-fingertip versus wrist-to-palm), yet the time interval was just

10 weeks! They observed alterations in the blood supply to the corpuscle, and this may explain the delayed phagocytosis and fibrosis they found.

In summary, very little experimental work has been conducted on the reinnervation of Pacinian corpuscles. The work reviewed above suggested that these corpuscles were reinnervated with difficulty, probably because of "mechanical factors." My own observations (see Chapter 7) indicate that Pacinian corpuscles are reinnervated in humans, but they are the last in the time sequence to be reinnervated. Although "mechanical" obstruction may block axonal regeneration to the corpuscle, I feel the basis for the above observations lies in the low probability of a regenerating axon making the proper peripheral connection where the nerve fiber to receptor ratio is 1:1 (see Chapter 7).

MEISSNER CORPUSCLES

In 1970, Wong and Kanagasuntheram,[43] in the study described in the preceding section, observed "early" Meissner corpuscle "reinnervation" 8 weeks following a nerve crush several centimeters proximal to the observation site. "The reinnervation of Meissner's corpuscles forty weeks after nerve crush was almost complete, but after nerve section (32 weeks) and nerve ligature (40 and 47 weeks) the process was less complete" (silver stain). Both nonspecific and acetylcholinesterase staining reactions were normal, with the latter having recovered normal staining characteristics first in the crush specimens.

Jabaley et al.[46] observed "reinnervated" Meissner corpuscles in 12 of 17 patient fingertip biopsies done an average of 24 months after nerve repair.

In a more detailed investigation of the effects of nerve repair upon the Meissner corpuscle, I did fascicular repairs upon the median and ulnar nerves of a deafferent primate hand (rhesus).[36] Sequential histologic studies, including ultrastructural studies, were done up to 9 months after nerve repair, with the contralateral fingertips serving as controls. Because of the lack of physiological or functional correlates, cholinesterase stains were not employed. In addition to refining earlier

observations, this study attempted to determine whether a regenerating axon reinnervated a pre-existing but degenerating corpuscle, reversing this process, or whether the regenerating axon reached the epidermal-dermal region and induced *de novo* Meissner corpuscles. The conclusion was that "in the rhesus monkey, axons of regenerating sensory nerves reinnervate the denervated Meissner corpuscle . . . there was no evidence of Meissner corpuscles regenerating *de novo*." The results of that study follow and are reported and illustrated in greater detail:

Controls. The histologic sections of the pre-operative biopsies of the control and operative fingertips, as well as the contralateral fingertip controls throughout the postoperative period, contained normal Meissner corpuscles, as demonstrated by both connective tissue and nerve staining techniques. The Meissner corpuscle showed segmentation into two to three lobules, each of which contained a lamellar arrangement of plump cells or spaces with many collections of pink-staining material believed to be axoplasm. The nuclei of the lamellar cells usually were located peripherally. The entire Meissner corpuscle was large and almost filled with dermal papilla on a section taken near the Meissner corpuscle's longitudinal axis (Fig. 5.3, A). On silver staining, at least one and usually three or more medulated axons reached the Meissner corpuscle and arborized within it by looping between the lamellae. Axon endings appeared as coils or sprays of fine twigs under the magnification employed (Fig. 5.4, A).

Two Days after Nerve Suture. In the sections stained for connective tissues, early signs of degeneration were apparent; the lobular subdivisions were blurred, the usually distinct internal lamellar pattern was obscured, and the collections of pink-staining material were less apparent (Fig. 5.3, B). With silver staining, the axon terminals were no longer present, with the exception of a few argyrophillic fragments (Fig. 5.4, B). Dermal nerve trunks demonstrated Wallerian degeneration.

Four Weeks after Nerve Suture. By both connective tissue and nerve stain techniques, the Meissner corpuscles in these control biopsies were denervated, demonstrating that the innervation to these fingertips had been divided. Without successful nerve repair, progressive Meissner corpuscle degeneration could be expected.

Six Weeks after Nerve Suture. The Meissner corpuscles stained for connective tissue (Fig.

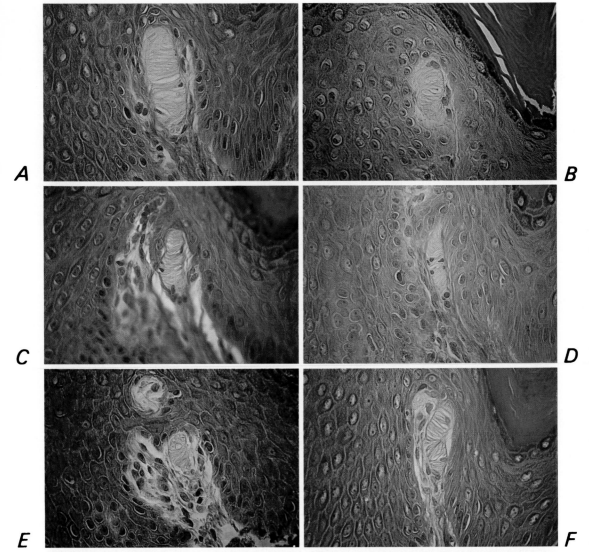

Figure 5.3. Reinnervation of denervated Meissner corpuscle. Mallory trichrome stain, ×160 *A*, Normal. Other sections are the following intervals after nerve repair: *B*, 48 hours; *C*, 6 weeks; *D*, 3 months, *E*, 6 months; *F*, 9 months. See text for description. (Reproduced with permission from A. L. Dellon: *J Hand Surg* 1:98–109, 1976.[36])

5.3, C) showed more advanced signs of degeneration. There was some diminution in overall size and there were no lobulations or collections of pink-staining material, but rather the entire Meissner corpuscle was bluish, flattened, ovoid, nearly devoid of internal architecture. The few detectable lamellar cells were not plump. With the silver staining technique (Fig. 5.4, C), most were devoid of argyrophillic material, except for the nuclei of the lamellar cells; the entire Meissner corpuscle was pale. An occasional Meissner corpuscle, however, had a thin axon inside. The dermal nerve trunks were now primarily empty endoneural sheaths, although an occasional sheath contained a thin regenerating axon.

Three Months after Nerve Suture. With connective tissue staining, most of the Meissner corpuscles appeared as they had at 6 weeks after nerve suture, except that most of the Meissner corpuscles were diminished in overall size (Fig.

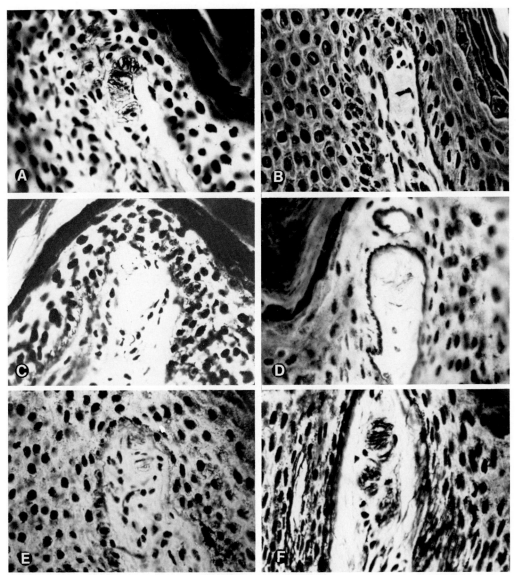

Figure 5.4.   Reinnervation of denervated Meissner corpuscle. Silver stain, ×160 *A*, Normal. Other sections are the following intervals after nerve repair: *B*, 48 hours; *C*, 6 weeks; *D*, 3 months; *E*, 6 months; *F*, 9 months. See text for description. (Reproduced with permission from A. L. Dellon: *J Hand Surg* 1:98–109, 1976.[36])

5.3, D). The silver staining method demonstrated about one third of the Meissner corpuscles to be aneuritic. The remaining Meissner corpuscles, however, definitely contained axons. These were single or multiple thin axons intertwined between the lamellar cells (Fig. 5.4, C). Most dermal nerve trunks contained thick and thin regenerating axons.

Six Months after Nerve Suture. About 70%

of all Meissner corpuscles contained plump lamellar cells with collections of pink-staining material. Meissner corpuscles were increased in size and a few Meissner corpuscles were lobulated (Fig. 5.3, E). With silver staining, about 80% of the Meissner corpuscles contained axons, many of which were now of normal thickness (Fig. 5.4, E). Dermal trunks appeared to be normal.

Nine Months after Nerve Suture. By both

connective tissue and silver staining techniques, virtually all Meissner corpuscles appeared normal, i.e., identical with the controls (Fig. 5.3, F and 5.4, F). About 5% of the Meissner corpuscles remained without signs of innervations, i.e., they showed progressive denervation. Whereas the control biopsies contained one Meissner corpuscle every

two to three papillary ridges, the operated hand biopsies contained one Meissner corpuscle every two to six papillary ridges, i.e., the Meissner corpuscle density following nerve suture was less than or equal to but never more than the control values.

Electron Microscopy. Electron microscopy at

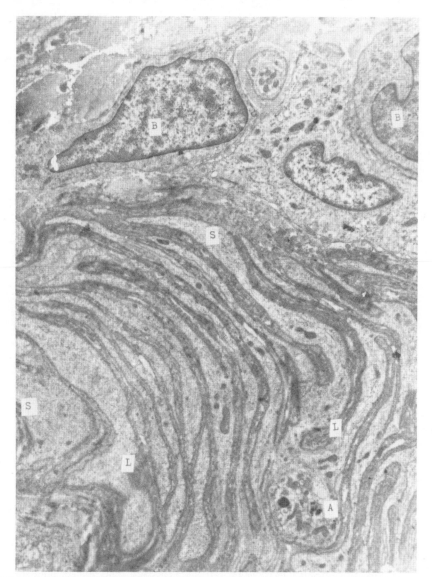

Figure 5.5. Reinnervation of denervated Meissner corpuscle. Electron micrograph, ×15,000: 3 months after nerve repair. Basal cells (*B*) are seen at top of dermal papilla. Note relative abundance of interlamellar substance (*S*) and short contracted lamellar cell processes (*L*) that characterize the degenerating corpuscle. But note the early reinnervation by the axon sprout (*A*). (Reproduced with permission from A. L. Dellon: *J Hand Surg* 1:98–109, 1976.[36])

3 months after nerve repair demonstrated a degenerated Meissner corpuscle in which new axonal sprouts were seen (Fig. 5.5). At 9 months after nerve repair, the Meissner corpuscle was indistinguishable from normal, with long, thin lamellar cell processes ensheathing thick axon terminals (Fig. 5.6).

MERKEL CELL-NEURITE COMPLEX

During investigations into the function of his "touch corpuscle" in the cat, Iggo[47] ob-served the effect of crushing the saphenous nerve. The corpuscles degenerated progressively. By 16 to 20 days after nerve crush, axonal branches reappeared among the capillary tufts and dermal papillae that represented the former touch corpuscles. By 25 to 30 days after crush, tactile cells are present again, and by 100 days the "tactile corpuscles appeared normal." By 30 days after the crush, mechanostimulation of the corpuscles and electrical recording from the saphenous nerve

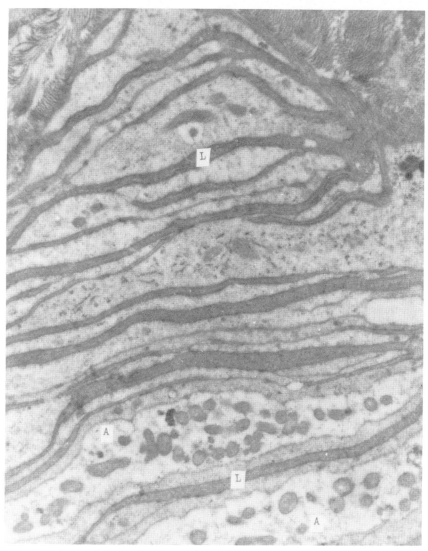

Figure 5.6. Reinnervation of denervated Meissner corpuscle. Electron microscopy, ×32,000: 9 months after nerve repair. Advanced reinnervation demonstrated by thick axon terminations (*A*) being ensheathed by lamellar cell processes (*L*).

demonstrated that a low threshold slowly-adapting fiber/receptor system had been re-established. (A low-threshold, quickly-adapting fiber/receptor system—the hair follicle—also was re-established.) This report was in the form of an abstract in the *Proceedings of the Physiological Society* in 1963 and received scant attention.

A decade later, Burgess and Horch et al.[48, 49] reported a series of carefully controlled neurophysiological and morphological investigations into the touch dome fiber/receptor system of the cat. Sural nerves were repaired and single unit recordings done after regeneration. These recordings were compared to the preoperative control recordings and dome population locations. Nineteen percent of control fibers were type I alpha fibers, innervating touch domes. The average fiber innervated two to four domes. Of the 445 regenerated fibers studied, just 11% were type I alpha fibers. Their mean conduction velocities were unchanged. Rates of adaption to maintained deformation were unchanged. The only difference observed was that the

regenerated fiber innervated just one dome, and its peripheral receptive field, instead of being confined exclusively to the dome, extended to the skin immediately surrounding the dome[48] (Fig. 5.7).

Burgess and Horch's next investigations[49] attempted to learn whether the pattern of domes following nerve repair was similar to that following nerve crush. The skin of the posterior thigh and the femoral cutaneous nerve was studied. Dome patterns were tatooed with ink under 25× magnification, and drawings made of the patterns. The femoral cutaneous nerve was electrically recorded, while this mapped area was tested to be sure no touch domes had been missed. One year later, the cats were studied again. Each touch dome was stimulated and the femoral cutaneous nerve recorded to demonstrate that the dome was actually innervated by that nerve. Control observations on dome "stability" demonstrated 87% of domes were in the identical position in which they had been observed 4 months previously. When touch domes that had been tatooed directly were

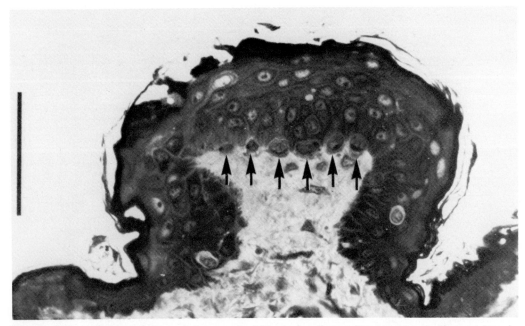

Figure 5.7.   Reinnervation of denervated Merkel cell-neurite complex in the cat touchpad. Following nerve crush, the degenerated Merkel cell-neurite complex becomes reinnervated and histologically is indistinguishable from normal (for comparison see Fig 4.7). (Reproduced with permission from Burgess et al.: *J Physiol* 236:57–86, 1974.[48])

evaluated, a 91 to 95% "stability" of the population was found. In the nerve *crush* study, one animal, retested 689 days after nerve crush, had all femoral cutaneous domes in the original femoral cutaneous field, while all other domes were outside the field (Fig. 5.8). Following nerve transection in five animals, the areas were retested between 393 and 1010 days after the surgery. The average preoperative field had 69 domes, the average postoperative field had 46. But in one field, there were actually more domes postoperatively (50 before versus 76 after). Eliminating this animal, the average animal recovered just 51% of its domes. Only 71% of the domes present at the postoperative test, however, were innervated by the regenerated femoral cutaneous nerve! This suggested that new domes had appeared due to activity of adjacent cutaneous nerves. Many of these new, noncoincidental domes were part of a "cluster." These clustered domes were smaller, had a closer interdome distance, and frequently the domes in the cluster were inner-

vated by more than one nerve. These "new" domes had normal morphology by light and electron microscopy.

The most recent study utilizing the cat touch dome model from the University of Utah Physiology Department, extends the analysis to the relationship of individual nerve fibers to their touch domes.[50] In the nerve crush type experiment, virtually all nerve fibers regenerated to the same two to four touch domes originally innervated (Fig. 5.9). In the nerve transection experiment, an average of only 60% of the fibers regenerated and each fiber reinnervated only half the number of previously innervated domes (Fig. 5.10). The dome to fiber ratio after nerve transection dropped from 2.6 to 1.3. The overall number of reinnervated domes was 35% of the original number.

In summary, it is clear that *in the cat*, the Merkel cell-neurite complex recovers virtually completely after nerve crush and to a lesser extent after nerve repair. The high coincidence between the location of the re-

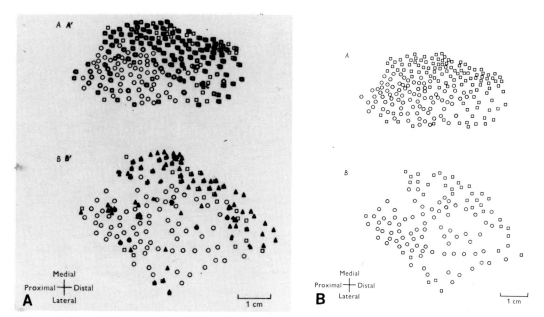

Figure 5.8. Reinnervation of denervated Merkel cell-neurite complex in the cat touchpad. Following nerve crush, the pattern of touch domes originally present (*B*) is almost completely recovered (*A*). In *A*, A' and B' is an overlay of the regenerated pattern onto the preoperative pattern of two separate cats, A and B. The nonfemoral cutaneous nerve was the nerve crushed. (Reproduced with permission from Burgess et al.: *J Physiol* 236: 57–86, 1974.[49])

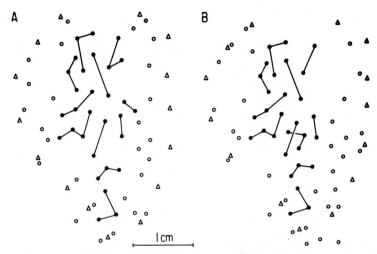

Figure 5.9.   Reinnervation of denervated Merkel cell-neurite complex in the cat touch-pad. Individual nerve fiber recordings before (*A*) and after (*B*) nerve *crush* demonstrate that not only are patterns of domes almost identical postregeneration, but also the relationship of individual fibers to touch domes is almost identical post-regeneration. (Reproduced with permission from K. Horch: *J Neurophysiol* 42:1437–1449, 1979.[50])

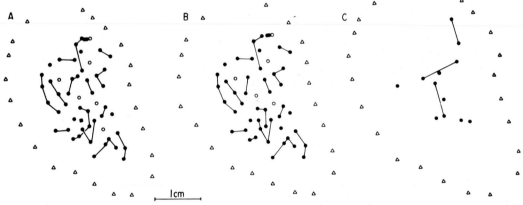

Figure 5.10.   Reinnervation of denervated Merkel cell-neurite complex in the cat touch-pad. Crush versus nerve division. Note difference in number of recovered domes (just 23%) and number of fibers (40%) relating to domes in *B* versus *A* (crush versus normal) and *C* versus *A* (division versus normal). (Reproduced with permission from K. Horch: *J Neurophysiol* 42:1437–1449, 1979.[50])

covered touch dome and its location prior to nerve injury and the relationship between the regenerating fiber after transection and the dome it reinnervates after nerve transection, suggest a specificity in the pattern of the end organ recovery. In the cat, by 1 month, the denervated dome essentially "disappears," including the apparent loss of the Merkel cell. In the nerve crush study, the 100% co-incidence pattern reflects the rapid regeneration of axons to the periphery before the complete degeneration of domes and therefore 100% complete reinnervations. In the nerve transection studies, the slowly regenerating axon has no end organ left to reinnervate. To explain the coincidence of recovered domes in this case, an "intrinsic specificity" may be hypothesized, in which only certain areas of the skin can differentiate into domes. Axons regenerate down the pre-existing Schwann tubes to the periphery area, and via some "trophic" influence this specific area is induced to form another dome. This is a borderline position between reinnervation of a denervated structure and "*de novo*" origin of the end organ. (Burgess et al.[49] rejected the *de novo* hypothesis because they found domes recovered in areas of previously excised domes following nerve transections. However, they, as Boeke before them, failed to realize that wound contracture could have pulled an area of "intrinsic specificity" into that excised area.) The alternative hypothesis, "extrinsic specificity," which Burgess et al.[49] favor, implies that a regenerating axon can induce a dome anywhere. This seems to me, at least in primate glabrous skin, to be untenable. If this hypothesis were so, the number of recovered domes in each of their animals should have been near 100%, with simply a low coincidence. They found the opposite: only half the original number of domes recovered and among these recovered domes the percent coincidence was high (average 63%). I believe these results in cat hairy skin are compatible with "intrinsic specificity."

One additional finding from Burgess et al.[49] deserves comment. Recovered touch domes were found within the peripheral field of the regenerating femoral cutaneous nerve fibers that were not innervated by the femoral cutaneous nerve. They suggested that axons "sprouted" from adjacent nerve territories to account for this. This is consistent with the earlier discussion in this chapter and previous observations.[40-42]

In primate, glabrous skin, the analog of the touch dome, the Merkel cell-neurite complex is found only beneath intermediary ridges. The time course of degeneration following nerve division in primates has not been documented, but, extrapolating from the above, the Merkel cell-neurite complex probably degenerates more quickly than the Meissner corpuscle. Therefore, it would less likely be present to be reinnervated by a regenerating axon. Since we know that constant touch is recovered following nerve repair, we may assume, in the absence of any previous documentation, that Merkel cell-neurite complexes are reinnervated after repair. We feel

the "intrinsic specificity" theory is consistent with this observation, in that a regenerating slowly-adapting fiber emerges from the subpapillary plexus and moves "at random" toward the epidermis. Trophic factors, either from the once apparent Merkel cell, or from the axon, or both, result in the regeneration of this fiber/receptor system in the specific regions about sweat ducts in the intermediate ridge. (For further discussion of trophic neural mechanisms, refer to Werner[15] and Drachman[51] reviews.)

CROSS-REINNERVATION STUDIES

Among Cross-Reinnervation Studies the intriguing questions of sensibility is whether a nerve fiber that once innervated one type of sensory end organ could innervate a different type of sensory end organ *and* result in a functional fiber/receptor system; if it could, which function, that of the fiber or of the end organ, would result? I feel that this question has never been answered clearly. I will review the few types of studies that have been done, suggest explanations for their results based upon the neurophysiologic and morphologic principles developed so far in this text, and suggest some definitive avenues of investigation.

One of the earliest studies demonstrated an interaction between the central neuron of a regenerating axon and the distal Schwann sheath into which it was regenerating.[52] Ventral rami of spinal nerves, containing large myelinated fibers in the rabbit, were sutured distally to the anterior mesenteric nerve, which had contained small *un*myelinated fibers. Small myelinated fibers appeared following the nerve repair. Suture of the ventral rami to the greater sphlanic nerve, which had contained small myelinated fibers, resulted in regenerating axons of intermediate thickness and myelinated. Thus, the neuron and its regenerating axon could induce myelination by the Schwann cells distally and even cause some enlargement of the endoneural sheath, while the sheath, in general, did restrict regenerating axon diameter below normal.

The first clinical experiment was war-inspired and involved transferring the proximal radial sensory nerve into the distal median nerve at the level of the wrist for irreparable median nerve loss.[53] Turnbull[53] reported four clinical cases, three of which were nerves repaired by the fibrin clot technique of Tarlov. The patients had their final reported evaluation at 16, 29, 34, and 52 months, respectively, after nerve transfer. All regained the perception of pain, temperature, and sudomotor function (sweating). The two patients followed the least amount of time could not perceive "touch." In all, point localization was poor. In all, most stimuli were interpreted as being from the radial innervated area, although some central transfer had occurred. Recently, Chacha et al.[54] reported results of this operation in six monkeys: two had the superficial radial sensory, two had dorsal ulnar sensory, and two had both nerves transferred into the distal median nerve in otherwise deafferented hands. At 3 weeks, the animals' median nerves and thumb and index fingertips were biopsied. They were stained with specific and nonspecific cholinesterase, as well as silver staining. Reinnervated Meissner corpuscles were observed and their cholinesterase staining reaction (specific and nonspecific) were normal. Reinnervation occurred in the two monkeys in whom both nerves were transferred into the distal median nerve. No observations were made on Merkel cell-neurite complexes, Pacinian corpuscles, or dermal nerve networks. No single unit nerve recordings were done.

One of the most frequently cited references is Lowenstein's[44] in which the proximal segment of the greater sphlanic nerve of the cat was "united" with the distal segment of a transected inferior mesenteric nerve in the cat. The "autonomic nerve" regenerated distally along the mesenteric axonal sheaths and subsequent histologic evaluation of the Pacinian corpuscles demonstrated that about one-third had been reinnervated. These corpuscles, when given mechanostimulation, were demonstrated by single unit neurophysiologic analysis to function like the normally innervated Pacinian corpuscle.

More recently, Paul, Merzenich, and Goodman[55,56] have reported a series of studies in which the brain's somatosensory area, the postcentral gyrus, was mapped in terms

not only of individual finger-area representation but also of slowly- and quickly-adapting nerve fiber/receptor systems in the monkey. A duplicate hand representation (as discussed in more detail in Chapter 3) was found (Fig. 5.11). One area (Brodmann's area 1) on the rostral surface of the postcentral gyrus had very few slowly-adapting fiber/receptor spots (5%), whereas the other area (Brodmann's area 3) on the posterior bank of the central sulcus had a much higher percentage (56%) of these. In six monkeys, then, median and ulnar nerves were transected, and sutured, to their *own* respective ends, utilizing an 8–0 nylon, microsurgical (presumably epineural) repair. Although not a cross-union of nerves as described above, regenerating median (for example) axons did regenerate down a significant number of different endoneurial sheaths. Cortical mapping after nerve regeneration demonstrated a significant number of multiple field responses, not seen in the control hemispheres (Fig. 5.12). Thus, there were central neurons following nerve regeneration that could be stimulated by more than one peripheral receptive field (heterogenous submodalities). This mixed input was presumed due to "cross regeneration at the periphery." Of note is the greater incidence of multiple field responses in area 1 (rostral surface where 95% of responses are normally quickly-adapting) than in area 3, 31% versus 11%. There was also an absolute decrease in the number of slowly-adapting responses in area 3 from 56 to 28% while there was no significant change in percentage of quickly-adapting responses in area 1.

The most recent approach to cross-regeneration again comes not from suturing different peripheral nerves together but from comparing the neurophysiologic properties of regenerating fiber groups. The data of Dykes and Terzis[57] suggest that following nerve crush, a regenerating axon, by means of its multiple sprouts, may still enter two separate peripheral receptive fields, each of which has a different response characteristic (see Fig. 12.12). This peripheral nerve single unit data is exactly analogous to that described by Paul et al.[56] as central, multiple field responses of the heterogenous submodality type.

Other examples of cross-innervation in-

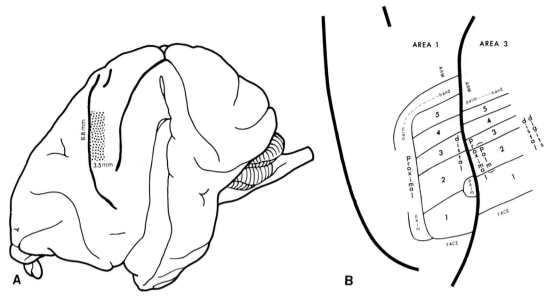

Figure 5.11. Dual representation of hand in sensory cortex. *A*, The sensory cortex, the postcentral gyrus, is posterior to the dark line, the central sulcus. The area of the gyrus within the sulcus is Brodmann's area 1. *B*, With the sulcus surface imagined as opened up, area 1 and area 3 are seen as dual hand areas. Area 1, however, was found to have mostly slowly-adapting receptors (56%), while area 3 was found to have mostly rapidly-adapting receptors (95%). (Reproduced with permission from R. L. Paul et al.: *Brain Res* 36:229–249, 1972.[55])

clude the classic taste bud studies. Cranial nerves carrying gustatory fibers could induce taste buds following cross-innervation, whereas nongustatory cranial nerves, autonomic nerves, and somatic sensory or motor nerves could not.[18,58] While these studies seem to demonstrate the absolute requirement of the specific axon, tongue germinal epithelium will develop taste buds when transplanted to the eye's anterior chamber.[59]

McLachlean, et al.[60] noted that denervated skeletal muscle is reinnervated at the site of the old (degenerated), motor end-plates. Bennett et al.[61] pursued this work using avian muscle. The fast muscle fibers were associated with "en grappe" type endings at the motor end-plates, while slow muscle fibers were associated with "en plaque" type. In the crossed nerve studies, regenerated fast muscle fibers grew into the slow muscle and formed "en plaque" type endings. Regenerating slow muscle nerve fibers grew into fast muscle and "en grappe" endings were found.

We may now try to infer the answers to the questions (1) can, for example, a regenerating axon from a slowly-adapting fiber/receptor system reinnervate a different type of receptor, for example, a Meissner corpuscle, and, if it can, (2) will it function as a slowly- or as a quickly-adapting fiber/receptor system? The studies reviewed suggest that for the fast/slow muscle groups, for the myelinated/unmyelinated axons regenerating into distal unmyelinated/myelinated sheaths and for taste bud systems, there is a mutual influencing of the cross-innervating structures. Taken together, these studies suggest that a regenerating axon can reinnervate a different type of end organ. The results of the studies on response characteristics of regenerating fiber populations and on cortical neuron responses after peripheral nerve regeneration suggest that the reinnervated end organs that were cross-innervated do function. I interpret the available data to mean that the function is determined by the end organ's original function.

The results of many of the studies referred

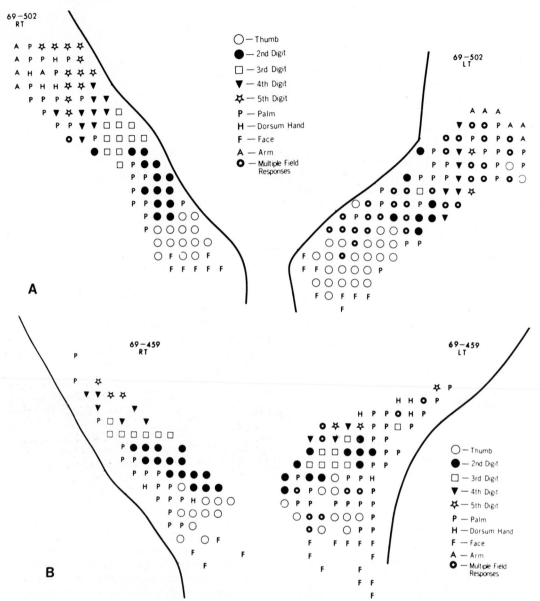

Figure 5.12. Central manifestation of cross-regeneration of peripheral nerve fibers. Median and ulnar nerves were transected and repaired. Central responses were later recorded by stimulating peripheral receptive fields. In both Brodmann's area 1 (*A*) and area 3 (*B*) the experimental hemispheric recordings (*right side* of diagram) demonstrated cortical neurons that responded to more than one peripheral field and were of both the slowly- and quickly-adapting response type. (Reproduced with permission from R. L. Paul et al.: *Brain Res* 39:1–19, 1972.[56])

to earlier may be better explained or reinterpreted by applying the neurophysiological correlates developed previously in this text. For example, Lowenstein's cross-innervation study is usually quoted as demonstrating that a receptor can be reinnervated by a different type of axon and yet function without change.[44] Actually, only one-third of the Pacinian corpuscles were reinnervated by the nerve that originally innervated the bladder. Was this because the results of the nerve "union" were poor, allowing only one-third of the axons to regenerate successfully? Alternatively, we know that the bladder innervation contains fibers that respond to stretch, relay muscle tone, etc. Is it not possible that some of these fibers are quickly-adapting and that these fibers reinnervated the Pacinian corpuscles and reproduced the functioning fiber/receptor system? If so, then Lowenstein's study did not demonstrate what it is usually cited as having shown.

The clinical cross-innervation studies of radial into median nerve showed overall poor recovery of functional sensation. Protective sensation was recovered. The relatively few fibers in the radial sensory branches were distributed to the entire median nerve territory. This had to result in too low an innervation density for tactile localization, no less discrimination. The free nerve endings, subserving pain and temperature, successfully reached the periphery, and needing no end organ, re-established protective sensation, albeit with false localization (stimuli referred back to the dorsoradial skin). The experimental cross-innervation studies of radial plus dorsal ulnar sensory into median provided a greater number of regenerating axons, and histologic confirmation of a sensory end organ reinnervation was achieved. The functional significance of this is unknown because the cholinesterase series of staining techniques is unrelated to sensory perception.

There are examples, however, of cross-finger flaps transferring dorsal skin, recovering good functional sensation when transferred to the (volar) fingertip.[55] How can this be explained? I believe that "hairy skin" has receptors (the hair follicles) that can be reinnervated by glabrous skin's quickly-adapting fibers and Haarscheibe, or follicles with a Merkel cell-neurite complex, that can be reinnervated by glabrous skin's slowly-adapting fibers to form functional fiber/receptor systems. Conversely, I believe that the quickly-adapting fibers that innervate hair follicles, and the slowly-adapting fibers that innervate Haarscheibe (or Merkel cell-neurite complexes about hair follicles) in the hairy skin, could reinnervate Pacinian/Meissner corpuscles or Merkel cell-neurite complexes, respectively, in the cross-innervation radial-to-median studies.

The radial nerve to median nerve cross-innervation provides the perfect model for experimental investigation of these problems. I suggest that all radial sensory fibers be

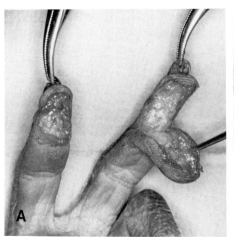 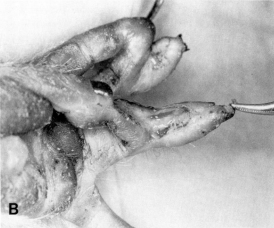

Figure 5.13. Monkey skin graft/flap study: *A*, Volar full thickness skin grafts were exchanged between the thumb and index finger. A hypothenar flap was done on the little finger. *B*, Dorsal view of the dorsal cross-finger flap from the middle finger to the ring fingertip. There is a forearm skin graft on the middle fingertip and dorsal flap donor site.

sutured to the volar digital nerves to a single finger. This maximizes the possibility that the fibers of the sensory radial nerve, which are fewer than the total number of sensory fibers in the median nerve, will have an innervation density sufficient to reinnervate the dense population of sensory receptors in the fingertip. Prior to fingertip biopsy, and obtaining light and electromicroscopy, single unit nerve recordings can be obtained from the sensory radial nerve at the wrist. This regenerated fiber population can be compared to the normal radial sensory and median sensory population. Peripheral mechanostimulation should incorporate moving and constant touch, as well as vibratory stimuli.

CLINICAL IMPLICATIONS

What is the ideal soft tissue resurfacing material for the fingertip? The results of this review suggest the following approach to this problem. Since normal fingertip sensory function requires the presence of peripheral mechanoreceptors capable of high fidelity transduction of sensory stimuli, it becomes clear that sensory axons must not only regenerate in maximum numbers into the donor tissue but also must reinnervate a suitable mechanoreceptor. There is no evidence that human mechanoreceptors, e.g., Meissner cor-

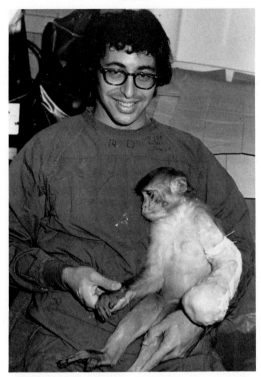

Figure 5.15. Monkey skin graft/flap study. The monkey's hand was protected with a cast of acrylic poured over plaster. (Reproduced with permission from A. L. Dellon and R. E. Terrill: *Hand* 8:165–166, 1975.[71])

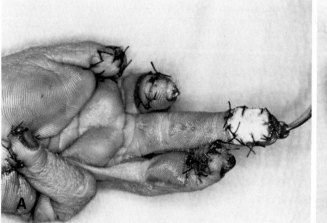

Figure 5.14. Monkey skin graft/flap study. *A*, Volar cross-finger flaps were done from the middle finger to the index fingertip, and from the ring finger to the thumb. *B*, Completed procedure showing also the hypothenar flap to the little finger.

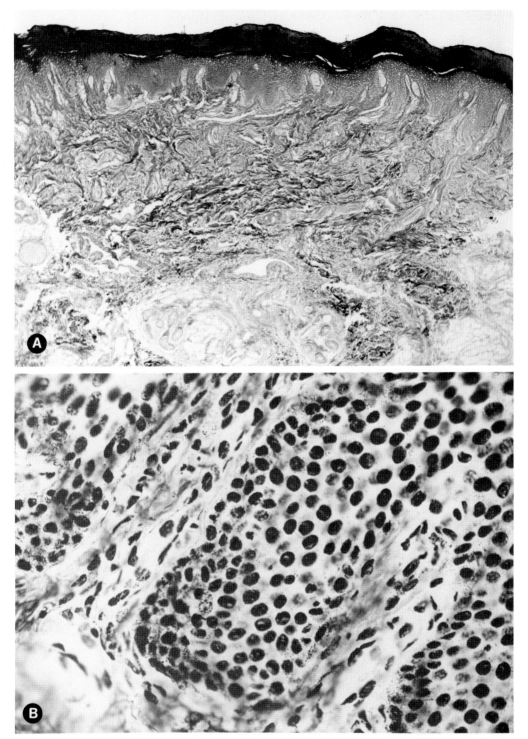

Figure 5.16. Monkey skin graft/flap study. Sensory end organs were best preserved in flaps where they were protected relatively from ischemia. *A,* Note row of innervated Meissner corpuscles (Silver stain, ×16). *B,* Note early reinnervation of two Meissner corpuscles and Merkel cell-neurite complex (Silver stain, ×300). Both are from a volar cross-finger flap in monkey biopsied 4 months after flap inset.

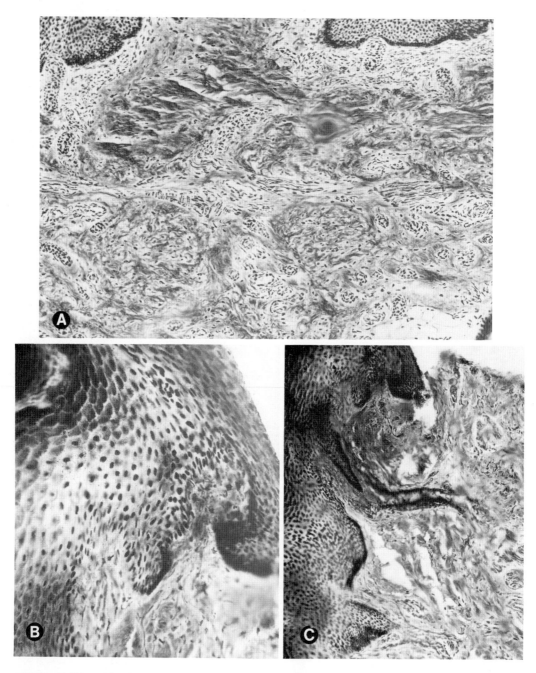

Figure 5.17. Monkey skin graft/flap study: The volar (glabrous) full thickness skin graft had excellent reinnervation of the dermal nerve networks (*A* and *C*), but the ischemic period before graft ''take'' resulted in significant, probably irreversible, loss of end organs. Note the ''ghost'' Pacinian (*A*) and ''ghost'' Meissner corpuscle (*B*). There was partial reinnervation of some remaining Meissner corpuscles in these biopsies taken 4 months after the graft (*C*) (Silver stain, ×150).

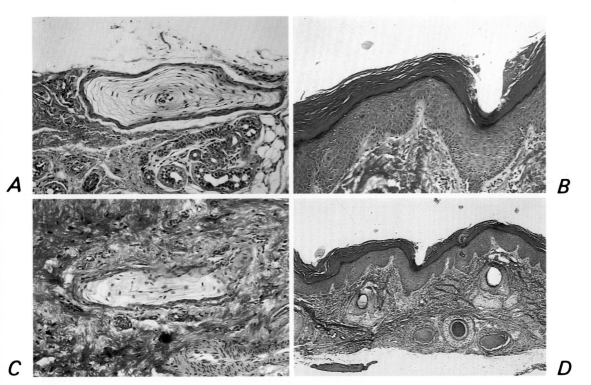

Figure 5.18.   Monkey skin graft/flap study: Dorsal finger skin contains Meissner-like corpuscles and hair follicles (Trichrome stain, ×64).

puscles, regenerate *de novo* after an axon regenerates into the dermis. To provide optimal potential for sensory recovery, therefore, it follows that the donor skin must contain the suitable mechanoreceptors. This implies that skin most resembling fingertip skin should be used. Such skin, i.e., hairless (glabrous) skin containing papillary ridges, is found only on the palm of the hand and fingertip and the sole of the foot and toes. A close approximation of this skin is dorsal fingertip skin which has modified papillary ridges and contains an occasional Meissner corpuscle.[63, 64]

I propose the following hypothesis: The highest potential for recovery of normal sensation is provided by skin with papillary ridges and the highest density of mechanoreceptors, i.e., distal glabrous skin. This hypothesis can be tested indirectly by reviewing the reported clinical experience with the treatment of fingertip injuries. The poorest recovery of sensation is found with distant pedicle flaps, e.g., abdominal and pectoral donor sites. Perhaps slightly better, but still poor, sensation is recovered when forearm or thigh thick split-thickness grafts are used. The best results are achieved with local pedicle flaps, e.g., thenar, hypothenar, and dorsal cross-finger flaps.[33,65–67] A recent report using dorsal cross-finger flaps combined with a program of sensory re-education (see Chapter 12) has resulted in recovery of virtually normal sensation subjectively and by two-point discrimination testing. With smaller pulp losses, of course, virtually normal sensation has been recovered using split thickness skin grafts[68] or conservative management.[69] In these cases, the normal skin surrounding the injury ultimately becomes the resurfacing "donor" tissue, by wound contracture in the latter case and by "graft" contraction in the former. The myofibroblast is probably at the "bottom" of both these processes and the distinction is probably already archaic.

Further support of the hypothesis that the degree of functional sensation recovered is

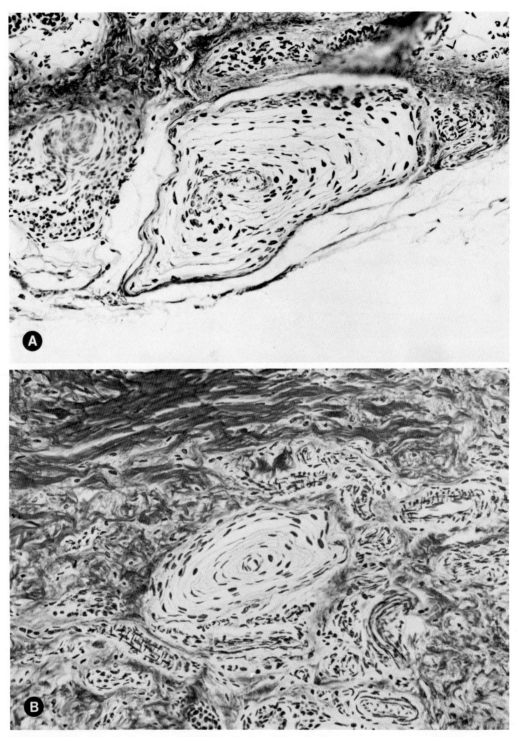

Figure 5.19.   Monkey skin graft/flap study: This partially reinnervated specimen permits statement that the pink component of the trichrome stains axoplasm. Reinnervated (*A*) and noninnervated (*B*) Pacinian corpuscle (*A*, Silver stain; *B* trichrome stain; ×64.)

proportional to the density of mechanoreceptors in the donor tissue comes from Kleinert's
study.[62] With dorsal cross-finger flaps, 90%
of his youngest patient group (6 to 13 years
old) recovered less than 6-mm two-point discrimination in contrast to just 40% of his
oldest patient group (greater than 40 years
old). I presume it is more than coincidence
that this result parallels the decline in sensory
end organ density with increasing age: the
Meissner Index (density of Meissner corpuscles) in the fingertip is more than twice as
high in a population less than 15 years old
than it is in a population greater than 40 years
old.[70]

In 1975, while a Clinical Associate in the
Surgery Branch of the National Cancer Institute, National Institutes of Health, I designed
a series of grafts and flaps in monkeys to test
the effect of ischemia and axonal regeneration upon the sensory end organ population.
The study has remained unpublished because
time constraints have prevented the necessary detailed evaluation of the thousands of
serial sections. In two monkeys, the operations consisted of: (1) full thickness volar skin
grafts switched between thumb and index
finger; (2) dorsal cross-finger flap from middle finger to ring fingertip; (3) hypothenar
flap to little finger; and (4) forearm skin grafts
to flap donor site on middle finger dorsum
and to middle fingertip (Fig. 5.13). In two
more monkeys, the operations were: (1) volar
cross-finger flaps from middle to index finger
and ring finger to thumb, and (2) hypothenar
flap to little finger (Fig. 5.14). Flaps were
divided and inset at 3 weeks and were protected until that time in acrylic casts[71] (Fig.
5.15). This study demonstrated reinnervation
of the dermal nerve networks in both grafts
and flaps (Figs. 5.16 and 5.17). No Meissner
or Pacinian corpuscles or Merkel cell-neurite
complexes were identified in forearm skin
grafted to the fingertip, although hair follicles
were reinnervated well. None of these sensory end organs were identified in dorsal
finger skin transferred to the fingertip, although hair follicles were reinnervated. An
occasional Meissner-like structure was identified as well as subpapillary plexus nerves in
search of end organs beneath the hairy skin
epidermal ridges (Fig. 5.18). Perhaps of greatest consequence were the two following ob-

servations: (1) the volar cross-finger flap was
the best reinnervated, with the best preser-
vation of pre-existing sensory end organs
(Fig. 5.16); and (2) the glabrous skin grafts
demonstrated ischemic damage to the sensory corpuscles (ghost Meissner and Pacinian
corpuscles) with poorer reinnervation than
the volar cross-finger flap (Fig. 5.17). One
partially reinnervated, serially sectioned
specimen allowed the following confirmation
of my earlier suspicion[36,72] that the pink-
staining component in the trichrome stain
identifies axoplasm (Fig. 5.19).

In summary, the preliminary results of this
monkey skin graft/flap study demonstrated
that skin containing sensory end organs is
the best resurfacing material, and that a local
flap of this tissue permits greater end organ
survival than a full-thickness graft, presumably because the end organs are relatively
protected from ischemia. Applications of
these concepts are illustrated at the end of
Chapter 12.

References

1. Remensnyder JP: Physiology of nerve healing and nerve grafts, in Krizek TJ, Hoopes JE (eds): *Sympo-sium on Basic Science in Plastic Surgery.* Saint Louis: CV Mosby, 1976, Ch 24.
2. Seddon, H: *Surgical Disorders of the Peripheral Nerves.* Baltimore: Williams & Wilkins, 1972, Ch 2.
3. Sunderland S: *Nerves and Nerve Injuries,* ed 2. Edinburgh: Churchill-Livingstone, 1978, Ch 8.
4. Sunderland S: *Nerves and Nerve Injuries,* ed 2. Edinburgh: Churchill Livingston, 1978, Ch 23,26.
5. Sunderland S: *Nerves and Nerve Injuries,* ed 2. Edinburgh: Churchill Livingstone, 1978, Ch 31,32.
6. Samders FK, Young JZ: The role of the peripheral stump in the control of fibre diameter in generating nerves. J Physiol 103:119–136, 1944.
7. Aitkens JT, Sharman M, Young JZ: Maturation of regenerating nerve fibres with various peripheral connections. J Anat 81:1–22, 1947.
8. Sanders FK, Young JZ: The influence of peripheral connections on the diameter of regenerating nerve fibres. J Exp Biol 22:203–212, 1947.
9. Boeke J: *The Problems of Nervous Anatomy.* Lon-don: Oxford University Press, 1940, pp 12–44.
10. Boeke J: On the regeneration of sensitive end-cor-puscles after section of the nerve. K Acad van We-tenschoppen (Amsterdam) 25:319–323, 1922.
11. Boeke J, Dijkstra C: De- and regeneration of sensible end-corpuscles in the duck's bill (corpuscles of Grandry and Herbst) after the cutting of the nerve, the removing of the entire skin or the transplantation of the skin in another region. K Acad van Weten-schoppen (Amsterdam) 35:1114–1119, 1932.
12. Miller SH, Rusennas I: Changes in primate Pacinian

corpuscles following volar pad excision and skin grafting. Plast Reconstr Surg 57:627–636, 1976.

13. Dellon AL: On changes in primate Pacinian corpuscles after volar pad excision and skin grafting. Plast Reconstr Surg 58:614–615, 1976.

14. Marshall AJ (ed): *Biology & Comparative Physiology of Birds*. New York: Academic Press, 1960, pp 33,44,210.

15. Werner JK: Trophic influences of nerves on the development and maintainance of sensory receptors. Am J Phys Med 53:127–142, 1974.

16. Farbman AI: Electron microscopic study of the developing taste bud in rat fungiform papillae. Dev Biol 11:110–135, 1965.

17. Biedler LM, Nejad MS, Smallman RL, et al: Rat taste cell proliferation. Fed Proc 19:302, 1960.

18. Guth L: Taste buds in the rat's circumallate papillae after reinnervation for the glossopharyngeal, vagus, and hypoglossal nerve. Anat Rec 130:25–37, 1958.

19. Fujimoto S, Murray RG: Fine structure of degeneration and regeneration in denervated rabbit vallate taste buds. Anat Rec 168:393–414, 1970.

20. Jabaley ME: Recovery of sensation in flaps and skin, in Tubiana R (ed): *The Hand*. Philadelphia: WB Saunders, 1981.

21. Terzis JK: Functional aspects of reinnervation of free skin grafts. Plast Reconstr Surg 58:142–156, 1976.

22. Kredel FE, Evans JP: Recovery of sensation in denervated pedicle and free skin grafts. Arch Neurol Psychiatry 29:1203–1221, 1933.

23. Davis L: The return of sensation to the transplanted skin. Surg Gynecol Obstet 59:533–543, 1934.

24. Davis, JS, Kitlowski EA: Regeneration of nerves in skin grafts and skin flaps. Am J Surg 24:501–545, 1934.

25. McCarroll HR: The regeneration of sensation in transplanted skin. Ann Surg 108:309–320, 1938.

26. Lofgren L: Recovery of nervous function in skin transplants with special reference to the sympathetic functions. Acta Chir Scand 102:229–239, 1952.

27. Reid DAC: Experience of a hand surgery service. Br J Plast Surg 9:11–16, 1956.

28. Barclay TL: The late results of fingertip injuries. Br J Plast Surg 8:38–43, 1955.

29. Adeymo O, Wyburn GM: Innervation of skin grafts. Transplant Bull 4:152–153, 1957.

30. Ponten B: Grafted skin: Observation on innervation and other qualities. Acta Chir Scand [Suppl] 257:1–78, 1960.

31. Fitzgerald MJT, Martin F, Paletta FX: Innervation of skin grafts. Surg Gynecol Obstet 124:808–812, 1967.

32. Hutchinson J, Tough JS, Wynburn GM: Regeneration of sensation in graft skin. Br J Plast Surg 2:82–94, 1949.

33. Mannerfelt L: Evaluation of functional sensation of skin grafts in the hand area. Br J Plast Surg 15:136–154, 1962.

34. Moberg E: Objective methods of determining the functional value of sensibility in the hand. J Bone Joint Surg [Suppl] 40-B:454, 1958.

35. Ridley A: A biopsy study of the innervation of forearm skin grafted to the fingertip. Brain 93:547–554, 1970.

36. Dellon AL: Reinnervation of denervated Meissner

corpuscles: A sequential histological study in the monkey following fascicular nerve repair. J Hand Surg 1:98–109, 1976.

37. Orgel M, Aguayo A. Williams HB: Sensory nerve regeneration: An experimental study of skin grafts in the rabbit. J Anat 111:121–135, 1972.

38. Celli L, Caroli A: La ripresa della sensibilita nei trapianti, ed. innesti cutanei della mano. Riv Chir Mano 8:23–62, 1970.

39. Terui A: Reinnervation in the free skin graft. Jpn J Plast Reconstr Surg 18:392–399, 1975.

40. Weddell G, Guttmann L, Guttmann E: The local extension of nerve fibres into denervated areas of skin. J Neurol Neurosurg Phychiatry 4:206–225, 1941.

41. Hoffman H: Local re-innervation in partially denervated muscle: A histo-physiological study. Aust J Exp Biol Med Sci 28:384–398, 1950.

42. Livingstone WK: Evidence of active invasion of denervated areas by sensory fibers from neighboring nerves in man. J Neurosurg 4:140–145, 1947.

43. Wong WC, Kangasuntheram R: Early and late effects of median nerve injury on Meissner's and Pacinian corpuscles of the hand of the Macaque. J Anat 109:135–142, 1971.

44. Lowenstein WR: Development of a receptor on a foreign nerve fiber in a Pacinian corpuscle. Science 177:712–715, 1972.

45. Krishnamurti A, Kanagasuntheram R, Vij S: Failure of reinnervation of Pacinian corpuscle after nerve crush: An electron microscopic study. Acta Neuropathol (Berl) 23:338–341, 1973.

46. Jabaley ME, Burns JE, Orcutt BS, et al: Comparison of histologic and functional recovery after peripheral nerve repair. J Hand Surg 1:119–130, 1976.

47. Brown AG, Iggo A: The structure and function of cutaneous "touch corpuscles" after nerve crush. J Physiol 165:28P–29P, 1963.

48. Burgess PR, Horch KW: Specific regeneration of cutaneous fibers in the cat. J Neurophysiol 36:101–114, 1973.

49. Burgess PR, English KB, Horch KW, et al: Patterning in the regeneration of type I cutaneous receptors. J Physiol 236:57–86, 1974.

50. Horch K: Guidance of regrowing sensory axons after cutaneous nerve lesions in the cat. J Neurophysiol 42:1437–1449, 1979.

51. Drachman DB (ed): *Trophic Functions of the Neuron*. New York: New York Academy of Sciences, 1974.

52. Simpson SA, Young JZ: Regeneration of fiber diameter after cross-unions of visceral and somatic nerves. J Anat 79:48–64, 1944.

53. Turnbull F: Radial-medial anastamosis. J Neurosurg 5:562–566, 1948.

54. Chacha PB, Krishnamurti A, Soin K: Experimental sensory reinnervation of the median nerve by nerve transfers in monkeys. J Bone Joint Surg 59A:386–390, 1977.

55. Paul RL, Merzenich M, Goodman H: Representation of slowly- and rapidly-adapting cutaneous mechanoreceptors of the hand in Brodmann's areas 3 and 1 of Macaca mulatto. Brain Res 36:229–249, 1972.

56. Paul RL, Goodman H, Merzenich M: Alterations in

mechanoreceptor input to Brodmann's areas 1 and 3 of the post-central hand area of Macaca mulatto after nerve section and regeneration. Brain Res 39: 1–19, 1072.

57. Dykes RW, Terzis JK: Reinnervation of glabrous skin in baboons: Properties of cutaneous mechanoreceptors subsequent to nerve crush. J Neurophysiol 42:1461–1478, 1979.

58. Zalewski AA: Combined effects of testosterone motor, sensory or gustatory nerves on reinnervation of regeneration of taste buds. Exp Neurol 24:285–297, 25:29–37, 1969.

59. Zaleski AA: Regeneration of taste buds after transplantation of tongue and ganglia grafts to the anterior chamber of the eye. Exp. Neurol 35:519–528, 1972.

60. McLachlean EM, Taylor RS, Bennett MR: The site of synapsis formation in reinnervation and cross-reinnervation mammalian muscle. Proc Aust Physiol Pharmacol Soc 3:62–69, 1972.

61. Bennett MR, Pettigrew AG, Taylor RS: The formation of synapsis in reinnervated and cross-reinnervated adult avian muscle. J Physiol 230:331–357, 1973.

62. Kleinert HE, McAllister CG, MacDonald CJ, et al: A critical evaluation of cross-finger flaps. J Trauma 14: 756–763, 1974.

63. Cauna N, Mannan G: Development and postnatal changes of digital Pacinian corpuscles (corpuscular lamellosa) in the human hand. J Anat 93:271–286, 1956.

64. Cauna N: Nature and functions of the papillary ridges of the digital skin. Anat Rec 119:449–468, 1954.

65. Sturman MJ, Duran RJ: Late results of fingertip injuries. J Bone Joint Surg 45A:289–298, 1963.

66. Smith JR, Bam AF: An evaluation of fingertip reconstruction by cross-finger and palmar pedicle flaps. Plast Reconstr Surg 35:409–418, 1965.

67. Porter RW: Functional assessment of transplanted skin in volar defects of digits: A comparison between free grafts and flaps. J Bone Joint Surg 50A:955–963, 1968.

68. Brady GS, Cloutier AM, Woolhouse FM: The fingertip injury–an assessment of management. Plast Reconstr Surg 26:80–90, 1960.

69. Holm A, Zacharias L: Fingertip lesions: An evaluation of conservative treatment versus free skin grafting. Acta Orthop Scand 45:382–392, 1974.

70. Ridley A: Silver staining of the innervation of Meissner corpuscles in peripheral neuropathy. Brain 91: 539–552, 1968.

71. Dellon AL, Terrill RE: A protective acrylic cast for use in experimental hand surgery. Hand 8:165–166, 1975.

72. Jabaley ME, Dellon AL: Evaluation of sensibility through microhistological studies, in Omer GE, Spinner M (eds): *Management of Peripheral Nerve Problems.* Philadelphia: WB Saunders, 1980, Ch 23.

SECTION 2

Evaluation of Sensibility

Chapter 6

IT'S ACADEMIC BUT NOT FUNCTIONAL

INTRODUCTION
MOBERG
WEBER TEST
PICKING-UP TEST
OTHER TESTS

INTRODUCTION

I believe hand surgeons have been handicapped at the start of their medical training. A person's perception of an event is conditioned by his prior training and experience. In medical school, our approach to evaluating sensibility in the hand is derived from our lectures or teaching in neuroanatomy and physical diagnosis. As we grapple with this "new language" of neuroanatomy, we begin to be "indoctrinated." We are told that, "the posterior white columns, the fasciculus gracilis and cuneatus constitute the principal path for conduction of discriminative sensibility related to cortical function, conveying impulses from proprioceptors regarding position sense and movement, from tactile discriminators necessary for the proper discrimination of two points simultaneously applied and from rapidly successive stimuli produced by application of a tuning fork to bone ... (and from) appreciation of differences in weight and ability to identify objects placed in the hand by feeling them."[1] The anterior spinothalamic tract "transmits impulses of light touch ... the sensation evoked by stroking an area of skin devoid of hair with a feather or wisp of cotton. This sensation supplements deep touch (pressure) conveyed in the posterior white columns."[1] The lateral spinothalamic tract is "of tremendous clinical importance ... temperature and pain fibers are located in this tract."[1]

We learned our sensory examination in the "neurology" or "nervous system" segment of Physical Diagnosis,[2, 3] and it is designed to localize lesions in the central nervous system. Thus, touch is to be evaluated by "the touch of a finger, a wisp of cotton or a camel's hair brush."[2] Position sense, temperature, pain (deep pressure is equated with pain), two-point discrimination and stereognosis (a test of "cortical integration") are also suggested.[2] Currier[3] suggests "the sensory examination is difficult to perform well and interpret correctly. His exam includes "vibration ... with a 128 cps tuning fork applied to a bony prominence ... pain with a sharp pin ... temperature sensation with any warm or cool object ... deep pain ... by squeezing, light touch by a wisp of cotton, two-point tactile sensation ... and stereognosis tested in the hands." It is, therefore, perfectly understandable that 10 years later, when the young surgeon attempts to evaluate a hand with a nerve injury or after a nerve repair, his approach is one vaguely recalled from his "academic" days. It is further perfectly understandable that while such an approach may localize a lesion in the central nervous system, it may have little relevance to evaluating the recovery of useful sensation in the patient's hand (Fig. 6.1).

"There is a real distinction between 'academic recovery' judged in terms of return of motor and sensory function and what may be termed 'functional recovery,' which is judged in terms of the patient's ability to return to complete social and economic independence."[4] This statement summarized the collective experience of the Nerve Injuries Committee of the British Medical Research Council after evaluation of their World War II

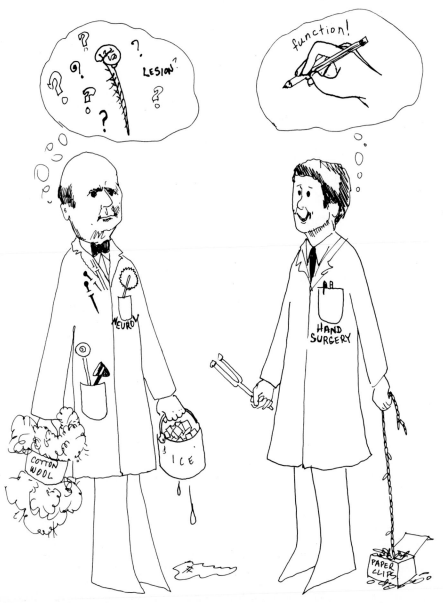

Figure 6.1. Academic versus functional. The neurologist's goal in evaluating sensibility is different from the hand surgeon's. Tests to evaluate spinal tracts and central nervous system pathways do not correlate with the ability of the hand to function.

studies. They chose the term "academic" to represent the classic or traditional neurologic approach to evaluating sensibility in the hand: pain was tested grossly with a pin or quantitatively with a spring-loaded, graded algesiometer; touch was tested grossly with a cotton wisp or quantitatively with calibrated, von Frey hairs. Tests for heat and cold "were not regularly employed since they did not provide any additional information of clinical significance."[5] Academic recovery was graded according to the outline originally proposed by W. B. Highet, and recorded by Zachary[6]*:

Stage 0: absence of sensibility in the autonomous zone of the nerve.
Stage 1. recovery of deep cutaneous pain sensibility within the autonomous zone.
Stage 2: return of some degree of superficial pain and tactile sensibility within the autonomous zone.
Stage 3: return of superficial pain and tactile sensibility throughout the autonomous zone with the disappearance of over-response.
Stage 4: return of sensibility as in Stage 3 with the addition that there is recovery of two-point discrimination within the autonomous zone.

"Functional recovery was judged by the use made of the injured limb by the patient."[4]

Although this approach indicates a recognition of the fact that the results of the classic physical diagnostic techniques were not predicative of a patient's ability to utilize his hand, the credit for bringing this to worldwide attention belongs to Eric Moberg. Although Moberg has said: "The distinction between academic and functional recovery is one of the important contributions to nerve surgery made by Seddon and his associates in Great Britain,"[8] Moberg, himself, has spent at least two decades[7-14] further emphasizing, refining, and demonstrating the importance of functional sensory testing.

MOBERG

Erik Moberg is one of the giants of Hand Surgery. His influence is felt in many spheres, and he continues, in "retirement," to be innovative and persuasive, for example, in the rehabilitation of the tetraplegic.[15]* His unceasing emphasis on the evaluation of functional sensibility for more than 2 decades deserves all our thanks. In 1958, the *Journal of Bone and Joint Surgery* gave 22 pages of text for Moberg's then iconoclastic and now classic paper on "Objective Methods for Determining the Functional Value of Sensibility in the Hand."[9] Written from the Hand Service, Sahlgren Hospital, Gothenberg, Sweden, this paper clearly stated the problem, "it has been borne home to me with the passage of years how little the results of the customary tests of sensibility in an injured hand correspond with the actual ability of the patient to use his hand." In this paper, Moberg described two new objective tests; the "picking-up test" and the ninhydrin test, now universally known. He further coined the terms "precision sensory and gross sensory grip." He resurrected the term "tactile gnosis" to replace "stereognosis." He also correlated results from using all the then known academic and functional tests on a series of patients. Moberg elaborated upon his work in the journal *Neurology*,[10] commenting in a footnote "when the investigation was completed in the main four years ago, it was realized that its results must entail a complete change in the attitude to the current methods of examination. For this reason, it was decided to delay publication of the results until after they could be checked still further. This was done on an extensive series

---

* This classification is often referred to as "Highet's Classification," yet we find it in Zachary's chapter and little else ever mentioned of Highet. Recently, I found the answer to this: Seddon[7] writes "W. Bremner Highet joined us at the outbreak of the Second World War. This talented young New Zealander was awarded the Jacksonian Prize by the Royal College of Surgeons of England for an essay on nerve injuries. The closure of the Mediterranean Sea left only the Cape route for the evacuation of men injured in the fighting in the Desert War. As a result of the shortage of transport shipping, many of them piled up in South Africa. Highet was chosen to look after those who had suffered nerve injury. He was sent by sea; the ship was torpedoed and there were no survivors."

---

* He prefers tetraplegic to quadraplegic (a mixture of Latin and Greek).

in regard to diagnosis, therapeutic measures and judgment of disability, and the results were corroborated in full."

On May 14, 1962, Erik Moberg gave the first Annual Sterling Bunnell Lecture to the American Society for Surgery of the Hand on "Aspects of Sensation in Reconstructive Surgery of the Upper Extremity."[8] Although I had associated the phrase "without sensation, the hand is blind," to Moberg, primarily from the emphasis in his writings, and his picture of a fingertip with an eye in its pulp (Fig. 6.2), Moberg credits Bunnell with writing that when sensory function is lost, "the so-called eyes of the fingers are blind." (In reading Bunnell's nerve repair paper for Chapter 11, I recently found this statement.[9])

That Moberg possessed that wonderful (and rare) character trait of critical review of one's own work is evident in the published Bunnell lecture.[8] Moberg described "limitations" then on the usefulness of his ninhydrin

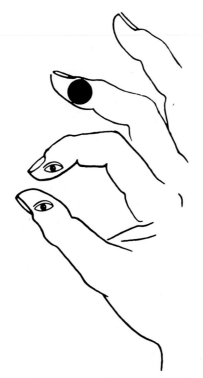

Figure 6.2. The eyes of the fingers. (Reproduced with permission from E. Moberg: *Hand Surgery*, ed 1, Flynn JE (ed.). Baltimore: Williams & Wilkins, 1966.[11])

test. While restating that it is the only objective test of recovery, of nerve fibers, therefore, making it valuable in "children and malingerers," it is "not useful in injuries to the brachial plexus or for skin grafts or flaps, it is useful after nerve suture only when prints are absent, and technical accuracy is necessary." The ninhydrin test essentially documented return of function to sweat glands, not a sensory function. Since sweat glands are innervated by very thin sympathetic fibers, the recovery of sweating should parallel recovery of pain and temperature (see Chapter 7). This observation, that recovery of sweating parallels recovery of protective sensation, has been confirmed again recently.[17] As Moberg, himself, demonstrated, perception of pain and temperature do not correlate with functional recovery.

Moberg was the first person, of whom I am aware, who attempted to correlate clinical sensory tests with hand function, and who recognized that certain clinical tests quantified the simple "yes" or "no" responses of other tests (see Table 6.1). Of interest is Moberg's comment that "I have not been able to find any report on a method of grading the function of the hand that could be used for the comparison."[10] Moberg began by defining hand function in terms of "what the hand can do," i.e., grips (Fig. 6.3). The precision-sensory grips included those necessary to screw on a bolt, wind a wristwatch, sew with a needle, knot a string, and button or unbutton. The gross-sensory grips included the ability to work with a heavy handle, like a wheelbarrow, use a spade, manipulate a doorknob, hold a bottle, or carry a basket. Utilizing the tests in Table 6.1, he studied 10 patients with previous median nerve injury who had recovered good motor function and were free of paresthesia. He studied the correlation between both the classic academic and his functional sensory tests with the patient's hand function as judged by sensory grips, the picking-up test, the patient's own opinion of his hand function, and the appearance of the hand (wear marks).[9, 10] Early in his study, Moberg chose to eliminate temperature testing because it "gives no more information than other methods," and vibration because "most joints of the hand are innervated from two sources."[10]

Table 6.1
Clinical Sensory Tests of Hand Function[a]

Quality	Testing Method	Quantitative Measurement
Touch	Cotton wool, strips of paper	von Frey hairs
Pain	Pin stick	Algesiometer
Localization	Localization of simple touch	Measurement of error
Temperature	Warm and cold objects	Degrees of temperature
Tactile gnosis	Writing digits on pulp, tactual recognition of objects, Seddon coin test, picking-up test	Weber two-point discrimination
Vibration	Tuning fork (128 cps)	

[a] Adapted from E. Moberg.[10]

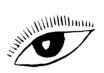 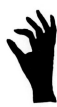

What	What	What
can the	can the	can the
eye	ear	hand
see?	hear?	do?

Figure 6.3. Functional sensation must be related to "what can the hand do?" (Reproduced with permission from E. Moberg: *Hand Surgery*, ed 1, Flynn JE (ed). Baltimore: Williams & Wilkins, 1966.[11])

Moberg's Conclusion

"It turned out that none of the known methods for examining the modality of touch or pain (or temperature or vibration) gave results which corresponded with the functional ability of the hand. Most of these tests were ... misleading. They are not good for grading disability and planning reconstructive surgery in the hand. The Weber two-point discrimination test proved to give accurate information on the functional value of the sensibility in the hand."[10]

Moberg's Specific Results

When two-point discrimination was 30 to 40 mm, there was "a certain capacity" for gross grip and a protective sensibility. Digit writing was found to give results that correlated with Seddon's coin test and two-point discrimination, but had practical shortcomings (clinically difficult to do and standardize). Seddon's coin test (an ability to distinguish whether a coin had a rough or smooth edge) correlated with two-point discrimination when two-point discrimination was "below 12 to 8 mm." But the coin test results "cannot be given in figures" and, therefore, it "cannot be used to distinguish between degrees of tactile gnosis lower than ... these figures."[10] Gross sensory grip was absent if two-point discrimination was greater than 40 mm. The picking-up test was possible if two-point discrimination was less than or equal to 12 mm. Von Frey's hair results only roughly correlated with two-point discrimination testing, e.g., all patients with two-point discrimination less than 15 mm had a touch threshold less than or equal to 1.0 gm (however, some fingertips with two-point discrimination greater than 40 mm also had touch thresholds of 1.0 gm). Moberg was later to write that "some tactile gnosis" equaled a two-point discrimination of 6 to 15 mm, whereas normal equaled a two-point discrimination of 3.5 mm."[8] Moberg was still later to write that gross grip required two-point discrimination "worse than 12 to 15 mm, but better than 30 to 40 mm, good tactile gnosis is hardly present if values are higher than 8 mm."

Neurophysiologic Basis for Moberg's Observations

A firm basis for understanding clinical observations on sensibility in the hand has been provided by Mountcastle and his colleagues in neurophysiology (see Chapter 3). Unfortunately, this basic scientific foundation has failed to reach most practicing surgeons and is only now beginning to be emphasized by those few who have realized what a powerful tool it is in interpreting clinical problems. (Indeed, this is one of the reasons for writing this book!)

In 1969, I made two simple lists: one was of extant clinical tests of sensibility and the other was of presumed neurophysiologic group of sensory fibers being tested (see Table 6.2). This list was "cut" from my earliest paper[18] by the reviewing editors, and did not appear until recently.[19] When I considered Moberg's "grips" as requiring primarily the ability to perceive an object that was in constant contact with the fingertip, such as holding the sewing needle or holding the milk bottle while pouring, it became clear that these static grips required an intact slowly-adapting fiber/receptor system. Fingerstroking and cotton wool wisps required perception of movement and, therefore, tested the quickly-adapting fiber/receptor system. Clearly then, the results of fingerstroking or moving a cotton wisp across the surface of the finger would not correlate with hand function as defined in terms of these grips. However, von Frey's hairs and the Weber test both required perception of an object in constant-touch with the fingertip, and therefore, did test the slowly-adapting fiber/receptor system. It would appear, at first, that both of these test results should correlate with hand function, whereas Moberg found

that only those of the Weber test did. My explanation for this is that the von Frey hair measures the threshold: a single nerve fiber may successfully regenerate, re-innervate a group of Merkel cell-neurite complexes, mature and, if that peripheral sensory field is tested, give a low or normal threshold for pressure. But, tactile gnosis, as defined by Moberg, required the ability to discriminate, and this requires, in Mountcastle's terms, (multiple) overlapping peripheral receptive fields, or a high innervation density. The Weber test measures the peripheral innervation density of the slowly-adapting fiber/receptor system. Therefore, Moberg's finding that only the results of the Weber two-point discrimination test correlated with hand function can be given a neurophysiologic rational if hand function is defined in terms of Moberg's static grips. The picking-up test (discussed in detail below) as practiced by Moberg, primarily required the performance of a static grip (Fig. 6.4), not object recognition.

In the remainder of the Chapter, I will review in detail the Weber test and other sensory tests, since, as Moberg[8] said, "the tools are still crude and must be improved." In Chapters 8 and 9, I will present two "improved tools."

Table 6.2
Sensory Tests Used to Evaluate the Various Nerve Fiber Populations[a]

Clinical Test	Sensation	Fiber/Receptor Population
Pin	Pain	Free nerve endings
Heat	Temperature	Free nerve endings
Cold	Temperature	Free nerve endings
Cotton wool	Moving-touch	Quickly-adapting
Finger stroking	Moving-touch	Quickly-adapting
von Frey hair	Constant-touch	Slowly-adapting
Weber test	Constant-touch	Slowly-adapting
Picking-up test	Constant-touch	Slowly-adapting
Precision sensory grip	Constant-touch	Slowly-adapting
Gross grip	Constant-touch	Slowly-adapting

[a] Reproduced with permission from A. L. Dellon: Contemp Orthrop 1:39–42, 1979.[19]

WEBER TEST

In 1853, Ernst Heinrich Weber, Professor of Anatomy at Leipzig, described a test of sensation distinguished by its ability to give a quantifiable test result. He described the use of calipers, whose points were held against the skin, at different distances apart, until a distance was found at which the subject could no longer distinguish one from two points in contact with the skin.[20] Weber emphasized that the compass ends should not be sharp, but rather be rounded (abgerundeten Spitzen). Weber also recognized that he was measuring what we call "innervation density." He wrote, "The more richly innervated and therefore, more sharply sensitive a piece of skin is, the more clear and correct one can sense the difference between two touched spaces." Weber found the most sensitive part

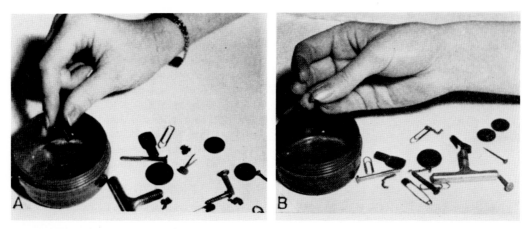

Figure 6.4. Moberg's picking-up test is primarily a static test, in which an object is picked up and then placed into a container. The patient is not asked to identify the object.

of the body for discrimination was the tip of the tongue, then the fingertip.

The ability to record a number after a test had scientific appeal, and we find many of the earlier careful and critical investigators using this test. For example, Silas Weir Mitchell,[21] in discussing his sensory testing techniques during the American Civil War, emphasized not only that the compass must have rounded tips, but also that the test could not be done in the presence of hyperesthesia or paresthesia. In Boeke's laboratory in the 1920's, Doctor Stenver, one of Boeke's co-workers, accidentally cut the dorsal sensory branch of his right ulnar nerve. This was "repaired" and the recovery of sensation followed: two-point discrimination, initially 50 mm decreased to 13 mm 12 months later.[22] In the late 1930's, McCarroll[23] studied sensory recovery in skin grafts: "Completeness of the return was also checked by a comparison of the two-point discrimination of the graft with normal skin." In the early 1960's, detailed results of the Weber test were reported by Mannerfelt[24] in his study of sensory recovery in skin grafts and flaps (see Chapter 5), and by Onne[25] in his study of sensory recovery following nerve repair (see Chapter 12).

Moberg[9, 10] recognized several limitations of the Weber test, and further refined its use. The test requires patient co-operation and careful application. The environment must be quiet and the patient's fingertip or tested area carefully positioned and supported to prevent movement. Patient motivation is a factor, e.g., the compensation case, and thus the test is very subjective. If the numerical value for the two-point discrimination test is close to the width of the tested area, the test most likely is evaluating sensibility in the normal adjacent area. Thus, to say that the two-point discrimination of a 1-cm skin graft is 9 mm is to say that there is *no* two-point discrimination within the graft. Most importantly, the ends of the testing instrument must be blunted. A sharp compass end will elicit the perception of pain, not touch. Similarly, a blunt tip, pressed hard, will elicit pain, not touch. Accordingly, Moberg[11] has emphasized that two-point discrimination testing be done with the least possible pressure: "making the skin blanch where the points are applied should be avoided." Most recently, he has emphasized this by demonstrating that pressure at the end of the testing instrument depresses the skin causing adjacent skin to be stimulated, and, therefore, the examiner is actually testing a wider area than he believes he is testing.[14] (The "correct" pressure to apply is discussed further in Chapter 10.) Moberg requires seven out of 10 correct responses for a given distance to be accepted as the two-point limen.

Representative values for two-point discrimination in the normal hand are given in Tables 6.3, 6.4, and 6.5, adapted from the writings of the credited authors. Each of these studies was an actual evaluation of two-point discrimination in normal or control popula-

Table 6.3
Normal Values for Two-Point
Discrimination (mm)

	Volar Finger			
	Distal Phalanx	Cal- loused Pulp	Middle Phalanx	Proxi- mal Phalanx
Moberg[11]	2–4	4–6		4–6
Parry[26]	0.5–4		1–6	4–6
Gellis and Pool[27]	2–4			
Millesi and Rin- derer[28]	1.5–6			

Table 6.4
Normal Values: Two-point Discrimination (mm)

	Dorsal Finger		
	Distal Phalanx	Middle Phalanx	Proximal Phalanx
Parry[26]	1–6	1–8	1–12
Gellis and Pool[27]		2–7	

Table 6.5
Normal Values: Two Point Discrimination (mm)

	Hand				
	Dorsum		Palm		
	"Dor- sum"	Thumb Web	Thenar	Mid	Hy- poth- enar
Moberg[11]	8–11				
Parry[26]			4–11	4–15	5–9
Gellis and Pool[27]		5–15	4–8		4–8

tion. Nevertheless, the accepted normal value for this classic two-point discrimination remains variously quoted. For example, Moberg[8] has written that a discrimination of 6 to 15 mm is required for "some tactile gnosis." Weiland et al.[29] have graded patients such that those with less than 10 mm had excellent function. Bell[30] has taken the 7 to 10-mm range as indicating "gross appreciation of two-point discrimination." Gelberman et al.[31] and Fess et al.[32] have listed the following classification, which is that accepted by the American Society for Surgery of the Hand: less than 6 mm is normal, 6 to 10 mm is fair, 11 to 15 mm is poor."[31] Millesi[28] has written that "although 80% of all persons (n = 80)

had two-point discrimination value up to 3 mm, one cannot say that a value of 4 and more is out of the normal range. More than 6-mm two-point discrimination would tend to be beyond the normal range." The most recent comment on this is from Poppen et al.[33] Greater than 8 mm is "the level above which tactile gnosis is hardly present." It appears that the classic two-point discrimination test results leave considerable room for interpretation of normal functional limits.

PICKING-UP TEST

In search of a test of hand function, Moberg[9] developed the picking-up test. The test was to answer the question, "What can the hand do?" He described the picking-up test in 1958:

The subject is asked to pick up a number of small objects on a table and to put them quickly as he can into a small box, first with one hand and then with the other. After he has done this a few times, he is asked to do the same thing blindfolded. It is then studied how rapidly and efficiently he picks up the objects: comparison is made between his right and left hand, and likewise between his performance when he is blindfolded and when he is not. The test with blindfolding can be made harder by asking him to identify the objects as he picks them up. If his hand possesses normal sensibility, it can "see" even when the subject has his eyes closed. If sensibility in the median nerve region is impaired, the subject grasps the objects with his thumb and the ring and little finger instead of with the thumb and forefinger as he normally would.

The objects to be picked up in Moberg's test are several coins of different sizes, paper clips, safety pin, nails, screws, and two forms of wing nuts or bolts, which I cannot otherwise name from photographs of his kit (Fig. 6.4). Moberg records the results of this test in his charts or results tables simply with a plus or minus.

In 1966, Parry[26] published a set of times required for blindfolded, normal Englishmen (and women) to recognize common objects. Parry utilized a "recognition time" activity as a routine part of his sensory rehabilitation program. This program is discussed in detail in Chapter 12. An abbreviated table of his normal values is given in Table 6.6.

Table 6.6
Average Time for Object Recognition in 40 Blindfolded Normal Subjects[a]

Object	Time (Sec)
Small coin	2
Large coin	3
Velvet	5
Plastic	4
Wool	5
Sandpaper	2
Rubber band	1
Screw	2
Safety pin	2
Key	2
Paper clip	2
Cork	2
Match stick	2

[a] Adapted from C. B. W. Parry.[26]

Modified Picking-Up Test

The picking-up test as Moberg employs it, has at least two different functions, the results of which cannot be compared on different occasions. The Moberg test, as he, himself, states, requires motor function and therefore, if the tested function is the *success of placing the object into the cup*, motor function is clearly a dominant component. The grip required in that situation is one for pinching and holding an object within the fingers and requires perception of constant-touch and pressure (the slowly-adapting fiber/receptor system). It was this component that Moberg found to correlate well with the results of the Weber two-point discrimination test and this is what we could predict (as discussed above). However, if the subject is asked to *identify what he is picking up*, then we are testing another thing! The patient will be noted to attempt to twist and turn and move the object to accomplish this task. (The critical role of "movement" is discussed in Chapter 8). Although this movement requires fine motor coordination, it also requires input from the quickly-adapting fiber/receptor system. The ability to identify objects is the essence of tactile gnosis. The time required for this recognition can be recorded for comparison at subsequent intervals to demonstrate progress or for comparison with normal.

I believe the goal of the picking-up test should be object identification, rather than object placement, and that the time required for recognition should be recorded with a stopwatch.[34]

The test can be made more meaningful by choosing objects of graded sizes, to present a series of graded difficulties. Furthermore, the objects are all metal to avoid object-temperature and texture as a distinguishing guide. In addition to size, each object has at least one other distinguishing feature. The objects I have chosen are illustrated in Figure 6.5 and listed in Table 6.7. The time required to identify each of these objects is listed for normal controls in Table 6.9. The patient is tested in two separate trials after first doing a timed, sighted, placement task to familiarize himself with the objects and their names (Fig. 6.5).

We begin the test by placing the objects on a desk top, which offers some resistance against movement (as opposed to placing the objects on glass or plastic where they may easily slide as the patient attempts to pick them up). The patient's ring and little fingers are gently taped to the palm of the hand to prevent their inadvertent use (cheating!) (Fig. 6.6). First, a timed, sighted picking-up test is done with the objects to be placed in a container. This familiarizes the patient with the test objects and gives the examiner a chance to evaluate motor function. If motor function is insufficient, the test cannot be used further at that time. The test result is the total aggregate time for the picking-up test and depositing of all the objects. Next, the patient is "blindfolded" by having him look away. The examiner then chooses an object and places it within the patient's three-point chuck grip for the patient's object identification. The test is run through twice until all objects are identified, or until 30 seconds has been spent unsuccessfully attempting to identify an object. Time for each object is recorded separately. This is acceptable because we are attempting to evaluate sensibility, not motor function. There will exist a time during recovery when the patient will be able to identify the object by moving it across the surfaces of his fingertips, but won't be able to keep it between his fingertips easily because he cannot perceive how tightly he is holding it. The (quickly-adapting fiber/receptor sys-

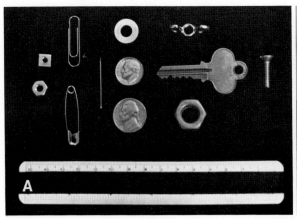
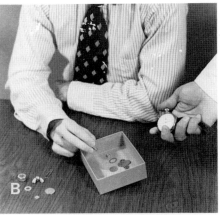

Figure 6.5. Modified picking-up test. *A*, Graded objects requiring increasing discrimination are used for object recognition. To familiarize patient with objects and allow patient and tester to agree on object names, a timed object placement test is run (*B*) prior to object recognition testing (see Tables 6.7 and 6.8). (Reproduced with permission from A. L. Dellon and B. Munger, in press 1981.[34])

Table 6.7
Modified Picking-Up Test: Example[a]

Task	Trial (sec)	
	I	II
Not blindfolded:		
(Patient picks up objects from desk top and places them into a box)		
Blindfolded:		
(Examiner places object between thumb, index and middle fingers for identification)		
1. Wing nut		
2. Screw		
3. Key		
4. Nail		
5. Large nut		
6. Nickel		
7. Dime		
8. Washer		
9. Safety pin		
10. Paper clip		
11. Small nut (hex)		
12. Small nut (square)		

[a] Reproduced with permission from A. L. Dellon and B. Munger, in press 1981.[34]

tem is functioning at a more advanced level than the slowly-adapting fiber/receptor system (Fig. 6.7). Normal values (10, normal adults) for this modified picking-up and timed object recognition test are given in Ta-

bles 6.8 and 6.9. Correlation of tests of sensibility and hand function are discussed further in Chapter 10.

OTHER TESTS

"Seddon's" Coin Test

Although Seddon[35] is credited with developing this test, he states "Although I have used this test fairly regularly, I did not—as has been stated—invent it; I learned it from Riddoch in 1940 and he made no claim to be the originator." In the preface to his book, Seddon says he "learned from George Riddoch, neurologist." Seddon described the coin test and the "precursor of the picking-up test."

The patient, whose eyes must be closed, is given a coin and asked to identify it. If he has a median nerve lesion . . . he must not cheat by pushing the coin towards an area of normally sentient skin.

I believe this test is now of historic interest, except that coin identification is included in the object recognition test.

Porter's "Letter Test"

In 1966, Porter,[36] then an Orthopaedic Registrar at King Edward VII Hospital in Sheffield, England, described a "simple objective test for fingertip sensation which is

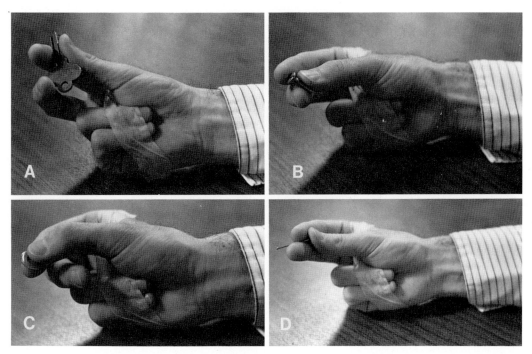

Figure 6.6. Modified picking-up test. To eliminate sensory input from ulnar innervation during timed object recognition, the ring and little finger are taped to the palm during the testing. Each object differs from another in the test series in a distinctive feature in addition to size (see Table 6.9). (Reproduced with premission from A. L. Dellon and B. Munger, in press 1981.[34])

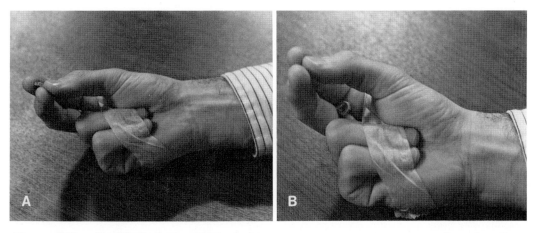

Figure 6.7. Modified picking-Up test. As sensory recovery progresses, there is a time when moving two-point discrimination has recovered and objects can be correctly identified (*A*), but because the slowly-adapting fiber/receptor system is poorly recovered (there is no classic two-point discrimination) the patient is unsure how hard to pinch (how much pressure to exert) to maintain the object between the fingertips and the object falls (*B*). (Reproduced with permission from A. L. Dellon and B. Munger, in press 1981.[34])

Table 6.8
Modified Picking-Up Test[a]

Normal Values for Object Pick-Up[b]			
Trial I		Trial II	
Mean (sec)	Range (sec)	Mean (sec)	Range (sec)
13	10–19	11	9–16

[a] Reproduced with permission from A. L. Dellon and B. Munger, in press 1981.[34]
[b] n = 8.

Table 6.9
Modified Picking-Up Test[a]

Object	Normal Values for Object Recognition[b]			
	Trial I		Trial II	
	Mean (sec)	Range (sec)	Mean (sec)	Range (sec)
1. Wing nut	1.7	1–3	2.0	1–3
2. Screw	1.4	1–2	1.5	1–2
3. Key	1.5	1–3	1.6	1–2
4. Nail	1.7	1–4	1.5	1–2
5. Large nut	1.8	1–3	1.4	1–2
6. Nickel	1.8	1–3	2.0	2
7. Dime	1.7	1–5	1.3	1–2
8. Washer	1.8	1–3	1.7	1–3
9. Safety pin	1.6	1–2	1.6	1–2
10. Paper clip	2.3	1–5	2.1	1–3
11. Small nut (hex)	2.1	1–3	1.6	1–3
12. Small nut (square)	1.6	1–3	1.6	1–3

[a] Reproduced with permission from A. L. Dellon and B. Munger, in press, 1981.[34]
[b] n = 8.

believed to be a more accurate index of tactile sensation and is less time-consuming than the conventional tests." Porter uses metal type-setting letters, H, O, U, V, Y of approximately 1.0 × 0.8 cm in size with the letters standing out in relief. The patient "runs his fingertip over the surface as a blind person would read braille (Fig. 6.8)."

Five letters are examined unhurriedly in one hand, and the patient then applies the letters himself to the pulp under test. Incorrect identification or failure to identify the letter after 30 seconds is recorded as an error, and a score is obtained out of five.

Porter tested 47 normal patients for two-point discrimination (mean of 0.33 cm longitudinally and 0.31 cm transversely over each fingertip, without any advantage radial versus ulnar), Moberg's picking-up test, and the letter test and compared them with 51 fingertip reconstructions (grafts and flaps). He found the results of the letter test "directly related to the two-point discrimination." Patients who could identify all five letters correctly had an average two-point discrimination of 4.5 mm, while those who could identify only one letter had an average of 7.5 cm. Of eight patients who had a "positive" result in Moberg's picking-up test, the average two-point discrimination was 7.3 mm and the average letter score was 2.3 compared to the 14 patients with "negative" results in the picking-up test whose averages, respectively, were 10 mm and .09 letters.

Although Porter's letter test offers another means of testing functional sensation, his results were not subjected to statistical tests of significance to demonstrate whether they offer an advantage in accuracy. To do the test requires the five letters. To compare any two authors' results would require the use of a similar set of metallic type. It would be interesting to know how Porter chose the five letters (out of 26 possible) and which one of the five was the most easily identified. His results do appear to confirm Moberg's value of two-point discrimination less than 12 being required for finer tactile discrimination. However, it is probably not strictly correct (as described further in Chapter 8) to equate the results of these two tests, since in the Weber test the ends are held in constant-touch with the fingertip, whereas in Porter's test, the letter is moved across the pulp, similar to digit writing. Thus, Porter's test is actually evaluating the quickly-adapting fiber/receptor system in addition to the slowly-adapting fiber/receptor system. I do not believe this test has practical clinical value.

Ninhydrin Test

This test was discussed earlier in this Chapter under "Moberg."

Plastic Ridge Device[33]

This device will be discussed in Chapter 8.

Wrinkle Test

It is common knowledge that our fingertips become wrinkled like prunes when we bathe.

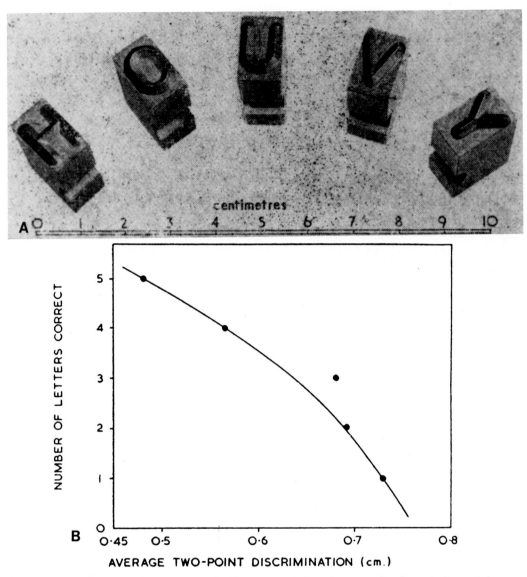

Figure 6.8.   Porter's letter test: *A*, The set of five letters. *B*, Correlation of letter identification and classic two-point discrimination in 51 fingertip grafts or flaps. (Reproduced with permission from R. W. Porter: *Br Med J* 2:927–928, 1966.[36])

In 1973, O'Rain[37] observed that denervated skin lost this ability. An attempt to study this phenomenon in patients with nerve injury and nerve compression, comparing wrinkling with classic two-point discrimination and ninhydrin, has been reported (Fig. 6.9).[38] Patients with complete nerve injury had no wrinkling, no two-point discrimination, and no sweating. Patients with nerve compression had no correlation among these tests, that is, two-point discrimination was abnormal

(greater than 15 mm), wrinkling was normal (in five of the eight patients), and ninhydrin staining was variable (normal in 3/8 and near normal in 5/8). I do not believe this test has clinical value.

von Frey Hairs (Semmes-Weinstein Monofilaments)

The development of von Frey's "hairs" is discussed in Chapter 1. They remain widely

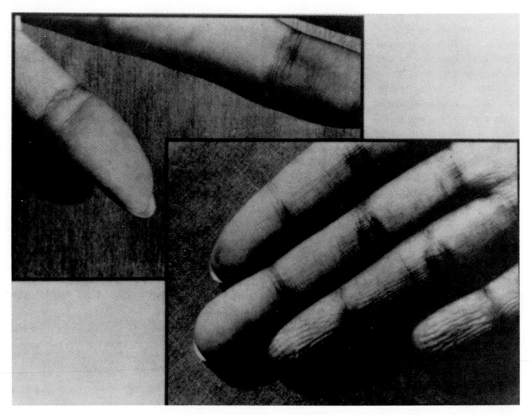

Figure 6.9. Skin wrinkling. Denervated skin, as seen in thumb at *upper left* and index and middle finger at *lower right*, loses the normal ability to wrinkle after emersion in water, as seen in little and ring finger *lower right*. (Reproduced with permission from P. E. Phelps and E. Walker: *Am J Occup Ther* 31:565–572, 1977.[38])

used, widely abused, widely misunderstood and controversial three quarters of a century later. For example, one center considers this test the cornerstone of their sensibility evaluation,[30] while a recent engineering analysis concluded[39]:

Variations in the buckling stress as high as a factor of eight are difficult to avoid. Gross errors arise from careless application, variations in the elastic modulus due to changes in temperature and humidity, and variations in the attachment of the fibers to handles and differences in the ends of the filaments. Interpreting results for this instrument (Semmes-Weinstein) requires an understanding of factors which can influence those results. Probes are simple to use but easy to misinterpret.

Weinstein[40] introduced the nylon monofilaments as an alternative to using hair. How-

ever, although nylon monofilaments are more aesthetic and seemingly more scientific than hairs, the filaments have irregularities in the shape of their contact surface and do not eliminate two problems discussed by Henry Head[41] in 1908. Although the object is to measure cutaneous pressure thresholds, high thresholds, in fact, are perceived not as pressure, but as pain.

Towards the end of our research we received a second set of hairs from Professor von Frey which were useful in measuring the punctate pressure capable of producing cutaneous pain. These so-called "pain-hairs" exercise considerably greater pressure than those used for testing cutaneous tactile sensiblity, and are graduated by calculating the pressure per unit area (see Table 6.10).[41]

The Semmes-Weinstein monofilaments (Fig. 6.10) are labeled with a numerical mark-

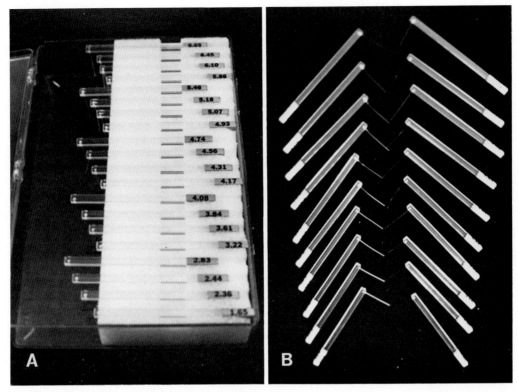

Figure 6.10. Semmes-Weinstein monofilaments for measuring cutaneous pressure thresholds. *A*, Numbers are not the force in milligrams but equal ($\log_{10}$ F mg). (Note how some filaments become bent with repetitive testing (*B*) invalidating their rating.

ing ranging from 1.65 to 6.65. This number is the log (10 F) where F is force in milligrams. As a further example of how easily this test's results are misconstrued, these numerical markings have been reported as the actual threshold values in grams (Fig. 6.11).[31] Rivers and Head attempted to distinguish the force applied from the stress (force per area) applied (Table 6.10). Levin et al.[39] also calculated these (Table 6.11), and these values were incorporated into her reporting system by Bell[30] (Fig. 6.11). Thus, Bell considers a normal threshold to be less than 0.068 gm. Poppen et al.,[33] however, without stating why, have chosen normal to be less than 1.0 gm.

There are at least four problems with the von Frey hair or monofilament type testing: (1) At which point does the upper limit of pressure actually test pain (2) In what terms should the end result be reported, i.e., numerical markings of Semmes-Weinstein monofilaments, force or stress? and (3) Dif-

ferent centers may report different results even using a "fully standardized series of von Frey hairs" (see Table 6.12).[42] In the World War II experience, "two hand centers deviated significantly, one greatly tended to report thresholds of 3 gm and another tended to almost never report thresholds of 50, 39, 10 and 3 gm."[42]

Perhaps the most significant problem with reporting end results of nerve repairs in terms of cutaneous pressure thresholds is that these do no correlate with hand function. This is discussed in Chapter 10 and is illustrated here from the Poppen et al.[33] recent detailed comparisons (Fig. 6.12). This figure from Poppen has the advantage of having included Onne's data.[25] It is clear that for any given cutaneous pressure threshold, the two-point discrimination values range from normal to complete lack of discrimination. For example, a pressure threshold of .75 gm (within normal limits for these authors) is consistent with a

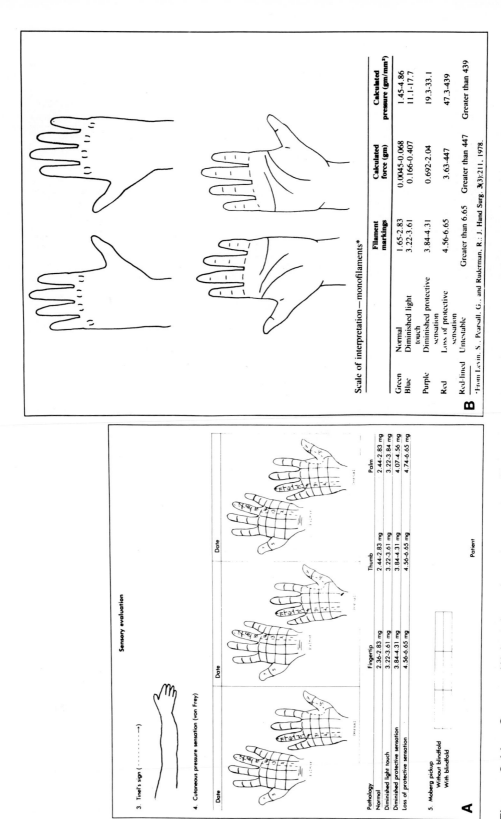

Figure 6.11. Semmes-Weinstein end-result reporting. The numerical markings on the instruments are logarithmic values of the force and should not be listed in milligrams (A)[31] but rather as correlated with force or pressure (B).[30]

Table 6.10
von Frey Hairs[a]

Number by Which Hair Is Known	Pressure (gm)	Hair Radius (μm)	Hair Area (mm²)	Radius of Circle of Same Area (μm)	Pressure per Unit Area	Tension
Tactile hairs						
1	0.04	30 × 54	0.005	40	8 gm/mm²	1 gm/mm
2	0.10	48 × 58	0.009	52	12 gm/mm²	2 gm/mm
3	0.21	55 × 90	0.015	70	14 gm/mm²	3 gm/mm
4	0.23	40 × 80	0.011	58	21 gm/mm²	4 gm/mm
5	0.36	60 × 90	0.017	74	21 gm/mm²	5 gm/mm
8	0.88	100 × 120	0.038	110	23 gm/mm²	8 gm/mm
Pain hairs						
35	1.4	100 × 130	0.041	114	35 gm/mm²	12 gm/mm
70	3.0	115 × 115	0.042	115	70 gm/mm²	26 gm/mm
100	3.5	80 × 140	0.035	110	100 gm/mm²	32 gm/mm
150	11.0	125 × 185	0.073	150	150 gm/mm²	73 gm/mm
266	12.0	115 × 125	0.045	120	266 gm/mm²	100 gm/mm

[a] Adapted from W. H. R. Rivers and H. Head.[41]

Table 6.11
Stress and Force Calculations and Measurements for a Semmes-Weinstein Pressure Aesthesiometer[a]

Manufacturer's Marking	Calculated Force (F', gm)	Diameter (D, mm)	Area (A, sq m)	Calculated Stress (S', gm/sq mm)	Slenderness (2L/R)	Measured Force (F, gm)	Standard Deviation (oF, gm)	Measured Stress (S, gm/sq mm)	Standard Deviation (oS, gm/sq mm)
6.65	448	1.142	1.02	439	130				
6.45	283	1.033	0.84	337	141				
6.10	126	0.805	0.51	243	180	86.5	4.3	171	16
5.88	76.0	0.732	0.42	181	200	73.2	1.9	175	13
5.46	28.0	0.582	0.27	107	251	22.3	1.5	82.0	9.6
5.18	15.2	0.525	0.22	69.1	280	18.6	0.8	84.9	7.9
5.07	11.8	0.475	0.18	65.6	312	17.0	1.5	94.9	13
4.93	8.53	0.423	0.14	60.9	341	10.6	0.5	76.1	7.4
4.74	5.51	0.322	0.081	68.0	453	3.14	0.07	38.9	2.8
4.56	3.64	0.313	0.077	47.3	473	2.81	0.06	36.6	2.6
4.31	2.05	0.284	0.063	33.1	520	1.85	0.06	29.5	2.4
4.17	1.48	0.244	0.047	31.5	593	1.58	0.06	33.7	2.9
4.08	1.20	0.228	0.041	29.3	650	0.977	0.030	23.9	1.9
3.84	0.693	0.214	0.036	19.3	689	0.562	0.011	15.7	1.1
3.61	0.408	0.171	0.023	17.7	851	0.213	0.004	9.29	0.64
3.22	0.166	0.137	0.015	11.1	1,050	0.112	0.007	7.50	0.84
2.83	0.068	0.132	0.014	4.86	1,090	0.091	0.005	6.52	0.68
2.44	0.0276	0.104	0.0085	3.25	1,400	0.034	0.002	4.02	0.43
2.36	0.229	0.075	0.0044	5.20	1,930	0.0094	0.0001	2.14	0.13
1.65	0.0045	0.063	0.0031	1.45	2,300	0.0040	0.0001	1.29	0.09

[a] Adapted from S. Levin et al.[39]

classic two-point discrimination of 4 or 32 mm. At 4 mm we could expect normal functional sensation. At 32 mm, we would expect sensations not even sufficient for gross sensory grip.

I believe that von Frey hairs, or Semmes-Weinstein monofilaments, or any new device that measures cutaneous pressure thresholds is severely limited in what it can tell us. Functional sensation depends on a critical

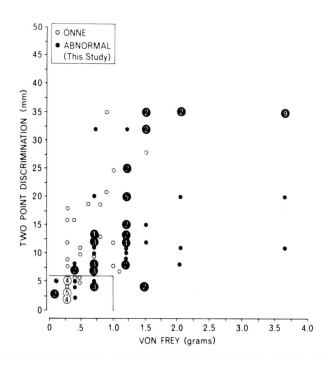

Figure 6.12. Correlation of von Frey and Weber testing after digital nerve repair. Note that for any given von Frey value there is a wide range of two-point discrimination values. Thus, there is no correlation between these two tests. *Black circles* are data from Poppen et al.[33] and *white circles* are data from Onne.[25] The graph is from Poppen et al.[33] The box in the *lower left corner* of the graph represents these authors normal limits (see text). (Reproduced with permission from L. Onne: *Acta Chir Scand [Suppl]* 300:1–70, 1962[25] and N. K. Poppen et al.: *J Hand Surg* 4:212–226, 1979.[33])

Table 6.12
Standardized Set of von Frey Hairs Employed at United States Hand Centers during World War II[a]

Hair Number	Threshold
0	>50 gm/mm²
1	50 gm/mm²
2	35 gm/mm²
3	25 gm/mm²
4	16 gm/mm²
5	5 gm/mm²
6	3 gm/mm²
7	>3 gm/mm²

[a] Adapted from Y. T. Oester and L. Davis.[42]

number of sensory fibers being present and connected to the appropriate mature receptor. A test that measures innervation density can supply the critical information. A test that determines thresholds alone cannot. Until then, I believe that determining innervation density is the most critical clinical test we can do of a given fiber/receptor system.

References

1. Truex RC, Carpenter MB. *Human Neuroanatomy*, ed 5. Baltimore: Williams & Wilkins, 1964, pp 203–212.
2. Major RH, Delp MH: *Physical Diagnosis*, ed 6. Philadelphia: WB Saunders, 1962, pp 320–323.
3. Currier RD: Nervous system, in Judge RD, Zuidema GD (eds): *Physical Diagnosis: A Physiologic Approach to the Clinical Examination*, ed 2. Boston: Little, Brown, 1968, Ch 20, pp 408–410.
4. Bowden REM: Factors influencing function recovery, in Seddon HJ (ed): *Peripheral Nerve Injuries*. London: Her Majesty's Stationery Office, 1954, Ch VII, pp 298–354.
5. Seddon HJ: Methods of investigating nerve injuries, in Seddon HJ (ed): *Peripheral Nerve Injuries*. London: Her Majesty's Stationery Office, 1954, Ch I, pp 1–15.
6. Zachary, RB: Results of nerve suture, in Seddon HJ (ed): *Peripheral Nerve Injuries*. London: Her Majesty's Stationery Office, 1954, Ch VIII, pp 354–388.
7. Seddon HJ: *Surgical Disorders of the Peripheral Nerves*. Baltimore: Williams & Wilkins, 1972, pp IX–X.
8. Moberg E: Aspects of sensation in reconstructive surgery of the upper extremity. J Bone Joint Surg 46A:817–825, 1964.
9. Moberg E: Objective methods of determining func-

tional value of sensibility in the hand. J Bone Joint Surg [Br] 40:454–466, 1958.

10. Moberg E: Criticism and study of methods for examining sensibility in the hand. Neurology 12:8–19, 1962.

11. Moberg E: Methods for examining sensibility in the hand, in Flynn JE (ed): *Hand Surgery*, ed 1. Baltimore: Williams & Wilkins, 1966, pp 435–439.

12. Moberg E: *Emergency Surgery of the Hand*. New York: Churchill Livingstone, 1968.

13. Moberg E: Future hopes for the surgical management of peripheral nerve lesions, in Michon J, Moberg E (eds): *Traumatic Nerve Lesions* New York: Churchill Livingstone, 1975.

14. Moberg E: Reconstructive hand surgery in tetraplegia, stroke and cerebral palsy: Some basic concepts in physiology and neurology. J Hand Surg 1:29–34, 1976.

15. Moberg E: *The Upper Limb in Tetraplegia*. New York: Grune & Stratton, 1978.

16. Bunnell S: Surgery of the nerves of the hand. Surg Gynecol Obstet 44:145–152, 1927.

17. Perry JF, Hamilton GF, Lachenbuch PA, et al: Protective sensation in the hand and its correlation to the ninhydrin sweat test following nerve laceration. Am J Phys Med 53:113–118, 1974.

18. Dellon AL, Curtis RM, Edgerton MT: Evaluating recovery of sensation in the hand following nerve injury. Johns Hopkins Med J 130:245–243, 1972.

19. Dellon AL: The paper clip: Light hardware for evaluation of sensibility in the hand. Contemp Orthop 1:39–42, 1979.

20. Weber E: Ueber den Tastsinn. Arch Anat Physiol, Wissen Med (Muller's Archives) 1: 152–159, 1835.

21. Mitchell SW: *Injuries of Nerves and Their Consequence*, 1872. American Academy of Neurology Reprint Series. New York: Dover, 1965, pp 179, 183.

22. Boeke J: *The Problems of Nervous Anatomy*. London: Oxford University Press, 1940, pp 12–44.

23. McCarroll HR: The regeneration of sensation in transplanted skin. Ann Surg 108:309–320, 1938.

24. Mannerfelt L: Evaluation of functional sensation of skin grafts in the hand area. Br J Plast Surg 15:136–154, 1962.

25. Onne L: Recovery of sensibility and sudomotor activity in the hand after nerve suture. Acta Chir Scand [Suppl] 300:1–70, 1962.

26. Parry CBW: *Rehabilitation of the Hand*, ed 2. London: Butterworths, 1966, pp 19, 107–108.

27. Gellis M, Pool R: Two-point discrimination distances in the normal hand and forearm. Plast Reconst Surg 59:57–63, 1977.

28. Millesi, H, Rinderer D: Sensory rehabilitation. Proc World Fed Occup Ther 7:122–125, 1979.

29. Weiland, AJ, Villarreal-Rios A, Kleinert HE, et al: Replantation of digits and hands: Analysis of surgical techniques and functional results in 71 patients with 86 replantations. J Hand Surg 2:1–12, 1977.

30. Bell JA: Sensibility evaluation, in Hunter JM, Schneider LH, Machin EJ, et al (eds): *Rehabilitation of the Hand*. Saint Louis: CV Mosby, 1978, Ch 25.

31. Gelberman RH, Urbaniak JR, Bright DS, et al: Digital sensibility following replantation. J Hand Surg 3: 313–319, 1978.

32. Fess EE, Harmon KS, Strickland, JW, et al: Evaluation of the hand by objective measurement, in Hunter JM, Schneider LH, Mackin EJ, et al (eds): *Rehabilitation of the Hand*. Saint Louis: CV Mosby, 1978, Ch 5.

33. Poppen NK, McCarroll HR Jr, Doyl JR, et al: Recovery of sensibility after suture of digital nerves. J Hand Surg 4:212–226, 1979.

34. Dellon AL, Munger, B: Correlation of sensibility evaluation, hand function and histology, in press 1981.

35. Seddon HJ: *Surgical Disorders of the Peripheral Nerves*. Baltimore: Williams & Wilkins, 1972, pp 53.

36. Porter RW: New test for fingertip sensation. Br Med J 2:927–928, 1966.

37. O'Rain S: New and simple test of nerve function in the hand. Br Med J 3:615–616, 1973.

38. Phelps PE, Walker E: Comparison of the finger wrinkling test results to established sensory tests in peripheral nerve injury. Am J Occup Ther 31:565–572, 1977.

39. Levin S, Pearsall G, Ruderman RJ: von Frey's method of measuring pressure sensibility in the hand: An engineering analysis of the Weinstein-Semmes pressure aesthisiometer. J Hand Surg 3:211–216, 1978.

40. Weinstein S: Tactile sensitivity in the phalanges. Percept Mot Skills 14:351–354, 1962.

41. Rivers WHR, Head H: A human experiment in nerve division. Brain 31:348, 1908.

42. Oester YT, Davis L: Recovery of sensory function, in *Peripheral Nerve Regeneration*. Washington DC: US Gov Print Office, 1956, Ch 5, pp 241–310.

Chapter 7

PATTERN OF SENSORY RECOVERY

INTRODUCTION
PATTERN OF RECOVERY
 FOLLOWING NERVE INJURY
HYPOTHESIS FOR THIS PATTERN
CLINICAL SUPPORT FOR PATTERN
 OF RECOVERY

INTRODUCTION

Following repair of a sensory nerve, the axons regenerate, reinnervate the distal tissue into which they have regenerated, and re-establish connection of the central nervous system with the external world. Are the various sensory submodalities all re-established simultaneously or is there a predictable sequence to this recovery of sensation?

One of the classic descriptions of the pattern of sensory recovery is that recorded by Head and his co-workers.[1, 2] Head's own superficial radial and lateral antebrachial cutaneous nerves were divided electively and the resultant sensory defect and pattern of recovery methodically noted. The standard neurologic tests (cotton wisps, pin, hot and cold, pressure) were utilized for the testing. The first returning sensations were unpleasant responses to the usually nonnoxious stimuli, and only extremes of stimuli, like heavy pressure, were perceptible. Head believed a separate population of nerve fibers mediated these sensations and he chose the term "protopathic," meaning "responsive to gross stimuli" for this type of sensibility. With time, the ability to be "more discriminating" re-

turned. Head believed this "epicritic" sensibility was due to a second population of nerve fibers, regenerating more slowly.

In 1934, John Staige Davis, who was the first Chief of the Division of Plastic Surgery at Johns Hopkins[3] and who authored the first textbook of Plastic Surgery in the United States,[4] reviewed published studies of sensory recovery in skin grafts up to that time. The few earlier reports had concluded that "speed of recovery depends upon the type of innervating nerve . . . touch, pain and temperature return in the order named after pressure."[5] The earliest observations of the pattern of sensory recovery were made most often in grafted skin and included the sequences (1) pain before touch before temperature[6]; (2) pain before temperature before touch[5]; (3) pain before touch[7]; and (4) pain and sweating cotemporaneously before temperature.[8]

Closely related to the observations made on grafted areas, were observations made on areas of normal skin being reinnervated following nerve injury. The classic tests of pain, temperature, cotton wool, and Tinel's sign, were utilized not to establish a pattern of sensory recovery but to attempt to establish a clinically reliable numerical value for the rate at which nerve fibers regenerated. Such a rate would enable the clinician to prognosticate, evaluate success of nerve repairs, judge the need for a "second look" or neurolysis, etc. Contemporary teaching is that "nerves regenerate at about 1 mm per day or an inch per month," usually "allowing two to four weeks for delay in crossing each suture line." Among the most fascinating studies to read are the classics by Seddon et al.[9] and Sunderland.[10] Every conceivable approach to arriving at this information, including sophisticated mathematics and meticulous longitudinal clinical studies following neuropraxia and nerve repair, for motor as well as sensory function, is utilized. Conclusions from their work are that we may never know the actual rate of axonal regeneration, because included in what we can clinically measure are (1) the "initial lag time" related to suture line crossing; (2) the advance of multiple axonal sprouts which may be stimulated (Tinel's) but are unrelated to functional or anatomic restoration; (3) the end or "terminal lag time" related to re-establishing (or failing to re-establish) the appropriate end organ connection; and (4) the end or "terminal lag time" related to recovery of a sufficiently low threshold of the fiber/receptor system. A series of observations from Seddon et al.[9] suggests the following rates:

Tinel's sign . . . advances at 1.71 mm/day
Motor radial
   nerve . . . . . . advances at 1.60 mm/day
Average, "all
   nerves" . . . . advances at 1.40 mm/day
Pain . . . . advances at 1.08 mm/day
Touch . . . . advances at 0.78 mm/day

In general, rates of recovery have been observed ranging from 1 to 4 mm/day. The final conclusions from both reviews may be summarized[9, 10] (Fig. 7.1):

1. The rate of sensory recovery may be calculated by measuring the advance of pain and touch sense in a long zone of cutaneous insensibility.
2. The rate of advance of Tinel's sign is of limited functional significance, but has some prognostic value.
3. The rate of recovery falls off progressively as the process nears completion.

4. The rate of regeneration diminishes as the distance increases between the axonal tips and the cell bodies, and this factor appears to be a variable independent from 3.
5. The factors affecting rate are: (A) the interval between injury and repair; (B) the state of stumps at suture line; (C) the postoperative stretching (suture line tension).

PATTERN OF RECOVERY FOLLOWING NERVE INJURY

On February 3, 1969, I presented a paper entitled "Correlation of Clinical Tests of Sensibility in the Hand with Recent Neurophysiological Evidence" to the meeting of the Johns Hopkins Medical Society. This was during my 3rd year of medical school. Shortly thereafter, the manuscript was submitted to the *Johns Hopkins Medical Journal* for consideration for publication. On July 30, 1969, the editor of the *Journal* wrote back, rejecting the paper. He wrote that while the manuscript was "an interesting review . . . there was no data which might support the opinions of the authors, and therefore, no real contribution was made . . ." Reviewers further felt I had "arbitrarily tested two sensory tests out of a dozen or more that might have been more sensitive." I added a series of patient examinations to the paper and resubmitted it in May, 1970. It included six tables and 10 figures and much theorizing. It was accepted pending revisions. After reworking and shortening, it was resubmitted in June, 1971, during my internship. It was accepted. It then contained just one table, six figures, and no theorizing. The paper was entitled "Evaluating Recovery of Sensation in the Hand after Nerve Injury."[11]

The pattern of sensory recovery was evaluated by serial clinical examinations. Evaluation included finger stroking and pressure with the examiner's finger on the patient's finger to stimulate perception of moving-touch and constant-touch, respectively, and tuning forks of 30 cps and 256 cps to stimulate perception of flutter and vibration (see Chapter 10). Twelve patients, six following nerve crush and six following nerve repair,

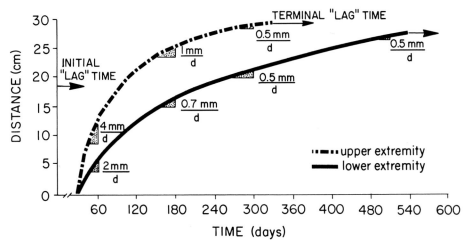

Figure 7.1.   Rate of regeneration of peripheral nerve. These are hypothetical curves of sensory recovery in an upper and lower extremity nerve, each repaired about 30 cm proximal to the distal phalanx, with curves being based on conclusion from Seddon et al.[9] and Sunderland.[10] Note: Initial lag time related to suture line crossing, terminal lag time related to attempted re-establishment of end organ connections, and receptor maturation. Due to increased distance of the lower extremity axon tip from its central neuron, its rate of regeneration is everywhere slower than for the upper extremity nerve. For both nerves, the rate of regeneration diminishes as the periphery is approached.

were evaluated. Injuries were to median (7), ulnar (2) and median plus ulnar (3) nerves. Following recovery of perception of painful stimuli, a consistent pattern was found for the touch "submodalities": perception that the 30 cps stimuli was the first to recover followed very closely by perception of moving-touch, followed in several months by perception of constant-touch, and finally by perception of the 256 cps stimulus (Fig. 7.2). The entire sequence occurred faster following crush injury than following nerve repair. Also noted in that study and illustrated with a figure (all of which was deleted from the published "edition" of the manuscript) was the orderly recovery of the normal threshold for both moving- and constant-touch: greater force was required with both test stimuli to achieve perception initially than it was later on in recovery; and at the time when greater force was being required to perceive the stimulus at the fingertip, less force was required over the proximal phalanx (Fig. 7.3).

The observations were made in that study that (1) patients appeared to improve in their perceptions during the test period, and that (2) deviations from the normal pattern of recovery, i.e., recovery of perception of 256-cps stimulus at the fingertip while perception of constant-touch remained at the palm, represented a "gap" or "failure" to achieve a given sensory potential, thereby laying the cornerstones for the development of sensory re-education (see Chapter 12).

HYPOTHESIS FOR THIS PATTERN

I propose that the basis for the observed orderly sequence of recovery of perception of stimuli in the fingertip following nerve injury (which is, first, pain and temperature, then touch, beginning first with 30 cps, then moving-touch, constant touch, and 256 cps) is related to nerve fiber diameter, primarily, and to the reinnervation of the sensory receptor, secondarily.

Given that the diameter of the unmyelinated C fibers and the thinly myelinated group A delta fibers is of the order of 1 to 2 μm, while that of the thickly myelinated fibers is of the order of 15 to 20 μm, these being the

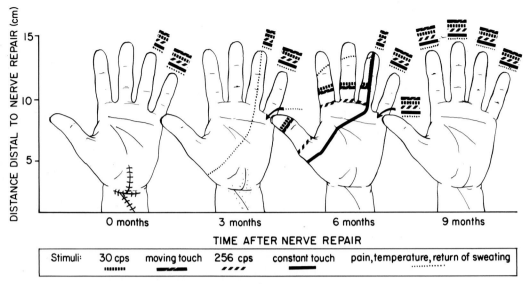

Figure 7.2. Pattern of sensory recovery following nerve injury. An orderly sequence occurs in return of perception of the touch submodalities. This sequence begins after reception of pain and temperature has recovered. As illustrated for a median nerve repair, the first to recover is perception of the 30-cps vibratory stimulus, followed closely by perception of moving-touch. Then, after usually a significant delay, comes perception of constant-touch, and finally the 256-cps vibratory stimulus. (Adapted from A. L. Dellon et al.[11])

groups mediating perception of pain/temperature and touch, respectively, there is an enormous difference in the volume of axoplasm of the nerve fibers in these two different groups. Following nerve injury, sufficient axoplasm must be produced to fill this axonal volume. Even though a regenerating axon regenerates as a thin axonal sprout, and even though the distal endoneural sheaths contract after nerve division, the total axoplasm required to re-establish continuity with the fingertip after a nerve division at the wrist must be greater for the touch fibers than for the pain and temperature fibers. Little is known about the ability of the dorsal root ganglia neurons, which are the cell bodies of these axons, to produce axoplasm. If we assume that a group A delta neuron can produce axonplasm as rapidly as group A beta neuron, it would take the group A beta neuron longer to produce its required axoplasm than group A beta because it has much more to produce.

For any given length, the volume of a cylinder is proportionate to the square of the radius of the cross-section of the cylinder, $V = 1 R^2$. For the A delta fiber, for example, radius of a 2 u fiber, is 1 u. For the A beta fiber, the radius for a 20 u fiber is 10 u. The ratio of volumes is therefore $(10^2):(1^2)$ or 100:1.

This hypothesis, which we call the "neuron pump" (Fig. 7.4), explains recovery of pain perception ahead of touch at the periphery on the basis of axoplasm production in a thinner fiber.

I propose that the basis for the observed sequence of recovery of touch submodalities is related to the nature of the sensory end organ. The sequence of 30 cps, moving-touch, constant-touch, 256 cps can be restated in terms of sensory receptor correlation as Meissner corpuscle, Meissner corpuscle, Merkel cell-neurite complex, and Pacinian corpuscle (see Chapter 3). Thus, the close proximity in time, which is often simultaneous, between recovery of 30 cps and moving-touch is explained on the basis that they both required the re-established integrity of the same fiber/receptor system. Recovery of 30

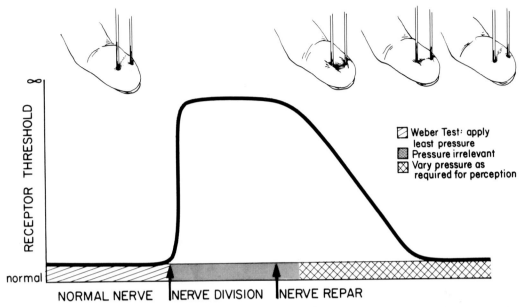

Figure 7.3. Recovery of sensory thresholds. The initial perception of a sensory submodality during recovery requires use of sufficiently high stimulus intensity. With time, the threshold for stimulus perception diminishes.

cps ahead of 256 cps relates to the relative ease of reinnervating a Meissner corpuscle compared to reinnervating a Pacinian corpuscle. (The pertinent references to this are discussed in detail in Chapter 5.) One group of investigators[12] believes that failure to clear myelin debris, or a similar "mechanical hypothesis," is the basis for poorer reinnervation of Pacinian corpuscle than Meissner corpuscle. I believe that a possibly more important basis is the intrinsic design of these two fiber/receptor systems. This hypothesis concerns the multiple fiber innervation of a Meissner corpuscle (three to nine axons may enter a single corpuscle) versus the single fiber innervation of a Pacinian corpuscle. Simply put, statistically there is a greater chance for a regenerating quickly-adapting fiber to reinnervate a Meissner corpuscle than a Pacinian corpuscle (Fig. 7.5). I cannot explain more specifically the order of constant-touch between these two extremes except as explained by an extension of the above hypothesis. The axon to corpuscle ratio of Merkel cell-neurite complex is less than one, whereas for the Meissner corpuscle it is greater than one (Fig. 7.5). Merkel reinner-

vation should occur after Pacinian. There is, however, apparently no "mechanical blockage" to regenerating slowly-adapting fibers growing beneath intermediate ridges and reestablishing contact with or inducing Merkel cells as there is with the reinnervation of a Pacinian corpuscle. Thus, constant-touch is perceived ahead of the 256-cps stimuli.

An alternative hypothesis regarding the recovery of the perception of constant-touch ahead of 256-cps stimuli may relate to receptor maturation or threshold recovery, rather than reinnervation of receptors, *per se*. Both a Merkel cell-neurite complex and a Pacinian corpuscle fiber/receptor system may re-establish continuity simultaneously, but perhaps the Merkel cell-neurite complex, where one fiber innervates many Merkel cells, reestablishes a lower threshold for stimulation earlier than does the single receptor Pacinian corpuscle.

CLINICAL SUPPORT FOR PATTERN OF RECOVERY

It seemed to take about a decade for the pattern of recovery of touch submodalities as

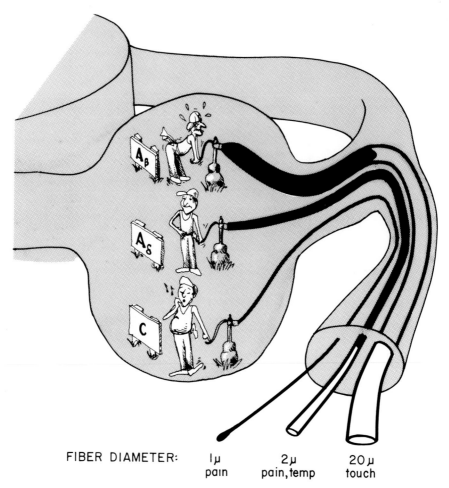

FIBER DIAMETER: 1μ   2μ   20μ
pain   pain,temp   touch

Figure 7.4. Neuron pump hypothesis. Assuming equal ability to produce axoplasm for dorsal ganglia neurons, axoplasm should reach the end of the lower volume, thinner fibers before the end of the higher volume, thicker fibers.

described to be disseminated, accepted, tested independently, and corroborated in print. My observations of the pattern described were made in 1969. In 1976, Jabaley et al.[13] reported detailed clinical testing, utilizing moving-, constant-touch, and 30- and 256-cps stimuli. These authors did not report longitudinal follow-ups on individual patients, but rather reported a series of findings on a series of patients at some time after nerve repair. Nevertheless, their observations confirmed my observed pattern in that they found a greater number of patients (13 of 17) able to perceive the 30-cps than the 256-cps stimuli, suggesting that 30-cps perception re-

covers ahead of the 256 cps. They found essentially the same number of patients (14 of 17) able to perceive moving-touch as 30-cps stimulus, again confirming my observations. They discovered that more patients perceived constant-touch (14 of 17) than 256 cps, again consistent with my observations. It was not possible from a review of their data to determine the relative recovery of moving- and constant-touch with respect to each other.

Two other studies have utilized this type of clinical testing in evaluating recovery of sensibility.[14, 15] These studies report observations consistent with my own.

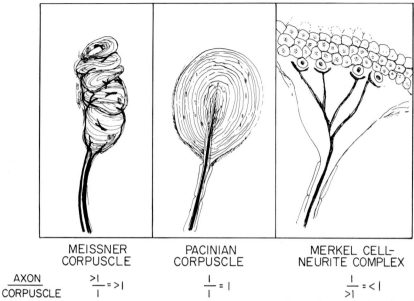

	MEISSNER CORPUSCLE	PACINIAN CORPUSCLE	MERKEL CELL- NEURITE COMPLEX
$\dfrac{\text{AXON}}{\text{CORPUSCLE}}$	$\dfrac{>1}{1} = >1$	$\dfrac{1}{1} = 1$	$\dfrac{1}{>1} = <1$

Figure 7.5. Relative ease of re-innervation hypothesis. Based upon observed axon to corpuscle ratios, it statistically should be easiest to reinnervate the Meissner corpuscle, and thus the first perceptions to be recovered are 30-cps vibratory stimuli and moving-touch. Perception of 256-cps vibratory stimuli are last to recover probably because of mechanical obstructions to Pacinian reinnervation and earlier threshold maturation of Merkel cell-neurite complexes.

My observation that once perception of a sensation has recovered, it becomes easier and easier to stimulate, i.e., threshold values are high at the time of initial recovery of the sensory submodality and then decrease with time toward normal, has been observed before,[16-18] but not applied to clinical sensory testing. Brown and Iggo[16] studied recovery of threshold in the slowly-adapting cat touch-pad fiber/receptor system. After nerve crush, this decreased from a threshold greater than 200 gm to one of 10 gm. Silver et al.[17] devised a "sensory index" based on a voltage threshold for electrical stimulation at a frequency of about 3 cps. They report a longitudinal observation after a median nerve repair of one patient in whom the index changes (threshold changes) as sensory recovery proceeds from proximal to distal. Recently, Dykes and Terzis,[18] in a baboon median nerve crush model, documented a progressive decrease in tuning curves for low frequency rapidly-adapting fibers; that is, at increasingly longer intervals after nerve in-jury, recordings from peripheral receptive fields demonstrated progressive decreases in threshold.

My own observations, over the past decade, have continued to confirm both the pattern of sensory recovery described above and the changing sensory threshold as the fiber/receptor system matures. Applications of these observations to the clinical evaluation of sensibility are presented in Chapter 10.

References
1. Head H, Sherren J: The consequences of injury to the peripheral nerves in man. Brain 28:116–337, 1905.
2. Rivers WHR, Head H: A human experiment in nerve division. Brain 31:323–450, 1908.
3. David WB: The life of John Staige Davis, M.D. Plast Reconstr Surg 62:368–378, 1978.
4. Davis JS: *Plastic Surgery, Principles and Practice.* Philadelphia: Blakiston, 1919.
5. Davis JS, Kitlowski EA: Regeneration of nerves in skin grafts and skin flaps. Am J Surg 24:501–545, 1934.
6. Kredel FE, Evans JP: Recovery of sensation in denervated pedicle and free skin grafts. Arch Neurol Psychiatry 29:1203–1221, 1933.

7. McCarrol HR: The regeneration of sensation in transplanted skin. Ann Surg 108:309–320, 1938.

8. Lofgren L: Recovery of nervous function in skin transplants with special reference to the sympathetic functions. Acta Chir Scand 102:229–239, 1952.

9. Seddon HJ, Medawar PB, Smith H: Rate of regeneration of peripheral nerves in man. J Physiol 102:191–215, 1943.

10. Sunderland S: Rate of regeneration in human peripheral nerve. Arch Neurol Psychiatry 58:251–295, 1947.

11. Dellon AL, Curtis RM, Edgerton MT: Evaluating recovery of sensation in the hand following nerve injury. Johns Hopkins Med J 130:235–243, 1972.

12. Krishnamurti A, Kanagasuntheram R, Vij S: Failure of reinnervation of Pacinian corpuscle after nerve crush: An electron microscopic study. Acta Neuropathol (Berl) 23:338–341, 1973.

13. Jabaley ME, Burns JE, Orcutt BS, et al: Comparison of histologic and functional recovery after peripheral nerve repair. J Hand Surg 1:119–130, 1976.

14. Gelberman RH, Urbaniak JR, Bright DS, et al: Digital sensibility following replantation. J Hand Surg 3:313–319, 1979.

15. Gelberman RH, Blasingame JP, Fronek A, et al: Forearm arterial injuries. J Hand Surg 4:401–408, 1979.

16. Brown AG, Iggo A: The structure and function of cutaneous touch corpuscles after nerve crush. J Physiol 165:28P-29P, 1963.

17. Silver A, Versaci A, Montagna W: Studies of sweating and sensory function in cases of peripheral nerve injuries of the hand. J Invest Dermatol 40:243–258, 1963.

18. Dykes RW, Terzis JK: Reinnervation of glabrous skin in baboons: Properties of cutaneous mechanoreceptors subsequent to nerve crush. J Neurophysiol 42:1461–1478, 1979.

Chapter 8

MOVING TWO-POINT DISCRIMINATION TEST

INTRODUCTION
PERFORMING THE TEST
NORMAL TEST VALUES
ABNORMAL TEST VALUES
CENTRAL NERVOUS SYSTEM
    CORRELATES
CHORAESTHESIA AND THE
    PLASTIC RIDGE
CLINICAL IMPLICATIONS

INTRODUCTION

In the past 2 decades, largely due to the urging of Erik Moberg,[1-5] the hand surgeon has abandoned the neurologist's pin and cotton wool, the goal of which was localization of a lesion within the central nervous system, and has embraced the paper clip, the goal of which is supposed to be measurement of the functional sensibility of the hand. Although the classic Weber "static sensory" two-point discrimination test does correlate with the hand's ability to perform static grips, critical observers have found that this classic two-point discrimination does not always parallel active hand function. Mannerfelt's[6] careful evaluation of skin grafted to fingertips revealed that two-point discrimination did not correlate with function, as judged by the coin test or Moberg's pick-up test. McQuillan[7] wrote that two-point discrimination "is entirely unreliable after nerve repair." Krag and Rasmussen's[8] analysis of neurovas-

cular island flaps revealed that half of the fingertips (with flaps) did well on the pick-up test, despite absent two-point discrimination. Parry and Salter[9] wrote that it is a "misconception to assume that two-point discrimination is a meaningful method of assessing stereognosis." As a clue to this paradox, Parry and Salter observed that *active movement* is fundamental to hand function and that a "static test," such as two-point discrimination, is "irrelevant to function." Instead, Parry and Salter use a timed object recognition test (see "pick-up test," Chapter 6) to measure hand function. Narakas[10] also has indicated that two-point discrimination is a static test, that tactile gnosis requires movement, and that "fair tactile discrimination can be present without valid two-point discrimination." Finally, Seddon[11] has written, "It is curious how elements of movement in tactile appreciation have been disregarded."

This series of criticisms of the classic Weber two-point discrimination test and of static tests seems recent. Yet more than a century ago, Silas Weir Mitchell[12] noted these essential criticisms. He wrote in 1872:

> In examining the sensibility, too much care cannot be observed, since there is a natural instinct which causes us to use any power of motion we may have in order to press upon and so examine the touching body ... The compass points, which ought to be rounded, ... should both come down with equal force and at once, since otherwise the succession of impressions informs the patient there are two points in use ... Above all, it is essential ... to see that the patient does not move the part during the time of testing it. There seems to be an almost uncontrollable prompting to do this in every instance where the sense of touch is puzzled; and if he be allowed to stir the part ever so little, the answer he will make will often prove correct, when in the absence of motion it would have been defective.

The sensation that something is moving across the surface of the fingertips is mediated by the quickly-adapting fiber/receptor system (see Chapter 3). Tactile gnosis, the ability to "see" with the fingertips, is possible to achieve through a series of discontinuous constant-touches, but this is awkward and inefficient. The natural approach to sensory exploration depends upon a continuous movement of the hand or fingertips. That our central nervous system and mechanisms are most effective when interpreting nerve impulses that vary over time has been demonstrated by the blind, who read most efficiently by moving their fingertips over the raised Braille dots, and by psychophysical investigations developing sight-substitute systems for the blind.[1, 13, 14] Until recently, however, there was no simple way to measure clinically the innervation density of this quickly-adapting fiber/receptor system.

It seemed to me that a test that could measure the innervation density of the quickly-adapting fiber/receptor system, if not the entire system of group A beta fibers and their receptors, would be a more valid measurement than the classic test, since the Weber test evaluates only the slowly-adapting fiber/receptor system. Such a new test must involve movement and be quantitative. Possible testing devices included screws with

different threads, materials with different textures, graded sandpaper, cloth with varied warps, etc., each of which would require standardizations, trials on normal and nerve-injured populations, dissemination of the test results, and, if the test's validity were accepted, the production of such a sensory tool for use by other clinicians. To be accepted and clinically used, the test instrument would have to be small, inexpensive, and readily available. It became apparent that the acceptance already achieved by the classic two-point discrimination test and the ubiquitous paper clip had laid the groundwork for a simple modification of Weber's test. The moving two-point discrimination test would be a test where the ends of the paper clip were moved across the surface of the fingertip at progressively narrower interprong distance until a two-point limen was reached.[15]

PERFORMING THE TEST

The moving two-point discrimination test is performed with a paper clip that is rearranged to form a testing instrument with two right-angle pointers (Fig. 8.1). These pointers may be adjusted so that the center of the tips vary from 2 mm to more than 30 mm apart. Due to the technique of the paper clip manufacture, a metallic barb usually is present on one edge of the paper clip tip (Fig. 8.1). The rearranged paper clip must be employed such that this barb is away from, i.e., does not stroke the fingertip surface.[15]

The fingertip to be examined is supported by the examining table or the examiner's hand. The paper clip is moved along the surface of the finger from proximal to distal. Just sufficient pressure is utilized for the subject to appreciate the stimulus (Fig. 8.2).

First the patient is oriented to the test. Just one of the two paper clip tips is moved along the finger length and the patient is asked what he perceives to have occurred. He is reinforced by being told "that was one moving point." Next both ends of the paper clip, separated by 5 to 8 mm, are moved along the surface of the fingertip. The patient is questioned again. He is then reinforced by being told "that was two."[15]

Next the fingertip is tested, beginning with

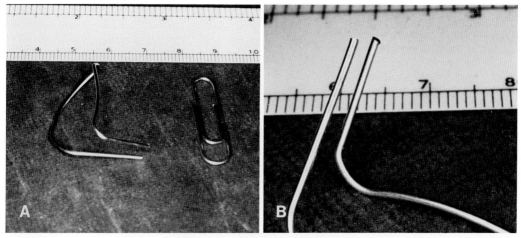

Figure 8.1.   The paper clip testing instrument. *A,* The paper clip is bent to form the test instrument. *B,* The process of manufacture results in a barb at the paper clip tip. Care must be taken to avoid stroking the fingertip with the barb. (Reproduced with permission from A. L. Dellon: *J Hand Surg* 3:474–481, 1978.[15])

the two ends 5 to 8 mm apart and proceeding in stages down to 2 mm apart. We do not attempt to measure moving two-point discrimination less than 2 mm. We always begin at a higher value and work down to a lower value to orient the patient to the testing procedure. We always move the paper clip parallel to the long axis of the finger, which generally means at an angle to the majority of the "fingerprint ridges."[15]

We randomly alternate the testing stimulus between the one and the two points. If the patient correctly perceives the changes, then we proceed to the next lower value. When the patient begins to answer slowly, and the moving two-point limen or threshold is being approached, we require seven of 10 correct responses before proceeding to the next lower value. Therefore, saying that the moving two-point discrimination of the thumb is 2 mm means that at least seven of 10 times the patient correctly identified whether the stimulus moving down the surface of the digit was one or both ends of the paper clip.

NORMAL TEST VALUES

The normal value for the two-point discrimination test was found by testing 39 hands in 32 people, ranging in ages from 4 to 83 years. These "normal" people all led active lives, which, for example, meant that one 83-year-old was self-sufficient, cared for her home, and gardened and painted as hobbies. The values are presented in Figure 8.3 for the thumb pulp of the dominant hand. There was no difference found between the dominant and nondominant hands or between the radial or the ulnar digits. There was no difference related to the patient's sex. Thus, the normal moving two-point discrimination may be taken as 2 mm in the distal fingertip.

ABNORMAL TEST VALUES

Invalids

Does the ability to discriminate diminish if the hand is not used. A clinical form of such sensory deprivation is represented by patients who, through diseases of discomfort in an extremity, fail to use it over a period of time. We studied six such patients; examples of the cause of their limited use are seen in Figures 8.5 and 8.6. Other causes were severe rheumatoid deformity, chronic alcoholism, osteoarthritis, and hip fracture with associated leg burn. The moving two-point discrimination test values were elevated (abnormal) in all six patients. In patients with disease in

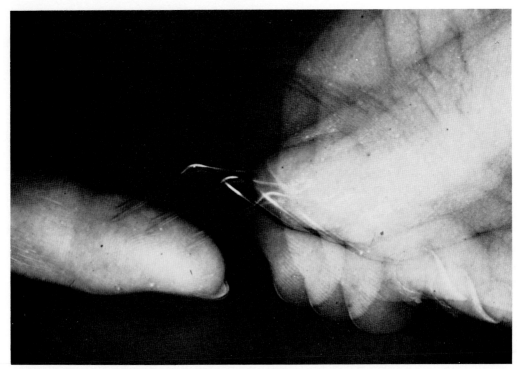

Figure 8.2. The moving two-point discrimination test. The two ends of the paper clip are pulled longitudinally from proximal to distal, along the fingertip, and across the papillary ridges. (Reproduced with permission from A. L. Dellon: *J Hand Surg* 3:474–481, 1978.[15])

each hand, this value was equal bilaterally. In one patient, one hand was immobile and had a moving two-point discrimination of 6 mm, whereas in the other fully mobile hand, the value was 2 mm.[15]

Nerve Compressions

In my early investigations with the test, 13 patients with 17 nerve compressions were evaluated.[14] These included 12 median, 4 ulnar, and 1 digital nerve compression. In general, when patients presented with intermittent numbness and tingling, moving two-point discrimination was normal. As degree and duration of compression increased to the point where there was persistent numbness, moving two-point discrimination values increased (became abnormal). These observations were confirmed in a later series of 36 patients with carpal tunnel syndrome.[16] In that series, loss of tactile discrimination was a late finding being preceded in order by a

positive Phalen's sign, a positive Tinel's sign, altered vibratory perception (see Chapter 9), and abnormal electrodiagnostic study (prolonged motor latency or antidromic sensory). Whenever the classic two-point discrimination was abnormal, the moving two-point discrimination was also abnormal. However, even a small increase in the value of the moving two-point discrimination test is significant. By this I mean a value of 4 mm for moving two-point discrimination is abnormal and indicates in our clinical and operative correlation intraneural fibrosis. Because the upper limit of normal for classic two-point discrimination is given as 3 to 5 or 4 to 6 mm, an "early" abnormal value is less easy to define. In contrast, the normal value for moving two-point discrimination is 2 mm, and a value of 3 mm is an early abnormal value. Extrapolating the Curtis and Eversmann work,[17] I have considered a moving two-point discrimination value of 4 mm to be an indi-

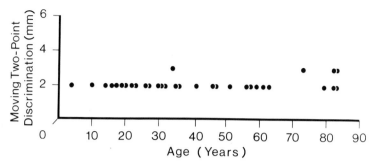

Figure 8.3. Control population. The normal value for the moving two-point discrimination test is 2 mm. There is essentially no change with age.

cation for internal neurolysis. Following carpal tunnel release and internal neurolysis, I have observed the abnormal moving two-point discrimination values return to normal.[15, 18]

A word of caution: In my experience, if the moving two-point discrimination is 3 to 4 mm in the thumb and index finger *bilaterally*, in patients being evaluated for nerve compressions, they have bilateral carpal tunnel syndromes with significant compression. If the thumb, index, and little fingers have values of 3 to 4 mm, there is compression of the ulnar nerve in addition to the median nerve; the ulnar area is usually compressed at the elbow. I confirm this by noting, almost invariably, a difference in sensation between the dorsal ulnar and dorsal radial surfaces of the hand to finger stroking and the 256-cps tuning fork (see Chapter 9). The combination of median nerve compression at the wrist and ulnar nerve compression at the elbow is not rare, especially in the rheumatoid population. (I don't test the middle or ring finger when evaluating ulnar or median nerve problems.)

Nerve Lacerations

In patients with complete division of a major peripheral nerve proximal to the palm, there is, of course, complete loss of sensation and therefore no tactile discrimination. However, in patients with a common volar digital nerve division or in patients with digital nerve injury, moving two-point discrimination in the autonomous zone of that nerve was usually 5 to 6 mm and two-point discrimination was usually 7 to 8 mm, depending on the width of the finger, as compared with 2 mm

on the uninjured side. If the digital nerve was cut proximal to its dorsal branch, moving two-point discrimination and classic two-point discrimination in the autonomous zone were more than 10 mm.[15] All but the very lightest moving-touch usually could be perceived over the injured autonomous zone while constant-touch could not.

Thus, one of the most common diagnostic errors, sticking a pin into the tip of a finger with a laceration, eliciting a pain response (ouch!) from the patient, and pronouncing the digital nerve "intact," can be avoided by careful tactile discrimination testing. Where the emergency situation doesn't allow this testing to be done (noise, children, uncooperative patient, intoxication, etc.), this diagnostic problem may be solved with the tuning fork (see Chapter 9).

Nerve Repair

The patients with nerve repair were evaluated at varying times after their surgery. They each received sensory re-education. When moving-touch and constant-touch perception returned to the fingertip, they entered late phase re-education and had moving two-point discrimination recorded at each subsequent visit. Twenty-three patients were studied.[15] The moving two-point discrimination progressed from near absent, i.e., 12 mm, toward normal over time. Moving two-point discrimination always returned prior to classic two-point discrimination (Fig. 8.4). Moving two-point discrimination was usually 12 mm, 2 to 5 months before classic two-point discrimination was 30 mm. When the moving two-point discrimination had recovered to

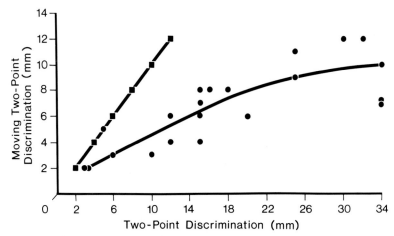

Figure 8.4. Recovery of classical and moving two-point discrimination. The fitted curve of observations (*black dots*) is below and to the right of the hypothetical curve (*black squares*) in which classic equals moving two-point discrimination. This indicates that during sensory recovery following nerve repair, moving two-point discrimination always is less (in mm), i.e., better discrimination than classic two-point discrimination. (Reproduced with permission from A. L. Dellon; *J Hand Surg* 3:474–481, 1978.[15])

the 5 to 8 mm range, two-point discrimination usually was in the 15 to 25 mm range. In those patients in whom sensibility returned nearly to normal, moving two-point discrimination reached 2 to 4 mm anywhere from 2 to 6 months before two-point discrimination reached 5 mm (Figs. 8.5 and 8.6). In two patients, the two-point discrimination never progressed below 8 mm, whereas the moving two-point discrimination was 2 or 3 mm. Those cases where moving two-point discrimination recovered to normal just 2 months ahead of two-point discrimination were in patients under 16 years of age. In every patient, as the moving two-point discrimination improved, hand function, as judged by patient opinion, observation of wear marks, and direct examination, improved too. By the time moving two-point discrimination was less than 5 mm, patients could, assuming motor function permitted, perform all of their usual activities (see Chapter 10).

CENTRAL NERVOUS SYSTEM CORRELATES

The "homunculus," the distorted body image stretched across the postcentral gyrus, is well-accepted as the organization of the somatosensory cortex. Within the hand area are two smaller areas which receive input from the cutaneous receptors and which differ histologically in their cytoarchitecture. Brodmann's area 1, on the rostral surface of the postcentral gyrus, and area 3, within the sulcus on its posterior wall, have been mapped with microelectrodes.[19] In area 1, 95% of the fields are quickly-adapting, whereas in area 3, 55% of the fields are slowly-adapting. Since a direct relationship exists between the stimulation of a quickly-adapting first order afferent (in the fingertip) and the eliciting of a quickly-adapting response in the sensory cortex,[20] I suggest that the brain has evolved an area differentially receptive to the perception of moving-touch stimuli. I suggest that Brodmann's area 1 primarily would receive sensory input generated by moving stimuli or the fingers moving about an object, whereas Brodmann's area 3 primarily would receive sensory input generated by objects in constant contact with the fingers and pressure.

This submodality segregation should also be present in the spinal cord, linking the specific sensory fiber/receptor systems of the fingertip to the cerebral cortex. Indeed, using

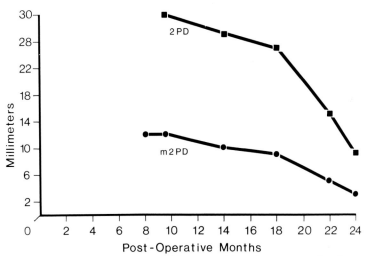

Figure 8.5. Clinical course. A 35-year-old man with primary repair of median nerve. Sensory re-education was given. Note: Moving two-point discrimination recovery was earlier and better than classic two-point discrimination. (Reproduced with permission from A. L. Dellon: *J Hand Surg*: 3:474–481, 1978.[15]).

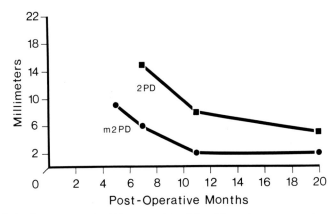

Figure 8.6. Clinical course. A 17-year-old girl with primary repair of ulnar nerve. Sensory re-education was given. Note: The moving two-point discrimination recovery was earlier and better than the classic two-point discrimination. (Reproduced with permission from A. L. Dellon: *J Hand Surg*: 3:474–481, 1978.[15])

precise recording and dissection techniques, this fiber sorting has been identified in the spinal cord.[21, 22]

My statement that the moving two-point discrimination test measures the innervation density of the quickly-adapting fiber/receptor system implies that this fiber/receptor system is capable, in neurophysiologic terms, of making fine discriminations. In 1967, von Prince and Butler[23] carefully studied patients following peripheral nerve repair and noted that even in the absence of classic two-point discrimination (low innervation density of the slowly-adapting fiber/receptor system), patients could distinguish textures, such as grades of sandpaper. In 1968, Vallbo and Hagbarth,[24] using percutaneous recording of peripheral nerves in awake human subjects, demonstrated increased quickly-adapting activity in response to increased roughness of a moving textured surface. In 1969, utilizing fine oscillators to stimulate the quickly-adapting fiber/receptor system, Bach-y-Rita's group[25] found what I would consider to be a moving two-point discrimination of 11 mm in comparison to the classic two-point discrimination of 78 mm. Thus the back, traditionally an area where static touch localizing ability is poor, could be utilized as a vision sensory substitute system with moving touch.

Perhaps the most sophisticated central nervous system correlates come from a series of studies by LaMotte and Mountcastle. In 1975,[26] they reported results of their investigation into the psychophysical ability of two primates, monkey and man, to discriminate fine differences in the sense of flutter-vibration. Both monkeys and humans were trained in amplitude and frequency discrimination to mechanical sinusoids (precise tuning forks). Subjective responses were obtained from the humans, while direct recording from the hand area of the postcentral gyrus (Brodmann's area 1) was obtained from the awake monkeys. Monkeys responded by opening or closing a microswitch adjacent to the forefinger of the stimulated hand: correct response activated a "reward" of apple juice.

Johnson had already demonstrated[27] that the Meissner afferents, those responsive to low frequency vibration had peripheral receptive fields of 1 to 2 mm and good frequency discrimination (in contrast to the Pacinian afferents, high frequency responsive, which have large receptive fields and poorer spatiotemporal patterning). Johnson suggested that the peripheral neural code (the pattern of neural impulses) for intensity (amplitude of the oscillation, "loudness of the vibration") is a spatial one, the number of actively responding Meissner afferents. This differs from the slowly-adapting system, where the neural code for intensity (pressure of the constant touch) is frequency of impulses generated in the single nerve.

LaMotte and Mountcastle,[26] in their psychophysical studies, extended Johnson's observation. Monkeys and men were comparable in the ability to discriminate between mechanical sinusoids differing in amplitude and frequency. That is, both species could detect differences in low frequency vibration

when those differences were either in the "loudness" of the vibrations or in their "pitch." Further, the detection system was exquisitely sensitive, being able to detect even very small differences in either of these qualities (differences of just 8 dB for amplitude or 1.8 Hz for frequency). They concluded that the ability to make subjective estimates of magnitude (amplitude) or frequency of these (moving) stimuli was based on spatial and temporal distribution codes, patterns of neural impulses that reflected the overall activity in the relevant neural population (the innervation system).

Utilizing a spatially textured stimulus, wire-wound cylinders of varying turns or nylon fabrics varying in weft and warp in a dual species psychophysical study, similar to that outlined above, LaMotte made the following observations. Movement of the wire-wound cylinder so that the movement of the fingertip pad back and forth along the cylinder length placed the transversely organized papillary ridges (fingerprints) parallel to the wire striations produced a sensation of vibration and texture. Discrimination of a difference of just 1.2 turns/cm was possible. If the fingertip moved in a direction perpendicular to the cylinder length, this discrimination wasn't possible. With the nylon yarns, lower yarn counts (a more open weave) were judged rougher and correlated with discharge rates of the Meissner afferent population. Thus, we see the ability of the quickly-adapting fiber/receptor systems to make fine discriminations where there is a high innervation density.[28]

In their most recently reported study,[29] LaMotte and Mountcastle ablated portions of the parietal cortex (postcentral gyrus) of monkeys previously trained in the above mechanical sinusoid discrimination. That ability to discriminate temporal-spatial patterning (movement) was lost following the ablation. This confirmed earlier clinical correlations between loss of tactile gnosis and loss of the middle third of the postcentral gyrus.[29, 30] In the first of these earlier studies,[30] 73% of patients with cortical lesions invading the postcentral gyrus could not identify common household objects (comb, bottle cap, key, spoon, pencil) with their contralateral hand.

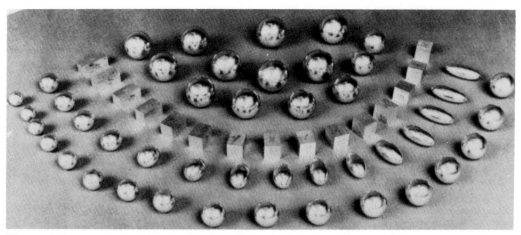

Figure 8.7.   Object recognition. Test objects used to evaluate tactile gnosis in patients with cortical lesions. (Reproduced with permission from P. E. Roland: *Arch Neurol* 33: 543–550, 1976.[31])

The more recent clinical study[31] attempted to define this loss of "tactile recognition," which, of course, is tactile gnosis, with a precisely defined object recognition test (Fig. 8.7). Ability to correctly identify these geometric shapes was correlated with the mapped cortical defect. Eight patients had significant impairment of this object recognition for each of the three sets of shapes, and each of these patients had a cortical defect invading the postcentral gyrus in its anterior and middle-third (Brodmann's area 1) (Fig. 8.8).

I propose that just as the Meissner corpuscle was the most recent sensory end organ to evolve (see Chapter 2), the specialization of Brodmann's area 1 for tactile gnosis is the most recent central manifestation of sensory evolution. Tactile gnosis depends upon movement detection. The moving two-point discrimination test, the most recent test of sensibility to evolve, determines the peripheral innervation density of this quickly-adapting fiber/receptor system.

CHORAESTHESIA AND THE PLASTIC RIDGE

The quest to quantify sensibility in a way that correlates with hand function better than the classic two-point discrimination test has led Poppen et al.[32] to conduct an extensive clinical trial with a "new" test instrument, the Plastic Ridge Device (Figs. 8.9 and 8.10). Their study was exceptional in that detailed evaluations of sensibility were conducted on a large number of patients (63) such that Semmes-Weinstein monofilaments, the Weber test, and the Plastic Ridge Device could be compared. In essence, they concluded: (1) von Frey hairs were the least predictive of a patient's tactile gnosis, and the results of von Frey testing correlated with neither the Weber test (see Fig. 6.12) nor the Plastic Ridge Device (see Fig. 8.11) and (2) the Plastic Ridge Device is better than classic two-point discrimination in detecting the presence of tactile gnosis (Fig. 8.12).

I have included the Plastic Ridge Device in this chapter because critical to its use, and essential to what it is testing, is the element of movement. The Plastic Ridge Device is a modification of Renfrew's "depth sense aesthesiometer."[33] The Plastic Ridge Device is moved across the area to be tested parallel to the longitudinal axis of the finger, at a rate of 10 cm in 10 seconds. The patient states when he perceives that something smooth is no longer moving across his fingertip. The Plastic Ridge Device is calibrated transversely in centimeters along the length of the ridge. The line passing the test site at the time the patient states his altered perception is taken as the recorded value for the device.

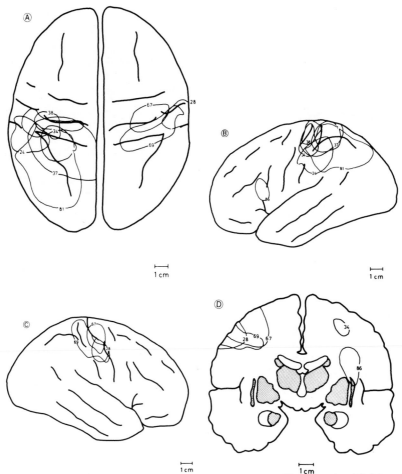

1 cm

1 cm

1 cm   1 cm

Figure 8.8. Cortical lesions correlating with absent tactile gnosis. Eight patients with significant impairment to recognize geometric shapes with their contralateral hand had these cortical defects in the anterior middle third of the postcentral gyrus (Brodmann's area 1). Section D, through the central sulcus, demonstrates that only four of the eight patients (Nos. 26, 69, 67, 34) had lesions that extended to area 3.[31]

The observations of Poppen et al.,[32] I believe, reinforce my impression that the ultimate test of tactile gnosis must be one that evaluates the quickly-adapting fiber/receptor system, i.e., incorporates a moving stimulus. After the appearance of their paper in May of 1979, I wrote a letter to the Editor of the *Journal of Hand Surgery*, which said, in part[34] "... (The observations of Poppen et al.[32]) are those we would have predicted based upon the neurophysiology of the involved nerve fiber/receptor systems."

The von Frey test tells us (conceptually) the

threshold required to stimulate a slowly-adapting fiber/receptor (group A, beta/Merkel disc). The Weber test tells us the innervation density of this slowly-adapting fiber/receptor system. Thus a small number of these fibers may have regenerated to the fingertip, reinnervated the appropriate receptors, and "matured" so that, at five years after repair, a low threshold (normal von Frey) might have resulted, but the number of fibers having regenerated might have been too few, i.e., a low innervation density, to give a normal Weber test. The dynamic plastic ridge device requires movement of the (device). Therefore, the test evaluates moving touch, which is mediated by the quickly-adapting fiber/receptor system (group A,

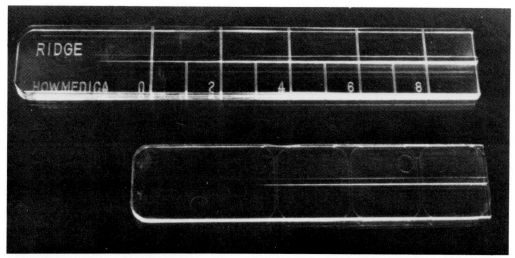

Figure 8.9.   Plastic Ridge Device. See text. (Reproduced with permission from N. K. Poppen et al.: *J Hand Surg* 4:212–226, 1979.[3])

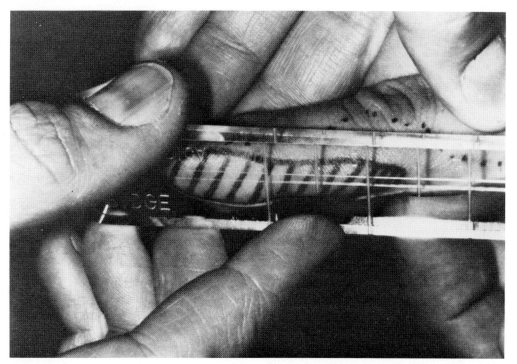

Figure 8.10.   Plastic Ridge Device testing technique. See text. (Reproduced with permission from N. K. Poppen et al.: *J Hand Surg* 4:212–226, 1979.[32])

beta/Meissner and Pacinian corpuscles). This is an entirely different fiber/receptor population, and therefore one would not expect the results of the von Frey or Weber (static) tests to correlate necessarily with those of this new dynamic test.

The principle behind the correlation of the plastic ridge test with tactile gnosis is identical to the principle behind the moving two-point discrimination test. Both tests evaluate the same fiber/receptor system.

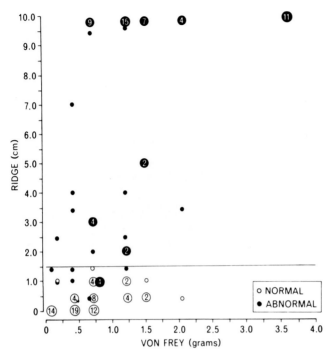

Figure 8.11. Relationship of Plastic Ridge Device and von Frey testing. There is no correlation between the results of these two testing techniques. For a given von Frey value, e.g., 0.75 gm, there is a wide range of Ridge values, e.g., 0.0 to 10.0. For a given Ridge value, e.g., 10.0, there is a wide von Frey value, e.g., 0.5 to 4.0 gm. (Reproduced with permission from N. K. Poppen et al.: *J Hand Surg* 4:212–226, 1979.[32])

There are, however, theoretical and practical problems with the Plastic Ridge Device. In their reply to my Letter to the Editor,[35] Poppen and McCarroll attempted to give the Plastic Ridge Device legitimacy, not by relating it to the known neurophysiologic basis of peripheral sensibility (see Chapter 3), but by relating it to the "somatic sense of space" ("choraesthesia") and to "space detection" instead of "gap detection." This is unfortunate. They cite the "tenfold increase in sensibility judgment made on the basis of overall dimension (disc threshold) when compared to gap detection (measured by disc-annulus or classic two-point discrimination) reported by Vierck and Jones.[36] It is true that Vierck and Jones found that their *four* normal subjects could detect differences in overall size between test objects (4 to 24 mm in diameter) *pressed* onto their *forearms* with a detection threshold of 2 to 6 mm. The classic two-point discrimination in this area was 25 to 35 mm. However, the purpose of that study was to develop a system to test areas *other than* the fingertip.[36]

Support for the Plastic Ridge Device on the basis that it measures the "somatic *sense* of space" suffers from the same criticism as the

development of the Palesthesiometer to measure the vibratory *sense*. There is no vibratory *sense*! Simply because someone demonstrated that (1) vibration can be perceived and (2) a central nervous system lesion can abolish that perception, a unique sense distinct from all others, warranting a name with a Greek prefix, has *not* been shown to exist. As is expounded in the next chapter, "pallesthesia" is mediated by the quickly-adapting fiber/receptor system. In 1960, Renfrew and Melville,[37] largely on a philosophical or introspective basis, and certainly without any direct neurophysiologic research, postulated the existence of the "somatic sense of space." Having postulated it, they named it "Choroesthesia." This does not prove its existence as a unique "sense." They attempted to distinguish the ability to perceive space changes occurring in a plane at right angles to the surface of the finger from space changes occurring in a plane parallel to the surface of the finger. As an example of the type of distinction they attempt to make regarding space, consider the following:[37]

Should a man look down a deep hole in the ground his statement that he can see the hole

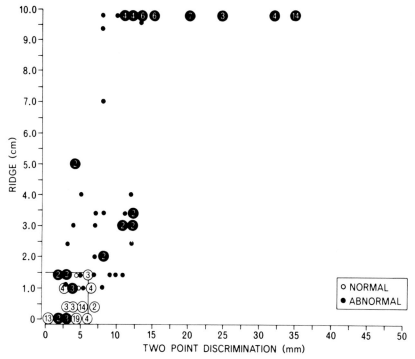

Figure 8.12.   Relationship of Plastic Ridge Device and classic two-point discrimination testing. There is no correlation. For a given classic two-point discrimination value, e.g., 7 mm, there is a wide range of Ridge values, e.g., 0.5 to 10.0. For a given Ridge value, e.g., 10.0, there is a wide range of discrimination, e.g., 7 to 35 mm. (Reproduced with permission from N. K. Poppen et al.: *J Hand Surg* 4:212–226, 1979.[32])

could be countered by the suggestion that since his retinal receptors are not stimulated, he does not really see the hole but only the ground around it, that is, he is permitted to see light space but not dark space.

Renfrew and Melville go on to discuss Kant's view of space, debate Realism and Idealism, and finally write "we have worked on the basis that a dermal touch feeling and a dermal space feeling are two different feelings. Our justification for this is based on introspection." They finally, although concluding the opposite, demonstrated direct correlation between their measured space sense and surface sense thresholds. They noted that space sense was lost with lesions of the parietal lobe and posterior spinal columns. They closed the paper with "speculation" as to the sensory receptors for this "sense": they thought these might be the Meissner corpuscle.[37]

I believe that choraesthesia, as such, is nonexistent. Tactile gnosis depends upon a profile of neural impulses peripherally generated at the fingertips as the fingertips move about, around, and over the object being recognized. These impulses reach the association cortex as they reach the conscious level, and thus, an identification is made. We must develop instruments that allow simple, unambiguous measurement of the group A, beta fiber's innervation density. The test instrument must be readily available, inexpensive, and understandable.

The Plastic Ridge Device has practical problems. For example, for more than a year I have been unable to obtain one to carry out my own series of studies with it! Once produced, it may become available in the hand center. Certainly it will not be as ubiquitous as the paper clip. Its calibration is a problem. You read it in centimeters of length, but it is really measuring how deeply the ridge goes into the pulp in millimeters!

The Plastic Ridge Device consists of an inclined plane which arises from a smooth surface at one end of the block of plastic (taper equal 1.5/100) to attain a height of 1.5 mm. at the other end (the 9.5 cm. mark on the linear scale). The ride values of 0.5, 1.5, and 2.5 cm. on the linear scale correspond to ridge heights of 0.15, 0.30 and 0.45 mm., respectively.[35]

Thus, one reports a value of 1.5 cm, which sounds like a poor result, but which really means a ridge height of 0.30, which is, of course, good. The state of sensibility evaluation is confused enough without a calibration that doesn't read out in terms of what is actually measured!

A real source of error in the use of the Plastic Ridge Device is determining the end point. To be sure, one examiner over time will give reproducible readings. But how fast does one move the device? If we move at 1 cm/sec, as suggested, and the patient takes some time to appreciate what he is feeling, and then more time to verbalize it, the calibration on the device has moved past the point at which the threshold was reached! So, a patient says "Now." You look at the device, and the 2.0-cm line is over the area. Now if you move the device faster there will be even more discrepancy between the recorded "ridge value" and the true "ridge depth" that was the threshold.

Furthermore, if the device isn't held flat, the patient will feel two moving edges; the ridge and the horizontal surface of the test device. This, rather than ridge depth, may cause him to respond. How hard do you press? If pressure is constant, the ridge will move along at the same depth! So you must increase pressure constantly as you move. Thus, stimulus intensity is also changing.

An additional practical limitation of the Plastic Ridge Device is using it on someone with a flexion contracture, for example, after combined tendon and nerve injury.[38]

Perhaps the most significant criticism of the study on the Plastic Ridge Device is the summary statement "... The Plastic Ridge Device detects the presence or absence of tactile gnosis in patients in the intermediate range of (classic) two-point discrimination

between 8 and 12 mm."[32] Tactile gnosis was never tested in that study. No specific functional testing or correlations, i.e., with the pick-up test or object identification, were performed!

In summary, I believe the *data* reported by Poppen et al.[32] support my general thesis, in terms of correlating sensory tests with the underlying neurophysiologic mechanism, as outlined above and in more detail in Chapter 10. I believe their study's theoretical basis, the "somatic sense of space," is most probably wrong. I believe the Plastic Ridge Device, when used by an experienced sensory tester, will give results that will parallel those of the moving two-point discrimination test. I am convinced that the lack of availability of the device, the confusion surrounding its calibration, the wide range of normal, and the potential pitfalls in its use will greatly limit its general acceptance.

CLINICAL IMPLICATIONS

The moving two-point discrimination test can determine the capacity of the hand to discriminate moving-touch stimuli.[15] Diminished function is detected early in nerve compression syndromes. Diminished sensation is detected in the finger with a lacerated digital nerve. Recovery of sensation is detected following release of nerve compression and following nerve repair.

The moving two-point discrimination test is easy to perform rapidly with equipment available virtually everywhere: a paper clip.

The moving two-point discrimination test offers several advantages compared to the classic two-point discrimination test. As the sensation of moving touch is recovered distally sooner than constant touch[8] (see Chapter 7), so too, moving two-point discrimination testing will give information concerning the results of nerve repair sooner than two-point discrimination testing. In the individual patient, the ability to discriminate two-points moving from one recovers not only sooner but also to a higher degree (lower moving two-point discrimination) than does constant-touch (Figs. 8.5 and 8.6). Therefore, if just classic two-point discrimination is tested, the individual's actual and potential sensory recovery are underestimated (Fig. 8.4). Expressed another way, the patient has a better functional result from his nerve repair than classic two-point discrimination testing suggests. The moving two-point discrimination test also is an accurate monitor of gains in function during sensory re-education.

Another advantage of the moving two-point discrimination test is that it is a "pure" sensory test. Moberg's pick-up test and Parry's timed recognition test depend on motor function; the sensation produced depends upon the motor system to manipulate the fingertips in moving-touch. The moving two-point discrimination test, a test done *to* not *by* the patient, permits the tester to assess purely sensory function.

Because the moving two-point discrimination test evaluates the fiber/receptor system that mediates moving touch, the moving two-point discrimination test overcomes the criticisms[6-11] of classic two-point discrimination in evaluating functional sensation. If the hand function to be predicted or correlated is purely a static one, i.e., precisely gripping a needle, then the two-point discrimination test will suffice. But if the sensory grip in fact requires movement, such as winding a watch or buttoning a button, or if the hand function requires the fingertips to move over an object, then the moving two-point discrimination test should be more appropriate. Recently, we have demonstrated that the moving two-point discrimination test is the only test of sensibility to correlate with the ability to recognize objects (tactile gnosis) (see Chapter 10).[39]

I propose a hypothesis to explain why the results of nerve repair as judged by classic two-point discrimination are so bad (see Chapter 11. Less than 1% of adults with median or ulnar nerve repairs at the wrist recover to level S4.), and why the moving two-point discrimination recovers sooner and to a better degree (Fig. 8.4). The critical components of this hypothesis relate to (1) the relative scarcity of slowly-adapting fibers (only about one-third of the group A beta fibers are slowly-adapting (see Chapter 3) and (2) the relative scarcity of slowly-adapting fibers to the Merkel cell (axon to receptor ratios are Meissner >1; Pacinian = 1, Merkel <1, see Fig. 7.5). Thus, following a nerve

repair, the absolute number of axons reaching the fingertip is reduced by attrition at the suture line, axonal misdirection down the wrong endoneurial sheath, and terminal connection mismatches. It is given that some minimal peripheral innervation density is critical for tactile discrimination. If only a third of fibers are slowly-adapting, and only, say, half the total number of fibers regenerate to the periphery, the critical innervation density for slow-adapters is more likely not to be met than for the quick-adapters. Furthermore, the degenerating Meissner corpuscle can be reinnervated by any one of the three to nine quickly-adapting axons that normally innervate it, while two to four degenerating Merkel cells are less likely to be reinnervated by the one slowly-adapting fiber that normally innervates them. Compounding this is the experimental observation that the Merkel cell degenerates more rapidly than Meissner corpuscle (Chapter 4). In essence, it is statistically highly more probable to reinnervate the Meissner corpuscles, the fiber/receptor system primarily tested by the moving two-point discrimination test.

There are two experimental studies that, in retrospect, support this hypothesis. Following nerve repair, there was a reduction in the number of slowly-adapting neuronal responses from 56 to 29% in Brodmann's area 3 while there was essentially no loss in the percentage of quickly-adapting neuronal responses in Brodmann's area 1 (see Fig. 12.18).[40] Following nerve repair, an average of only 60% of the slowly-adapting fibers regenerated, and each fiber reinnervated only half of the Merkel cells it previously reinnervated.[41]

Finally, a comment about what fiber population is actually stimulated when the paper clip is moved along the surface of the fingertip. As the paper clip moves across the papillary ridges, it sets up not only a sequence of brief touches, but also a vibration within the area of its movement, similar to the disturbance the passenger in a car feels crossing railroad tracks. These low-frequency pertubations of the resting state in the fingertip pulp stimulate the entire Meissner afferent group of quickly-adapting fibers. Almost certainly, however, the remaining quickly-adapting fibers (the Pacinian afferents) will be stimulated as will the slowly-adapting fiber/receptor systems. But as the paper clip moves along the fingertip due to the phenomenon of "recruitment," increasing responses will come from the quickly-adapting fiber/receptors. The slowly-adapting fiber/receptors, always in the minority, probably make only a functionally insignificant contribution to our perception of the two moving points. Therefore, I believe it is effectively correct to speak of this test as one that evaluates the innervation density of the quickly-adapting fiber/receptor system in general, and the Meissner afferents in particular.

References

1. Moberg E: Objective methods of determining functional value of sensibility in the hand. J Bone Joint Surg [Br] 40:454–466, 1958.
2. Moberg E: Criticism and study of methods for examining sensibility in the hand. Neurology 12:8–19, 1962.
3. Moberg E: Methods for examining sensibility in the hand, in Flynn JE (ed): *Hand Surgery.* Baltimore: Williams & Wilkins, 1966.
4. Moberg E: *Emergency Surgery of the Hand.* New York: Churchill, Livingstone, 1968.
5. Moberg E: Future hope for the surgical management of peripheral nerve lesions, in Michon J, Moberg E (eds): *Traumatic Nerve Lesions.* New York: Churchill Livingstone, 1975.
6. Mannerfelt L: Evaluation of functional sensation of skin grafts in the hand area. Br J Plast Surg 15:136–154, 1962.
7. McQuillan W: Sensory recovery after nerve repair. Hand 2:7–9, 1970.
8. Krag K, Rasmussen KB: The neurovascular island flap for defective sensibility of the thumb. J Bone Joint Surg [Br] 57:495–499, 1975.
9. Parry CBW, Salter M: Sensory re-education after median nerve lesion. Hand 8:250–257, 1976.
10. Narakas A: Personal communication, 1978.
11. Seddon HG: *Surgical Disorders of the Peripheral Nerves.* Baltimore: Williams & Wilkins, 1972, p 43.
12. Mitchell SW: *Injuries of Nerves and Their Consequences.* American Academy of Neurology Reprint Series. New York: Dover, 1965, pp 84, 184.
13. Bach-y-Rita P, Collins CC, Saunders FA, et al: Vision substitution by tactile image projection. Nature 221:643–644, 1969.
14. Collins CC, Bach-y-Rita P: Transmission of pictorial information through the skin. Adv Biol Med Phys 14:285–315, 1973.
15. Dellon AL: The moving two-point discrimination test: Clinical evaluation of the quickly-adapting fiber/receptor system. J Hand Surg 3:474–481, 1978.
16. Dellon AL: Clinical use of vibratory stimuli in evaluation of peripheral nerve injury and compression neuropathy. Plast Reconstr Surg 65:466–476, 1980.
17. Curtis RM, Eversmann WW Jr: Internal neurolysis as an adjunct to the treatment of the carpal tunnel syndrome. J Bone Joint Surg 55A:733–740, 1973.
18. Dellon AL: Results of internal neurolysis in peripheral nerve compression, in press 1981.
19. Paul RL, Merzenich M, Goodman H: Representation of slowly- and rapidly-adapting cutaneous mechanoreceptors of the hand on Brodmann's area 3 and 1 of Macaca mulatta. Brain Res 36:229–249, 1972.
20. Powell TPS, Mountcastle VB: The cytoarchitecture of the post-central gyrus of the monkey Macaca mulatta. Bull Johns Hopkins Hosp 105:108–131, 1959.
21. Horch KWM, Burgess PR, Whitedorn D: Ascending collaterals of cutaneous neurons in the fasciculus gracilis of the cat. Brain Res 117:1–17, 1976.
22. Schneider RJ, Kulies AT, Ducker TB: Proprioceptive pathways in the spinal cord. J Neurol Neurosurg Psychiatry 40:417–433, 1977.
23. von Prince K, Butler B Jr: Measuring sensory function of the hand in peripheral nerve injuries. Am J Occup Ther 21:385–395, 1976.
24. Vallbo AB, Hagbarth KE: Activity from the skin mechanoreceptors recorded percutaneously in awake human subjects. Exp Neurol 21:270–289, 1968.
25. Eskilden P, Morris A, Collins CC, et al: Simultaneous and successive cutaneous two-point threshold for vibration. Psychon Sci Sect Hum Exp Psychol 14:146–147, 1969.
26. LaMotte RH, Mountcastle VB: Capacities of humans and monkeys to discriminate between vibratory stimuli of different frequency and amplitude: A correlation between neural events and psychophysical measurements. J Neurophysiol 38:539–559, 1975.
27. Johnson KO: Reconstruction of population response to a vibratory stimulus in quickly-adapting mechanoreceptive afferent fiber population innervating glabrous skin of the monkey. J Neurophysiol 37:48–72, 1974.
28. LaMotte RH: Psychophysical and neurophysical studies of tactile sensibility, in Hollies N, Goldman R (eds): *Clothing Comfort: Interaction of Thermal, Ventilation, Construction and Assessment Factors.* Amer Arbr Sci, Amer Arbor, 1977, by report to the international union, LaMotte R, Mountcastle B: Symposium on "Active Touch," Beaune, France, 1977.
29. LaMotte RH, Mountcastle VB: Disorders in somesthesia following lesions of parietal lobe. J Neurophysiol 42:400–419, 1979.
30. Corkin S, Milner B, Rasmussen T: Somatosensory threshold: Contrasting effects of post-central gyrus and posterior parietal lobe excision. Arch Neurol 23:41–58, 1970.
31. Roland PE: Asterognosis: Tactile discrimination after localized hemisphere lesions in man. Arch Neurol 33:543–550, 1976.
32. Poppen NK, McCarroll HR Jr, Doyle JR, et al: Recovery of sensibility after suture of digital nerves. J Hand Surg 4:212–226, 1979.
33. Renfrew S: Fingertip sensation: A routine neurological test. Lancet 1:396–370, 1969.

34. Dellon AL: The Plastic Ridge Device and moving two-point discrimination (Letter to the Editor). J Hand Surg 5:92, 1980.
35. Poppen NK, McCarroll HR Jr: Reply. J Hand Surg 5:92–93, 1980.
36. Vierck CJ Jr, Jones MB: Size discrimination on the skin. Science 163:488–489, 1969.
37. Renfrew S, Melville ID: The somatic sense of space (choraesthesia) and its threshold. Brain 83:93–112, 1960.
38. Carter P: Personal communication, April, 1980.
39. Dellon AL, Munger B: Correlation of sensibility evaluation, hand function and histology, in press 1981.
40. Paul RL, Goodman H, Merzenich M: Alterations in mechanoreceptor input to Brodmann's areas 1 and 3 of the post-central hand area of Macaca mulatta after nerve section and regeneration. Brain Res 39: 1–19, 1972.
41. Horch K: Guidance of regrowing sensory axons after cutaneous nerve lesions in the cat. J Neurophysiol 42:1437–1449, 1979.

Chapter 9

VIBRATORY SENSE AND THE TUNING FORK

INTRODUCTION
PREVIOUS CLINICAL STUDIES
TUNING FORK
VIBROMETER
POSITION SENSE
CLINICAL APPLICATIONS
VIBRATORY TESTING

INTRODUCTION

"Pallesthesia," the sense of vibration. What is it? Is there a distinct vibratory "sense" as there is a sense of smell? Is the perception of a vibratory stimulus mediated by its own submodality-specific neuroanatomic pathway, such as the perception of sound or light? The answer to these questions is "No."

From the time the doctor or therapist begins health care studies, he (she) is taught from the anatomist's archives and by the neurologist's classic approach. The perception of vibration, or vibratory sense, is taught as if it were a separate sensory submodality, such as pain, temperature, and touch. This is further confounded by being termed "bone conduction." Tuning forks are applied to bone prominences like the lateral malleoli, the frontal bone and the mastoid process. The final step in this subliminal indoctrination is the constant association of this "vibratory sense" with known spinal cord anatomy; "vibratory sense" is destroyed with lesions to the posterior white columns, the fasciculus cunneatus and gracilis.[1-5]

Vibration, or the "sense" of flutter-vibra-tion is simply another touch submodality. Perception of a vibratory stimulus is the same as perception of successive, brief touch stimuli. As the neurophysiologists now have demonstrated clearly, the nerve fibers that mediate the perception of vibratory stimuli are the large myelinated fibers, the group A, beta fibers, and they are characterized as belonging to the quickly-adapting fiber group.[6-8] Thus, vibratory stimuli are mediated by the same nerve fiber population that mediates the perception of moving-touch!

The perception of low frequency vibratory stimuli, about 30 cycles per second (30 cps) is mediated by a quickly-adapting fiber/receptor system, the Meissner corpuscle in glabrous skin, and the hair follicle lanceolate endings in the hairy skin. The perception of high frequency vibratory stimuli, about 256 cps, also is mediated by a quickly-adapting fiber/receptor system, the Pacinian corpuscle in glabrous skin, and the hair follicle lanceolate endings in the hairy skin (see Chapter 3).

The clinical evaluation of vibratory perception tests the same neural pathways as moving-touch. These do go from the fingertip to the brain via the posterior spinal white columns. Vibratory stimuli, however, offer unique possiblities in evaluating peripheral sensibility. Testing is readily done with the tuning fork, an instrument almost as prevalent as the ubiquitous paper clip. Patients are generally naive in tuning fork experiences. A tuning fork stimulus, therefore, is usually a new experience, and the patient need not involve his "association" cortex in an attempt to label or name his perception. He need only answer whether or not he perceives "something" and compare it to another fingertip's perception of the same stimulus. Vibratory perception is nonnoxious: drunks are awakened by it, children laugh at it, the acutely injured patient is not further discomforted by it.

PREVIOUS CLINICAL STUDIES

Diabetes mellitus was among the first disease states to be studied with vibratory stimuli. Williamson[9] was the first to note diminished vibratory perception in diabetic neuropathy. Observations by others soon followed[10] and continued to be refined.[11] Clinical evaluation of other forms of peripheral neuritis included those associated with tabes and pernicious anemia.[12, 13]

Investigations into vibratory perception in the normal population demonstrated decreasing perception with increasing age, with this loss being due primarily to changes in threshold.[11, 13–15]

Reports of vibratory stimuli used to evaluate peripheral sensibility in the hand are few (Table 9.1). Minor[16] may have been the first to note abnormal vibratory perception following nerve injury (1904). In 1936, Gilmer[17] briefly reported a patient with a palm laceration who had divided the common volar digital nerves to the middle, ring, and little fingers. The injury was followed for 2 years. A nerve repair is not stated explicitly. The earliest perception to return was low-frequency vibratory perception with high amplitude at the fingertip. At 2 years, thresholds were returning to normal and higher frequencies could be perceived.[17]

In 1970, McQuillan[18] tested a "mechanical vibrotactile stimulator" in which he varied stimulus amplitude and frequency to get a "sensogram" similar to an audiogram. His subsequent report[19] compared these sensograms with classic two-point discrimination in 13 uninjured "controls" and in seven patients following median nerve repair. He concluded that "sensibility to vibratory stimuli is lost after median nerve division. The loss diminishes with the passage of time after nerve repair. The degree of loss of vibratory sensibility can be accurately measured," and that vibrotactile threshold assessment is "superior to two-point discrimination as a method of assessment of results of nerve repair." However, the "sensogram" calculations require the determination of the difference between vibratory thresholds for successive tuning curves during the course of sensory recovery. Though perhaps highly accurate, I feel this method is cumbersome and not readily applicable.

In 1972, I reported the use of two tuning forks, 30 and 256 cps in evaluating recovery of sensation following nerve repair.[20] These frequencies related to the maximum sensitivities of the two subpopulations of quickly-adapting fibers as determined by Mountcastle,[8] and were believed to be related to the Meissner and Pacinian end organs, respectively. Tuning forks were subsequently reported useful in determining when to initiate sensory re-education[21] (see Chapter 12). Eval-

Table 9.1

Diagnosis of Bilateral, Carpal and Cubital Tunnel Syndromes[a]

Vibratory Stimuli	Right		Left	
	Thumb	Little Finger	Thumb	Little Finger
256 cps	±	±	±	±
30 cps	±	±	±	±
t_{120}	.36	.50	.36	.50
Two-point				
Classic	6	8	6	8
Moving	4	4	4	4
Hand-dorsum				
Ulnar vs radial	↓		↓	

[a] These carpal and cubital tunnel syndromes were in a 20-year-old woman with rheumatoid arthritis.

uating sensory recovery with tuning forks has since been used by Jabaley et al.[22] in attempting to correlate the clinical results of nerve repair with the histologic pattern of reinnervation and by Lindblom and Meyerson[23] in evaluating the functional results of digital replantation.

Most recently, I reported our clinical experience with the use of vibratory stimuli to evaluate peripheral nerve injury and compression neuropathy.[24] The study evaluated 148 injured nerves in 101 patients, and demonstrated that the tuning fork is an acceptable, convenient, simple and quick test of nerve integrity in the emergency milieu. The study further demonstrated that altered vibratory perception is possibly the earliest clinical finding in peripheral compression neuropathy, and may, therefore, be the best sensory test with which to monitor compartment syndromes. The results of the study will be discussed in detail below.

TUNING FORK

The earliest observations on vibratory perception are those of Valentin from 1852. He was studying the "sense of touch impression." He modeled his test instrument after clockworks or small thin wheels with teeth. He called his instrument a "Tastscheibe," a touch disc, or cogwheel. By knowing the number of teeth on the wheel and how fast he was moving it across the fingertip, he could calculate touch frequencies. In an analogy to the flicker-fusion phenomenon in optics, he was interested in when the perception of many small touches became altered, and in the capacity of nerves to transmit these rapid frequency stimuli.[25]

von Wittich's work, reported in 1869, is cited by both von Frey[26] and in the review by Fox and Klemperer[27] as using this cogwheel to study vibration. von Wittich also reportedly[26] employed organ pipes for his vibratory studies.

Rumpf[28] introduced the tuning fork into clinical use in 1889. He employed a set of 14 tuning forks with frequencies ranging from 13 to 1000 cps. He reported normal values and observations on a case of syringomyelia. In 1899, Gradenigo[29] modified the tuning

forks for auditory testing. By adding a calibrated black and white triangle to the vibrating prongs, he could calibrate amplitude, and thus stimulus intensity. Symms[30] introduced the tuning fork into neurology in 1918.

Of interest is von Frey's comment[26] that prior investigations (before 1915) used the tuning fork by striking its prongs and placing the single stem end against the test area. He believed that vibratory perception was mediated through receptors in the skin. He believed that vibration was repetitive touch stimuli and not a separate vibratory sense. To test vibration, he attached a "sensory hair" to the prong of a 100-cps, electromagnetically driven, tuning fork. I believe, therefore, that von Frey was the first to use the pronged end of the tuning fork as the stimulus end.

To appreciate von Frey's contribution in this area it must be recalled that "bone conduction" a term still with us, originated with Max Egger in 1899.[31] Egger believed that the receptor for vibratory perception was bone and that the tuning fork was the best instrument to test "skeletal sensibility." This theory was challenged by Rydel and Seiffer in 1903. Their clinical observations led them to conclude vibration was perceived not only of bone, but also by the fine nerve fibers beneath the skin.[31] Minor also argued against bone being the receptor of the vibratory "sense."[16] During his investigations, von Frey actually anesthetized the skin with a novocaine solution containing adrenalin ("suprarenin"). He found vibratory perception diminished only in the "white" skin areas. He believed cutaneous receptors perceived vibration and that bone was a simple mechanical conductor of the vibratory wave to other areas of skin.[26]

Today, the tuning fork has left the realm of curiosity. Indeed, it has become almost commonplace, and, perhaps as such, almost ignored. Although virtually every second year medical student arms himself with a tuning fork before entering the clinical arena, the progessively parochial training course toward medical specialist reduces the ranks of those armed with tuning forks to those in the neurosciences. Nevertheless, tuning forks are standard hospital equipment and are found routinely in the drawer in the examining

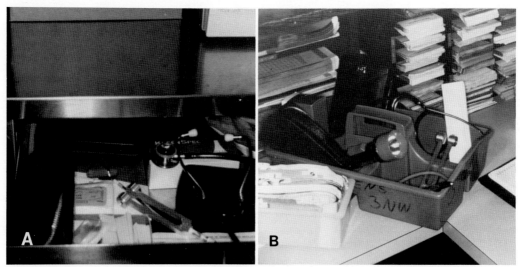

Figure 9.1. Tuning forks are standard hospital equipment. They can be found in the drawer of the consultation room (*A*) and in the physical exam tray or basket on the ward (*B*).

room, in the physical exam box in the nurses station, and in the emergency room (Fig. 9.1). The available tuning fork is usually one capable of vibrating in the midfrequency range, 128 or 256 cps.

The technique of tuning fork application that is taught traditionally in medical school contrasts to the technique I suggest for evaluating sensibility in the hand (Fig. 9.2). Traditionally, the base or the nonpronged end of the tuning fork is applied to a thin-skinned bony prominence:

The examination was conducted in the following manner: The same force of blow being used each time, the fork was struck and the *base* in contact with the styloid process of the ulna. The patient was asked to describe what he felt. If his description did not indicate a distinct perception of the vibration, he was tested with the nonvibrating fork and asked if there was any difference between the two contacts. If he did not perceive any, he was not examined further. If he gave a clear description, the fork was struck again, and he was asked to state the instant the sensation ceased. Then the prongs were touched to stop the vibration, and if he did not reply instantly, the examination was discontinued. If his reply was simultaneous with the cessation of vibration, the fork was struck again and the length of time the vibration was felt was estimated with a stopwatch. Five such examinations were made on each of the

following bony points: styloid process of the ulna, styloid process of the radius, olecranon process, internal malleolus, external malleolus, tibia and patella. If there was a considerable discrepancy in the results obtained from any one point, ten trials were made at that point. The results presented are the averages of at least five trials for each point tested. In order that the element of fatigue might be excluded as much as possible, two successive examination were not made at one place.[27]

I believe that when the tuning fork is employed to evaluate peripheral sensibility in contrast to cranial nerve VIII or the posterior spinal tracts, the prolonged ends of the tuning fork should be employed. The fingertips have significant subcutaneous tissue interposed between the skin and bone, and the prongs, having greater amplitude of vibration than the base of the tuning fork, provide a more intense stimulus. The normal threshold for vibration varies with the stimulus frequency. The lower frequencies have a higher threshold, and therefore require a greater amplitude for perception.[8] In the normal hand the threshold values are all low, and the vibrating tuning fork base certainly can be perceived. However, in nerve compression and following nerve repair, the thresholds are significantly increased. Accordingly, I feel that the greater amplitude available at the pronged end makes the pronged end the stimulus of choice in evaluating peripheral sensibility. The examiner will be using a supramaximal stimulus. The patient's altered perception, therefore, cannot be due to using a stimulus of insufficient intensity (Fig. 9.2).

Which frequency tuning fork should be chosen? As discussed in Chapter 3, the 30-cps tuning fork is best to evaluate the Meissner afferents, the quickly-adapting fiber/receptor system located in the superficial dermis. The 256-cps tuning fork is best to evaluate the Pacinian afferents, the quickly-adapting fiber/receptor system located in the deep dermis and subcutis. Both are needed if you are (1) following the recovery of sensation after nerve injury; (2) deciding the appropriate timing and phase of sensory reeducation; and (3) investigating peripheral sensibility. However, for clinical evaluation of nerve injury, either nerve compression or nerve division, both appear to be equally valid and, as a matter of convenience, I use the small 256-cps tuning fork. Any available tuning fork may be used in the range between 30 and 256 cps. I have no experience with the 512-cps tuning fork, but feel that it may not stimulate enough of the low-frequency responsive Meissner afferent to reflect accurately the status of the entire quickly-adapting fiber population.

How do you evaluate the patient's perception of the tuning fork stimulus? This can only be done qualitatively. Precisely for this reason, that is, in order to have a quantitative evaluation of vibratory sensibility, the "pallesthesiometers" were developed (see next section). For most clinical evaluations, however, a qualitative assessment is both accurate and sufficient.

Testing

In order to achieve a vibratory stimulus of sufficient intensity (amplitude) to evaluate the compressible, spongy fingertip pad, we hold the tuning fork's prong tangentially to the fingertip. The area to be tested is always compared to its contralateral area. Additionally, the area is compared to an ipsilateral noninvolved area. For example, if the patient, by history, has a right carpal tunnel syndrome, the right thumb and index finger are tested and compared to the right little finger (ulnar versus median innervated) and to the left thumb and index finger. If the patient reports altered perception of either of the vibratory stimuli in either thumb or index finger in the test areas in contrast to any control areas, the evaluation is recorded as "abnormal." For example, if the patient, by inspection, has a laceration over the radial side of the right index finger's proximal phalanx, the radial side of the right index finger just distal to the interphalangeal joint (but not the fingertip) is tested and compared to the finger's ulnar digital nerve "autonomous zone" and to the radial side of the left index finger. Again, if the patient reports altered perception of either of the vibratory stimuli in comparison to either the ipsilateral ulnar digital or contralateral radial digital area, the evaluation is recorded as abnormal. The tuning fork is struck anew between each test area. The examiner uses his own acoustic perception of the resultant vibration. as well as his own tactile feedback of the striking force (and the pain generated in his patella), to judge roughly equivalent supramaximal stimulus intensities.

If an altered perception is elicited, the stimulus is repeated again. Perception is judged "altered" if the patient answers affirmatively to the question, "Did those *two* feel *different*?" This is followed by the question, "How did they feel?" Response examples judged "positive" for an abnormal perception are: "I didn't feel anything," "it felt softer, or "louder, or "quieter", or "as if my finger were covered with a layer of cloth," etc. Not asked is the question: "Did you feel *that*?" The patient, whose eyes are shut when the tuning fork is applied to the test area, is also asked to localize the perception. Often with a digital nerve divided at the middle phalanx or a median nerve division, a vibration is perceived when the fingertip is stimulated but the perception is localized to the finger's dorsum. This occurs not because the nerve being tested is functioning, but because the vibratory wave travels down the finger, stimulating a nerve innervating an adjacent nerve territory.

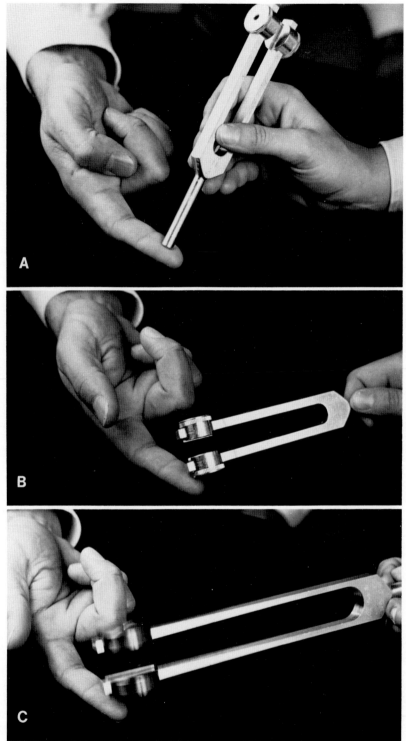

Figure 9.2. Method of tuning fork use. *A*, Traditional techniques as applied by neurologists and otorhinolaryngologists to bony prominences. *B* and *C*, Technique suggested for evaluating peripheral sensibility. The prong end has greater amplitude and is more suitable to test the fingertip pulp in patients with altered vibratory threshold.

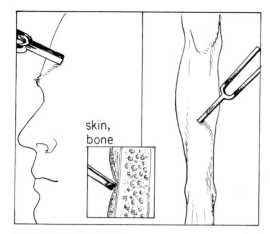

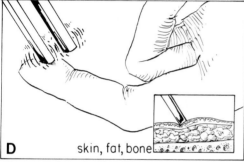

Figure 9.2. *D*, Traditional areas of tuning fork application are in close proximity to bone. The fingertip has greater volume of subcutaneous tissue.

VIBROMETER

The need of basic scientists and clinical investigators to quantitate the vibratory threshold led to the production of various "pallesthesiometers." Many of the early investigators believed that vibration was not touch, but a separate sense. In 1890, Tomson,[33] described the "extraordinary" ability of two deaf people to know of changes in their immediate environment by perceiving transmitted vibrations. He wrote vibration ". . . almost assumes the dignity of a special sense." Treitel[34] was a strong advocate of vibration being a separate sense. He observed in 1897 that 128-cps stimulus was not well-perceived in the lips and cheek, places which were very sensitive to touch. Furthermore, in cases of syphyllitic and alcoholic neuritis, vibration could be perceived while perception of touch was lost. Thus, Rydel[32] felt it

appropriate to name this special sense of whirring from the Greek word for quivering: the term "Pallesthesia" was born. The instrument to measure this "sense" would be termed, of course, a "pallesthesiometer." Because, as discussed in this chapter's introduction, "vibratory sense" is not a separate sense, the term "vibrometer" will be used throughout the remainder of this section. (A good historical review of this "separate sense" question is available by Geldard.[35])

The most quantitative a tuning fork assessment could be was to count the seconds from the stimulus perception to stimulus fade out, as recommended by Williamson,[9] or the so-called "alternate displacement method," recommended by Head.[36] In this latter method, the lapsed time is measured between the cessation of vibratory perception on one side and the moment when the fork, still vibrating, is no longer perceived on the contralateral side.

To quantitate vibratory threshold, the vibratory stimulus had to be controlled. An electrically controlled "rheocord" was described in 1902,[37] and an electromagnetically driven fork in 1904.[16]

Two basic vibrometer variations were developed ultimately: frequency could be varied with amplitude constant, such as the model that was utilized to test Helen Keller,[38] or amplitude could be varied, with a constant frequency, usually chosen as 120 cps, because of the 60-cycle alternating current circuit.[39, 40] Cosh[13] has described a vibrometer in which both frequency and amplitudes can be varied. Recently (1977) Daniel et al.[41] with a uremic population reported on the value of the "Biothesiometer", a variation on the amplitude-variable model. Our experience with this model has been reported, and will be summarized below (Fig. 9.3).[42]

I believe the vibratory threshold stands in relation to the moving two-point discrimination test as the von Frey hair measurement does to the classic two-point discrimination test. The vibratory threshold, determined at a given frequency and at a given "spot" on the fingertip, tells you the functional status of a given quickly-adapting fiber/receptor, or its peripheral receptive field. If the threshold is low (normal), a single fiber and its peripheral receptive field are either (1) normal or (2) recovered from the injury, compression or repair. However, a single functioning nerve fiber and its peripheral field are insufficient for tactile gnosis. Tactile gnosis requires a "large number" of overlapping peripheral receptive fields. Evaluation of this capacity requires a measurement of the innervation density of this system: which is provided by the moving two-point discrimination test. Thus, a patient may perceive a 30-cps and 256-cps stimulus, have a normal vibratory threshold at 120 cps at his fingertip, but still be unable to identify an object placed within his fingertips (see Chapter 10 for these functional correlations of sensory testing).

Vibratory threshold determinations are useful occasionally in diagnostic dilemmas. The patient with bilateral nerve compressions deprives the clinician of his normal "contralateral control." In these instances, having available an "absolute" such as the vibratory threshold can be helpful. For example, with a bilateral carpal tunnel syndrome, the tuning fork test demonstrates usually an equal perception of the stimulus between both thumbs. The perception is nearly always considered much better or "louder in the little fingers." However, the situation may arise with bilateral carpal and bilateral cubital tunnel syndromes (I've seen this three times) where vibratory thresholds can demonstrate that although vibratory perception is uniform in all fingers, it is really uniformly reduced. However, in my experience, by the time this has occurred, the moving two-point discrimination test is also abnormal (Table 9.1).[42] Of course, electrodiagnostic studies are also available (though not "on the spot" and they are "invasive" and expensive).

The vibratory threshold is abnormal in peripheral nerve compression syndromes such as carpal tunnel and cubital tunnel syndromes. With surgical decompression of the involved nerve, these abnormal high thresholds return to normal.[42] Although vibratory threshold determinations are not required for diagnosis in the routine situation, the observed improvement in threshold values can be useful in monitoring the patient postoperatively. In the patient following ulnar nerve release at the elbow, for example, where there is loss of tactile discrimination preoperatively, often the postoperative hyperesthesia or slow course of recovery are taken by the patient as signs that the operation was not "successful." In such circumstances, demonstration that the vibratory threshold has improved provides the "objective proof" needed for patient (as well as physician) reassurance. The not infrequent combination of median-at-the-wrist and ulnar-at-the-elbow compression offers another situation for reassurance. Relief of the carpal tunnel symptoms is often quick and dramatic, while the little finger paresthesia persists. In complex hand injuries, neurolysis follow-up is also aided by threshold monitoring (Table 9.2).

In summary, I have found[41] vibratory threshold measurements are accurate, easy to do, and quick. They give values whose interpretation, allowing for age-variance, is in agreement with our standard sensory evaluation techniques (the paper clip and tuning fork). Vibratory threshold measurements rarely have been required for diagnosis. Vibratory threshold measurements have been of value in the office setting, primarily in longitudinal studies, where progressive improvement in the threshold has proven reassuring at a time prior to recovery of moving two-point discrimination.

POSITION SENSE

In many ways, the "position sense" is similar to the "vibratory sense." We again have been conditioned early in our training to believe that there is a "sense" that deals with keeping us informed of the location, in three-dimensional space, of one part of our body with respect to another. Again, like vibration, we are told that this "sense" is conveyed by fibers traveling in the posterior spinal tracts, whose impulses are generated by joint receptors and musculotendenous junctures.

Erik Moberg[43, 44] deserves the credit for bringing to our attention the very important observation that "position sense" or proprioception is primarily related to cutaneous sensibility. The realization came during his work with tetraplegics. I thank him for reminding me of the work from the Depart-

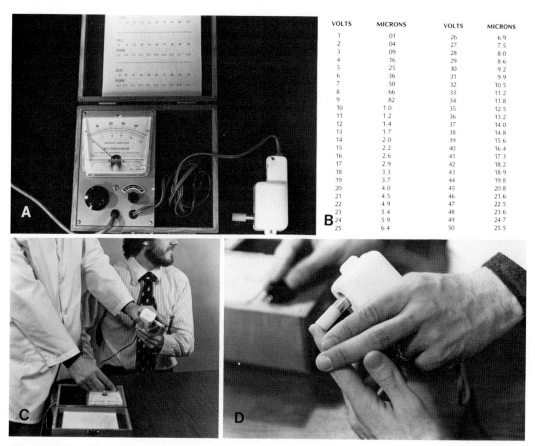

This table shows the Vibratory Amplitude of your Bio-Thesi-ometer vibrator button in MICRONS OF MOTION at 120 cycles per second. (A micron is 10 to the -4th cm.) at different voltage readings on the meter dial. See the page on "Vibratory Thresholds in Normals" which is given in Microns of motion.

VOLTS	MICRONS	VOLTS	MICRONS
1	.01	26	6.9
2	.04	27	7.5
3	.09	28	8.0
4	.16	29	8.6
5	.25	30	9.2
6	.36	31	9.9
7	.50	32	10.5
8	.66	33	11.2
9	.82	34	11.8
10	1.0	35	12.5
11	1.2	36	13.2
12	1.4	37	14.0
13	1.7	38	14.8
14	2.0	39	15.6
15	2.2	40	16.4
16	2.6	41	17.3
17	2.9	42	18.2
18	3.3	43	18.9
19	3.7	44	19.8
20	4.0	45	20.8
21	4.5	46	21.6
22	4.9	47	22.5
23	5.4	48	23.6
24	5.9	49	24.7
25	6.4	50	25.5

Figure 9.3. The vibrometer. Illustrated (*A*) is the Biothesiometer, an amplitude-variable, fixed frequency (120 cps) instrument. *C* and *D*, End of vibrator is held in contact with the fingertip while the stimulus intensity is gradually increased. The threshold is read as the voltage required to deliver the perceived stimulus. Voltage is converted to microns of displacement (stimulus intensity) from the calibration chart (*B*).

ment of Orthopedics at Johns Hopkins in which patients who had total hip replacements were still able to demonstrate good hip position sense.[45] Previously, Gelfan and Carter[46] had demonstrated that there is no "muscle sense" in man. A pull on tendons at the wrist did not cause awake volunteers to perceive finger movement. Only finger movement did this.

Certainly there are quickly-(Pacinian) and slowly-(Rufini) adapting endings within joint capsules, but they appear to initiate impulses at the extremes of their joint's range of motion, acting more in a protective way than for true proprioception.[47, 48]

There is a close relationship between "vibratory sense" and "position sense," both of which are conveyed via the group A beta

Table 9.2
Neurolysis Ulnar Nerve in Wrist and Palm Six Months Following Electrical Burn and Skin Grafting[a]

Date	Thumb				Little Finger			
	m2PD (mm)	2PD (mm)	256	t_{120}	m2PD (mm)	2PD (mm)	256	t_{120}
Preoperation 11/13/79	2	3	nl	.16	6	18	↓↓	1.0
Operation 1/10/80								
Postoperation								
2/22/80	2	3	nl	.16	4	10		.36
3/14/80	2	3	nl	.16	3	5	nl	.25
5/30/80	2	3	nl	.16	2	4	nl	.16

[a] Abbreviations used are: m2PD, moving two-point discrimination; 2PD, classical two-point discrimination; 256, vibratory stimuli at 256 cps; t_{120}, vibratory threshold at 120 cps in micrometers.

fiber population. In 1936, Newman and Corbin,[49] in a paper primarily concerned with describing a variable-amplitude, 60-cps vibrometer, noted that vibratory threshold increased with age and was increased in "arthritics." They went on to conclude: "This would seem to imply that arthritic patients have a greater loss of proprioceptive fibers than a similar age group of normals." In 1942, Fox and Klemperer[27] evaluated vibratory threshold in the hands of patients with brain lesions.[27] Although they did not comment directly on their observations, the three hand diagrams in which impaired position sense was designated for each finger, clearly show a direct correlation between elevated vibratory threshold and impaired position sense. In each of these patients, stereognosis was also severely impaired.

Moberg has found an excellent correlation between two-point discrimination and proprioception in the hand; that is, the best predictor of who will be able to identify correctly the position change of his finger is the two-point discrimination test.[43]

Most recently, Clark et al.[50] have published a study involving percutaneous single-unit nerve recording in awake human subjects. One group of volunteers had intraarticular (knee) local anesthesia and another had a local block of the skin in a 15-cm band about the knee. With either or both types of block, subjects could still correctly identify lower leg position. Does this mean that cutaneous sensibility is not needed for proprioception?

No! The band of skin anesthetized was too narrow. Skin of the entire thigh and lower leg has traction exerted upon it with knee flexion/extension.

Another recent study, utilizing percutaneous single-unit nerve recordings, defined the extent of activation of the different mechanoreceptive afferents during finger movement.[51] In brief, all four categories (Meissner and Pacinian groups of quickly-adapting, and types I and II slowly-adapting) were excited by voluntary finger movements. Slowly-adapting units were active during static finger positions. Few true joint receptors (fibers where activity was present only with joint movement and for which there were no peripheral receptive cutaneous field) could be found. Thus, the mechanism of cutaneous sensibility has the capacity to mediate position sense.

In summary, I believe that position sense is a complex function comprised of afferent impulses from three sources (1) the musculotendinous afferent which may affect primary synergistic/antagonistic muscle balances and impact minimally at the conscious level; (2) the joint receptors, which appear to begin entering the conscious level only as potentially injurious joint activity (extremes) is approached; and (3) the large, myelinated nerves subserving cutaneous sensibility (probably the slowly-adapting fiber/receptor system) which appears to be primarily responsible for the awareness of joint position in the functional range.

CLINICAL APPLICATIONS

Nerve Division

Most clinicians feel they can diagnose an acute nerve injury, certainly a completely divided nerve in the upper extremity. And the vast majority of clinicians could, easily, make the diagnosis of a divided median or ulnar nerve at the wrist. But how about a partial nerve injury? How about the same evaluation in a child? And what of the more distal hand injuries, say, in the palm, through a small wound not associated with tendon injuries? The isolated digital nerve injury, without associated tendon injury is, perhaps, the most difficult to diagnose, even for experienced examiners.

I feel the tuning fork offers several advantages in the diagnosis of nerve locations. The vibratory stimulus is gentle, nonthreatening, noninvasive, and accurate. Children accept it. Drunks accept it. The patient in pain accepts it. The tuning fork can be applied to a bandaged hand without having to unwrap it. It is quick. These advantages were demonstrated[42] in patients with upper extremity lacerations potentially involving nerves.

In 48 patients with 78 nerves at risk for potential division, evaluation of sensibility with vibratory stimuli was correlated with anatomic findings at surgical exploration. This included six median, five ulnar, two radial, and 65 digital nerves. Altered vibratory perception correlated in all cases with conduction block in the nerve. There were 0% false positives (Fig. 9.3). We use the term "conduction block" because in four of the 52 nerves evaluated for which diminished vibration was perceived, the nerves (digital) were still intact: in two they were stretched and lax, having sustained a "stretchy palsy" (snow blower injury) and in two they were contused and hemorrhagic (having had epineurium stripped) (Fig. 9.4). The other 26 nerves although lying directly below a deep skin laceration, were judged to be intact on the basis of the patient's perception of the vibration (Fig. 9.5). In each of these cases, at surgical exploration the nerves were intact. There were 0% false negatives (Table 9.3).

Evaluation of the puncture wound to the palm with associated sensory change is a challenge. The offending agent is commonly a knife or a piece of glass. Conceivably, the numbness or paresthesia over the web space (most usually the ring/little finger web) could be from a contusion to the nerve. Often the patient is not agreeable to exploration of "such a small hole." In these instances, the tuning fork examination usually demonstrates diminished vibratory perception over the distribution of the digital nerve or common volar digital nerve in question. I advise waiting 4 to 6 weeks and begin tetanus/antibiotic prophylaxis. I follow them at regular, close intervals. In only one of our patients has vibratory perception returned to normal, accompanied by a progressive decrease in palmar pain over 4 weeks, with ultimate complete recovery. Five other patients had persistent decrease in vibratory perception and palmar pain. These patients were explored. Three had complete divisions, requiring secondary repair or grafting. Two had incontinuity neuromas, requiring secondary repair (Fig. 9.6). I repaired the nerve as much to relieve the palmar pain as to restore peripheral sensibility.

Evaluation of the isolated digital nerve injury is so difficult because there is overlap at the fingertip. The autonomous zone is proximal to the fingertip and doesn't extend to the volar midline (Fig. 9.7). Some authors[52, 53] have suggested this overlap in the pulp doesn't exist. Wallace and Coupland,[53] for example, carried out an anatomic dissection on 25 thumbs and 25 index fingers. They found that "no evidence of cross-over of nerve supply to the other side of the thumb . . . (or) of the pulp was apparent." However, these were gross dissections done on embalmed specimens. The appropriate study would involve nerve-staining a serially sectioned finger pulp from a patient with a single digital nerve injury. If such a possibility were encountered, that histologic investigation would be important. There is no doubt, clinically that such pulp overlaps occur: often patients have been referred to me who "could feel the needle stick in the fingertip" when examined in the emergency room, who later required repair of their digital nerve injury (Fig. 9.8). Weckesser[54] tested two-point discrimination before and after a digital nerve

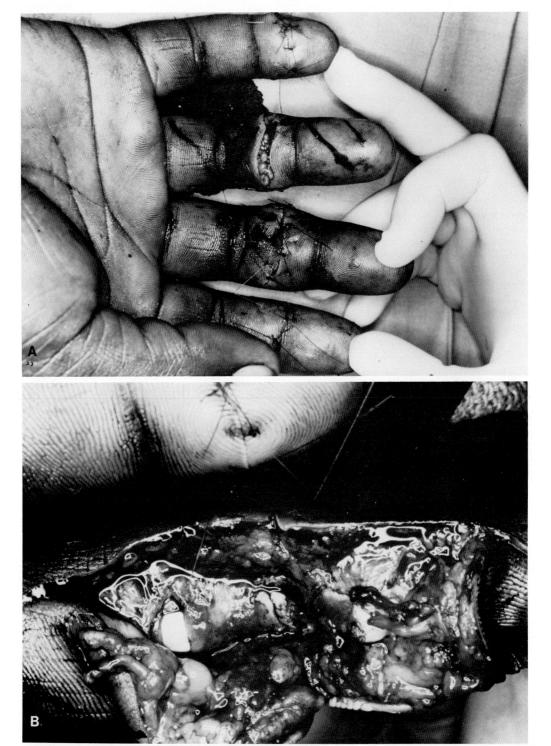

Figure 9.4. Evaluation of potential acute nerve injury. *A*, Patient had lacerations to fingers sutured and was then referred for "tendon injury to middle finger." Preoperative tuning fork evaluation was abnormal. *B*, Intraoperative evaluation demonstrated complete division of ulnar neurovascular bundle and radial digital nerve in addition to tendon injury.

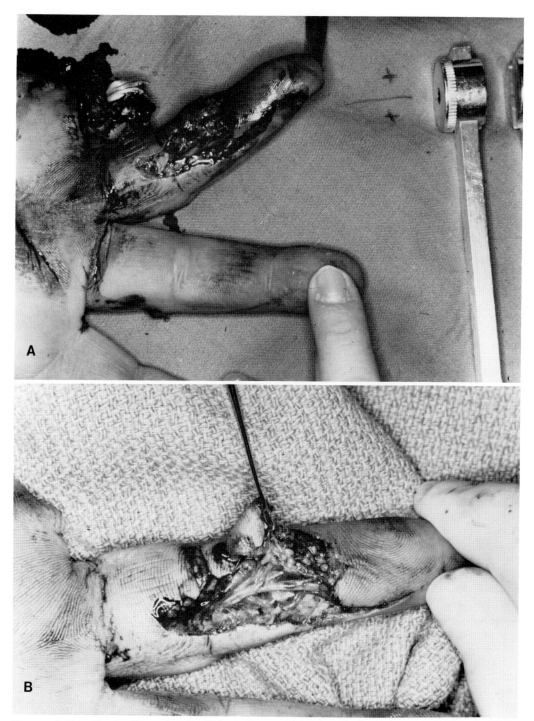

Figure 9.5. Evaluation of potential acute nerve injury. *A*, Radial saw injury amputated little finger and avulsed segment of soft tissue from side of ring finger. Vibratory perception was normal. *B*, At exploration, digital nerve was found intact, without either contusion or stripped epineurium.

Table 9.3
Evaluation of Potential Acute Nerve Injuries[a]

Vibratory Perception	Clinical Evaluation	Operative Findings (%)	
Normal (n = 26)	Nerve functioning	Nerve intact	100
Abnormal (n = 52)	Nerve conduction blocked	Nerve divided	92
		Nerve stretched	4
		Nerve contused	4

[a] n = number in group.

block in patients after digital nerve repair. In the majority of patients, the value changed after nerve block, demonstrating function overlap (Fig. 9.9). Poppen et al.[55] have again emphasized the problem of diagnosing and evaluating recovery in a single digital nerve injury precisely because of this overlap at the pulp. A recent (1975) description of how to diagnose a digital nerve injury demonstrates the inadequacy of most current approaches to this problem.[56]

The examination may be confined to testing the reaction to pain either by pain-pinch or by pinching the skin of the the finger and fingertip with a forceps. Sometimes nerve damage can be diagnosed by inspection of the wound. During the convalescent period, a more detailed examination is necessary including two-point discrimination of tactile gnosis, but these tests are often difficult to do successfully on digital nerve lesions.[56]

I studied 20 fingers which had a single completely divided, digital nerve, and evaluated them for the perception of constant-touch, moving-touch, 30- and 256-cps stimuli, and classic and moving two-point discrimination. In every case, the patient stated he could feel the examiner's fingers moving over the so-called autonomous zone of the divided nerve. Testing done to the finger's tip was usually normal. In every case, the patient stated he could feel something touch him when the examiner's finger pressed, with any but the lightest touch, upon this same area. Classic two-point discrimination was greater than or equal to 8 mm (transversely across the finger), and moving two-point discrimination was greater than or equal to 6 mm in comparison to the 2 to 3 mm discrimination on the noninjured side of the finger. If the digital nerve was divided proximal to

the branch to the dorsum of the finger, then the two-point discrimination tests were each greater than or equal to 10 mm. Perception of either 30-cps or 256-cps stimuli was always perceived as diminished over the test area when compared to the noninjured side.

In summary I feel that tuning fork testing, in which a perceived difference in vibration exists between the two tested autonomous zones of the digit, is a highly accurate diagnostic test for digital nerve injury. In acute injuries, I feel it is the method of choice.

Nerve Compression

Mechanisms/Diagnosis

Basic to the diagnosis of nerve compression is the pathophysiology. Understanding the mechanism of compression neuropathy gives insight into the best diagnostic approach. For example, after 25 years experience with 1,201 cases of chronic nerve compression (carpal tunnel syndrome), Posch and Marcotte,[57] make the diagnosis as follows:

On examination, dryness over the thumb and first 2.5 fingers leads one readily to a diagnosis of carpal tunnel syndrome. Examination with pin prick for decreased sensation is extremely important. Thenar atrophy is noted in long-standing cases.

Dryness, due to loss of function of the sympathetics, and analgesia, due to loss of function of the pain fibers, are related to the thinnest nerve fibers in the median nerve. Are the thinnest fibers the first fibers to lose function? Surely, muscle atrophy is diagnostic, but what should the earliest signs be? It was only a generation ago that before the surgeon (Learmonth) was called by the neurologist (Woltman) at the Mayo Clinic, the diagnosis required "the tips of the second and third digits . . . with vesicles and ulcers . . . and complete anesthesia" to be present.[58] Present knowledge of pathogenesis and neurophysiology should allow a different approach today.

Recall that the peripheral nerve is a mixed nerve having fibers varying in size from 1 to 2 μm. (c fibers) to 25 μm. (A-alpha fibers, motor). In the sensory component of the mixed nerve, a very large percentage of fibers are the large, 15 to 20-μm. A-beta fibers, the

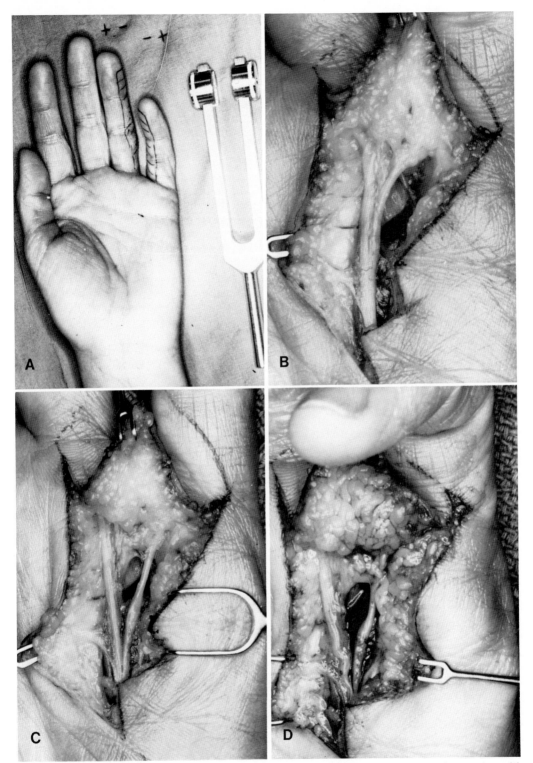

Figure 9.6. Evaluation of potential acute nerve injury. Puncture wound to palm with minimal but definite decrease in vibratory perception over ulnar half of ring finger and marked decrease over ulnar half of little finger. *A*, At surgery a large neuroma was found (*B*). Neurolysis of scarred digital nerve to ring and nerve suture to digital nerve to little finger after resection of neuroma (*C* and *D*).

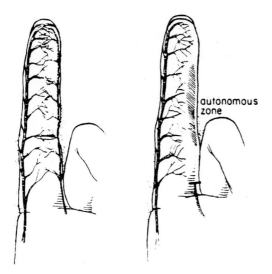

autonomous
zone

Figure 9.7. Overlap of digital nerve peripheral receptive fields at the fingertip, so that testing at the fingertip, itself, is misleading when evaluating the single digital nerve injury. Test the autonomous zone.

"touch fibers." When a local anesthetic is injected around a mixed nerve, it crosses the epineurium via diffusion, and via diffusion into each component nerve fiber. The thinnest nerves are therefore affected first, and, as each surgeon has usually had a chance to learn for himself, the first perceptions lost are those related to the thinnest fibers, temperature and pain. Loss of "touch", movement, and pressure are the last perceptions to be lost (see Fig. 9.10).[59]

When neural ischemia is produced by an upper arm tourniquet, for example, oxygen tension is reduced in the vessels supplying the nerve. The oxygen gradient from inside the vaso nervosum to the axoplasm decreases. The large nerves, with more axoplasm, are affected by the decreased gradient sooner than the thin nerves, whose smaller diameter allows the available oxygen still to supply its needs at a time when the large fibers cease to function. Thus with ischemia, the first perceptions to be lost are those of the large fibers: touch. Pain perception is lost last. The patient experiences "pins and needles"[60] (see Fig. 9.10).

When direct pressure is applied to a nerve, the overall force applied to the epineurium is distributed throughout the fascicles to the axons within. Some unequal distribution will occur as a gradient from directly beneath the two pressure points toward the nerve areas farthest away. But within a given fascicle, the largest axons will directly press upon the nearest axon neighbor. Large axons will abut large axons, creating, at least at the initial pressure gradient levels, microinterstices. Within the small sheltered spaces will lie then the thinnest nerves (see Fig. 9.10). Thus, with direct pressure upon a nerve, the first perceptions to be lost should be those of the larger nerves: touch. Pain perception should be lost last. Indeed, experimental and clinical observations support this sequence.[61, 62]

It may be argued that direct pressure on a nerve has its effect, in pathogenesis, by diminishing blood flow (Fig. 9.10). Direct pressure induces neural ischemia. This is the postulated mechanism in the acute compartment syndrome.[63, 64] However, the critical observation coming from this pathoneurophysiology, is that with compression neuropathy, acute or chronic, the first sensory component to become affected and therefore the first perception to become altered is touch, not pain. We should direct our diagnostic testing not with a pin or needle, but with techniques to evaluate the perception of touch. I suggest the tuning fork.

Carpal Tunnel Syndrome

The clinical presentation and anatomical basis of the carpal tunnel syndrome are well known and have been described extensively, if not exhaustively. Perhaps the most thorough and well referenced treatment of this subject is Spinner's.[65]

The purpose of this section is to present the value of vibratory testing in nerve compression problems, beginning with the most common. I believe that abnormal vibratory perception in the thumb and/or index finger, in comparison to ipsilateral little finger, is the earliest possible nonprovocative sign (and often positive when the provocative signs are negative) in the carpal tunnel syndrome and therefore deserves a place in the clinical examination.

Comprehensive sensibility evaluation was performed on 36 patients with a history compatible with the carpal tunnel syndrome.[42] In

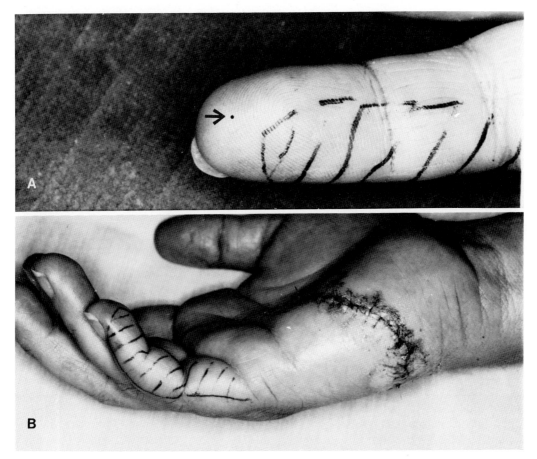

Figure 9.8. Evaluation of potential acute nerve injury. *A*, Note dot at fingertip pulp where first examiner found a normal response to needle stick and pronounced the digital nerve intact. Vibratory perception over autonomous zone was abnormal. *B*, Note sutured hypothenar laceration and outline of sensory defect. At exploration there was complete division of digital nerve to ulnar side of little finger.

28% of these patients, perception of vibratory stimuli was equal (normal) in the thumb and index finger of the affected hand in comparison to the ipsilateral little finger and contralateral digits (see Table 9.4). In this group with normal vibratory perception, both the classic and moving two-point discrimination were normal, and electrodiagnostic studies were normal (except for one patient with increased *motor* latency). The provocative type examinations demonstrated a normal Tinel's sign (negative Tinel) in 90% and a normal Phalen's test (negative Phalen) in 60% of this group (see Table 9.4).

In 72% of the patients with a history compatible with the carpal tunnel syndrome, there was an abnormal perception of vibratory stimuli. In this group, both classic and moving two-point discrimination were normal in 50% of the patients. In those patients with abnormal vibratory perception who were evaluated further, Phalen's test was negative (normal) in 30%, Tinel's sign was negative (normal) in 39%, and electrodiagnostic studies were normal in 37% (see Table 9.4).

Was either of the two tuning forks more discriminatory or less ambiguous than the other? No. Because it is smaller and, therefore, easier to use, the 256-cps tuning fork would appear to be the more preferable testing instrument.

All the patients studied following release

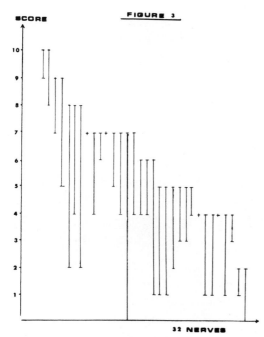

Figure 9.9. Demonstration of digital nerve overlap at fingertip. Note drop in "sensory score" (which included two-point discrimination) in 28 of 32 patients after single digital nerve block. (Reproduced with premission from E. C. Weckesser: *Clin Orthop* 19:200–207, 1961.[54])

of the carpal tunnel syndrome demonstrated return of vibratory perception to normal.

Cubital Tunnel Syndrome

The purpose of this section is not to describe the cubital tunnel syndrome, its pathogenesis or operative care. Again Spinner's[66] description is encyclopedic. I wish to emphasize here that vibratory testing has the potential to improve early diagnostic accuracy in peripheral compression neuropathy. Certainly when the patient presents with a hollowed thumb/index web space, or protruding metacarpal shafts with a carrot-tipped little finger, ulnar problems not only immediately are apparent but also are usually beyond the help of surgical decompression.

My earlier observation,[42] that vibratory perception is diminished in the little finger in contrast to the thumb volarly and over the ulnar half of the hand in contrast to the radial half dorsally, has been confirmed without

exception in our subsequent cubital tunnel patients. The return of vibratory perception to normal heralds the recovery of tactile discrimination. The finding over the dorsum of the hand is critical since it localizes the compression to a site above the wrist, and in my experience is usually present (or becomes abnormal) before weakness in the flexor profundus to the little finger.

Acute Compartment Syndromes

By acute compartment syndrome is meant the relatively sudden occurrence of a rise in pressure in a closed space through which space passes a nerve. If a leukemic has a bleeding episode within the carpal canal, an acute carpal tunnel syndrome results. This would be rare. Probably the most common use refers to the posttraumatic rise in pressure due to bleeding, for example, in the anterolateral compartment of the lower leg, often associated with fibula fracture. In the upper extremity, rapid pressure rises can, most commonly, place the median nerve in the forearm in jeopardy. Mechanisms are missile injury, crush, bleeding (brachial artery punctures for blood gasses), etc. In the wrist, of course, and in the small spaces of the hand, pressure rises also place the enclosed nerve in potential danger. Prolonged pressure rise will stop circulation, with ischemic damage to muscle, and ultimately with soft tissue loss. For the purposes of this discussion, the burn (extracellular fluid extravasation beneath an eschar) is included as an acute compartment syndrome.

Diagnosis of a compartment syndrome is taught traditionally to be made by the combination of symptoms and signs that include pain in the compartment, pain in the muscles passing through the compartment when insertion, e.g., toe, is moved (passive muscle stretch), loss of arterial pulses distal to the compartment, e.g., dorsalis pedis, and diminished "sensation", e.g., pin prick. However, based on the foregoing discussion, it should be clear that this traditional diagnostic complex is composed of relatively "late" signs and symptoms. The earliest symptom theoretically should be paresthesias distal to the compartment, coupled with pain or a sense of fullness within the compartment. The earliest sign should be diminished perception of

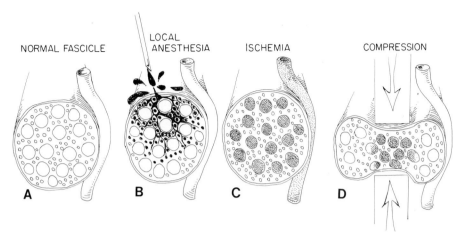

NORMAL FASCICLE   LOCAL ANESTHESIA   ISCHEMIA   COMPRESSION

A   B   C   D

Figure 9.10.   Relationship of fiber diameter to sequence of sensory loss. *A*, The normal nerve is composed of a wide spectrum of fiber diameters. With local anesthetics (*B*) or ischemia (*C*), the diffusion effect is paramount. Large fibers are the last to be affected by anesthetic and the first to be affected by decreased oxygen concentration. With direct compression (*D*), these fibers are initially sheltered from the force by the larger fibers. Thus, with pressure or ischemia, touch and vibratory perceptions are diminished first, and pain and temperature perceptions last. The reverse is true with local anesthetics.

touch which, I believe, in the conscious patient is best evaluated with vibratory stimuli. Interesting in this regard is the observation of Salisbury et al.[67] that digital survival following escarotomy in burned hands correlated better with diminished sensibility than with decreased digital artery (Doppler) flow.

The present state of the art, when a compartment syndrome is suspected, is to directly measure the intracompartmental pressure. Excellent techniques to measure the pressure, documented both experimentally and clinically, have been described recently.[68–73] All of these techniques are invasive and require varying degrees of sophisticated monitoring. However, a simple compartment pressure, close enough to reality to make the decision regarding surgical intervention, can be made by Whitesides' method.[68] Of critical importance to our thesis are the observations[69, 71] that diminished "touch and pain" preceded passive-stretch muscle pain and distal pulse loss and paralysis in the progression of the compartment syndrome (see Fig. 9.11).

Preliminary observations on the use of vibratory stimuli to evaluate acute compartment syndromes in the upper extremity sup-

Table 9.4
Carpal Tunnel Syndrome

Normal Values	Vibratory Perception	
	Normal	Abnormal
Provocative tests		
Phalen's sign	60%	30%
Tinel's sign	90%	39%
Electrodiagnostics		
Sensory latency	100%	37%
Two-point discrimination		
Classical	100%	50%
Moving	100%	50%

port the thesis that the tuning fork evaluation can make an early diagnosis.[42]

Nine patients with potential for acute onset of median nerve compression at the wrist were evaluated. All demonstrated altered vibratory perception. As examples, consider first two burn patients in whom the extremity burns were extensive. One patient had no perception of vibration on admission; escarotomies were done without recovery of vibratory perception (see Fig. 9.12). In this patient, all digits were lost. The other burn patient (see Fig. 9.13) had normal vibratory perception on admission, but during the fluid resuscitation phase had increased extremity swelling. The vibratory perception became diminished. Escarotomy and release of the

COMPARTMENT SYNDROME PROGRESSION

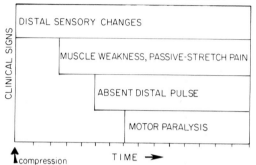

Figure 9.11. Compartment syndrome sign-symptom progression. The earliest symptoms are pain in the compartment and numbness and tingling distal to the compartment. The earliest sign is diminished touch perception, best tested with vibratory stimuli.

carpal tunnel were performed with subsequent return of normal vibratory stimuli. Ultimately there was survival of full digital length in all fingers.

Perhaps most important is the inference from the early observations[42] that a progressive diminution in vibratory perception might be used as a guide to time surgical intervention in the evolving acute compartment syndrome.

If perception of vibratory stimuli became abnormal at or before the critical increase in compartment pressure was recorded (and the exact pressure level remains a debated issue) then perhaps those who are either not familiar with the techniques or don't want to use an invasive technique would have a reliable alternative, i.e., the tuning fork. I have already initiated the clinical study to determine this: correlating perception of vibratory stimuli with compartment pressures in our patients, and include here the first three patients.

For the first patient (see Fig. 9.14), I thank Doctor Larry Leonard who, at the time the

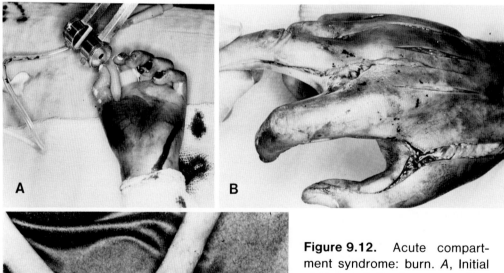

Figure 9.12. Acute compartment syndrome: burn. *A,* Initial absence of vibratory perception in severe burn. *B,* No recovery of perception postescarotomy. *C,* Ultimate full digital loss bilaterally.

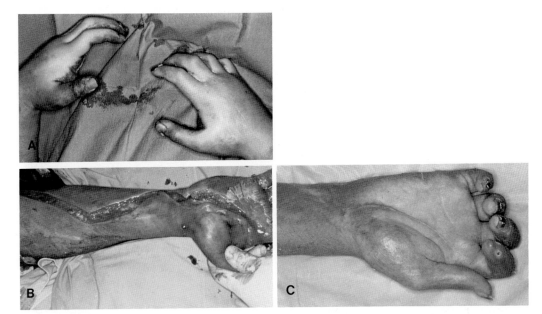

Figure 9.13. Acute compartment syndrome: burn. *A*, Initial good vibratory perception was lost during fluid resuscitation and escarotomy was performed (*B*). Ultimate full digital salvage (*C*).

patient was studied, was the chief resident in plastic surgery at Johns Hopkins Hospital. For the third patient (see Figure 9.16), I thank Doctor Russell Moore, who, at the time the patient was studied, was the Hand Fellow at Union Memorial Hospital's Raymond M. Curtis Hand Center.

The first patient was noted to have a markedly swollen, purplish and painful hand on the day following a coronary bypass procedure. The radial artery had been catheterized prior to the procedure to provide monitoring and the catheter removed in the intensive care unit prior to the hand becoming swollen. Because of the patient's critical condition, intraoperative exploration of the radial artery and pharmacologic manipulation of the peripheral vascular system were not possible. The patient had diminished (abnormal) vibratory perception. Compartment pressures were obtained using the technique described by Kingsley et al.[72] in which the I.C.U. pressure gauges are connected to the compartment, a small bolus of sterile saline injected into the compartment, and the pressure read at equilibrium. Pressures were 30 mm Hg and, in this low cardiac output state, were considered elevated. Dorsal space fasciotomies were done with good release of the pressure and ulti-

mate full tissue and hand function salvaged (Fig. 9.14).

The second patient (see Fig. 9.15) sustained a crush injury to his right hand and wrist 24 hours prior to his emergency consultation. On examination, he had a grossly swollen and ecchymotic palm and volar forearm. He had greatly diminished vibratory perception over his thumb, index, and middle fingers. Pain perception was still intact. Release of his carpal tunnel was advised and was refused. I elected then to follow him with compartment pressures while elevating his hand. Tuning fork perception improved concomitant with a decrease in compartment pressure. Over the next month, he recovered normal sensation.

The third patient, a drug addict, was seen in the emergency room 24 hours after the onset of hand pain. On examination, there were recent injection sites in the antecubital fossa, the hand was cold, swollen, bluish, and without radial or ulnar pulses. There was perception of pain on vibratory stimuli (Fig. 9.16). Compartment pressure in the forearm and carpal tunnel were 90 and 100 mm Hg. Despite extensive fasciotomy, the hand became gangrenous, requiring amputation.

These three cases suggest that vibratory perception becomes abnormal when the pres-

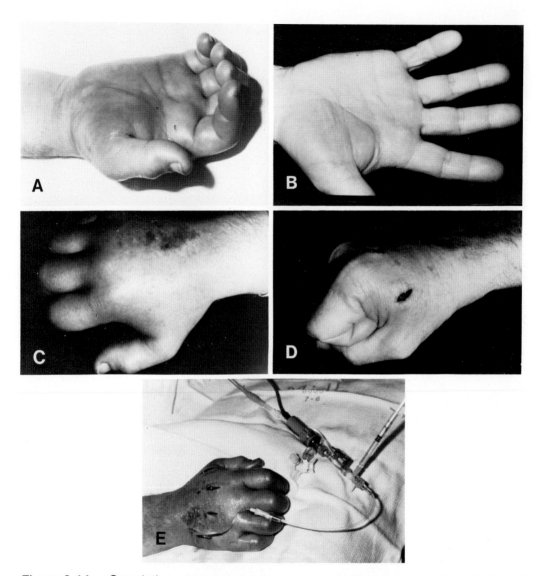

Figure 9.14. Correlating compartment pressure and vibratory perception. Before (*A* and *C*) and 1 week after (*B* and *D*) fasciotomy in a man who developed ischemia of his right hand in the immediate period following coronary bypass surgery. The right radial artery had been catheterized before the cardiac surgery and there was impending gangrene. Vibratory stimuli could be perceived but were abnormal in comparison with the left hand. *E*, Apparatus used for pressure monitoring.

sure in the compartment surrounding the nerve reaches 35 to 40 mm Hg. This is the pressure at which most advocates of compartment pressure monitoring are advocating fasciotomy. Further clinical experience with these correlations are, of course, needed. Furthermore, I am now directly investigating this in an animal model.

VIBRATORY TESTING

Tuning Fork Advantage

The tuning fork offers a significant advantage to the clinician evaluating a potential nerve injury. For example, in the child it has been observed that "lacerated nerves are fre-

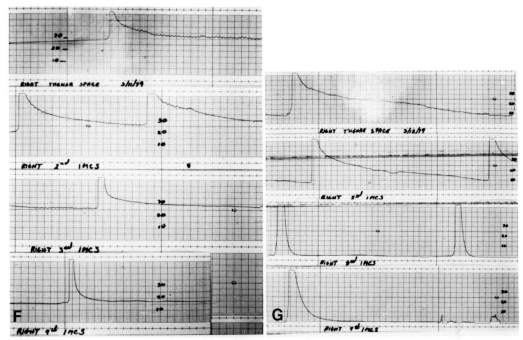

Figure 9.14. *F*, Pressure tracings before and (*G*) 8 hours after fasciotomy. Pressures dropped from 30 mm Hg. to 0 to 10 mm Hg. There was no tissue loss and full function restored. (Reproduced with permission from N. W. Kingsley: *Plast Reconstr Surg* 63: 404–408, 1979.[72])

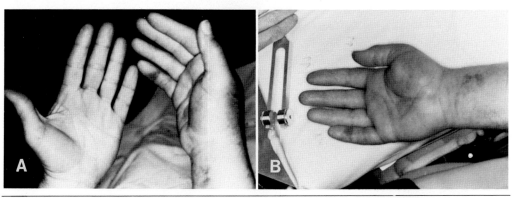

Time Postcrush	Perception of:			Compartment Pressure (mm Hg)		
	Needle Stick	256 cps	m2PD (mm)	Hypothenar	Thenar	Carpal Tunnel
24 hr	+	↓↓	>10	2	40	45
30 hr	+	↓	8	0	28	35
48 hr	+	nl	4	0	5	10
2 wk	+	nl	2	—	—	—

Figure 9.15. Correlating compartment pressure and vibratory perception. *A*, Ecchymotic and edematous right hand and wrist 24 hours after crush injury. *B*, Evaluation of sensibility. Note pain perception was always present. Vibratory perception was greatly reduced initially over thumb and index finger while normal over little finger. Compartment pressures were elevated in thenar eminence and carpal tunnel. Patient responded to continuous elevation of the hand with the clinical improvement noted in chart.

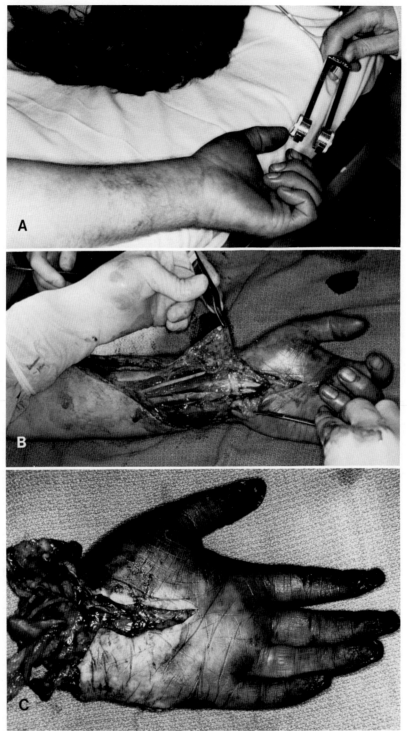

Figure 9.16. Correlating compartment pressure and vibratory perception. *A*, Drug addict 24 hours after brachial artery injection. There was no peripheral pulse, no perception of pain or vibration, and the hand was cold, swollen and bluish. Compartment pressures were 90 to 100 mm Hg and extensive fasciotomies were done (*B*). Gangrene developed, necessitating amputation (*C*).

quently missed" and that sensory loss is "difficult to test for."[74] The tuning fork, perceived by the child as a musical sounding toy, is readily accepted; the usual pin produces fear, if not future distrust. Once the tuning fork is introduced to the child, you simply obscure his view with your hand and apply the tuning fork: his perception of the vibration is signalled by a hand movement or a laugh. Another example is the emergency room encounter with the noncooperative, usually drunk, male patient. In this situation, a needle frequently evokes hostility while the tuning fork's vibrations seem to penetrate the inebriated stupor. In situations where repetitive testing is required, such as evaluating the progress of a nerve repair or recovery from neuropraxia, the tuning fork is an easily applied, noninvasive technique with high patient acceptance. Furthermore, vibratory stimuli are not ambiguous as it is the rare patient who has felt them before. Vibratory stimuli allow you to avoid the situation where you are touching a patient's finger following nerve repair and asking him if he feels your touch. Because the regenerating sensory fibers are often misdirected and always deficient in number, the patient may not interpret the altered profile of neural impulses he is receiving in a manner that lets him answer "yes" to your question. Since he may have no previous memory in his association cortex with which to identify this altered neural profile as "touch," he often will incorrectly answer a question calling for an identification, even though sensibility has been recovered. Vibratory stimuli circumvent this problem.

Potential Pitfalls

As with all diagnostic tests, the tuning fork has potential pitfalls. There are three. First, when evaluating a digital nerve, it is critical that the examiner ask the patient not whether he "feels anything" but whether he "feels the same thing on each side (not the tip) of the finger." If the patient answers "no," then the examiner must pursue the questioning with "how do they differ?" A "positive" test, indicating blocked nerve conduction in the examined nerve, is indicated by the patient's decreased perception of the vibratory stimu-

lus. If the possibility exists that both digital nerves have been injured in the finger, and the patient perceives the stimulus, it is then critical to compare this perception to the contralateral digit. In the case of nerve compression at the wrist, where the perception over the thumb and index are compared to that over the little finger, the contralateral fingertips must be tested for comparison because of the possibility of both median nerve and ulnar nerve compression.

The second potential pitfall is that perception of the stimuli may occur through an adjacent peripheral field of a noninjured nerve, e.g., radial nerve with a median nerve injury. The examiner must always conclude by having the patient localize the stimulus perception. "Where did you feel that?" If the patient points to the dorsal surface of the proximal phalanx of the index finger or thumb when you are testing in the territory of the median nerve, this "perception" should, obviously, not be considered normal. Such events occur, as discussed earlier, because the tuning fork sets up a traveling wave within the substance of the entire finger and this wave may have sufficient energy to stimulate receptors at a distance from the test area. Careful discrimination by the examiner can avoid these potential pitfalls.

Finally, the alteration in vibratory perception is not always a diminution. As I have been examining increasing numbers of patients with early nerve compression problems, I find that often the alteration is one of *hyper*sensitivity. For example, a patient with carpal tunnel symptoms of short duration may observe that the feeling caused by the tuning fork touching the thumb is "more sensitive" or "more electric." It is therefore possible that early in the course of neural ischemia a state of *hyper*esthesia is present. The critical examiner must be aware of this possibility.

References

1. Major RH, Delp MH: *Physical Diagnosis*, ed 6. Philadelphia: WB Saunders, pp 300, 320–322.
2. Currier RD: Nervous system in Zuidema GD, Judge RD (eds): *Physical Diagnosis: A Physical Approach to the Clinical Exam*, ed 2. Boston: Little, Brown, 1968, pp 409–410, 424–425.
3. Truex RC, Carpenter MB: *Human Neuroanatomy*,

Baltimore: ed 5. Williams & Wilkins, 1964, pp 149, 205.

4. Elliott FA: *Clinical Neurology.* Philadelphia: WB Saunders, pp 419-420, 1964.

5. Gilray J, Meyer JS: *Medical Neurology.* Toronto: MacMillan, 1969, pp 2,4,59,60.

6. Mountcastle VB: Physiology of sensory receptors: Introduction to sensory processes, in Mountcastle VB (ed): *Medical Physiology,* ed 12. Saint Louis: CV Mosby, 1968, Ch 61, pp 1345-1371.

7. Konietzny F, Hensel H: Response of rapidly and slowly-adapting mechanoreceptors and vibratory sensitivity in human hairy skin. Pfluegers Arch 368: 39-44, 1977.

8. Mountcastle VB, Talbot WH, Darian-Smith I, et al: A neural base for the sense of flutter-vibration. Science 155:597, 1967.

9. Williamson RT: The vibratory sensation in diseases of the nervous system. Am J Med Sci 164:715-727, 1922.

10. Woltman HW, Wilder RM: Diabetes mellitus: Pathologic changes in the spinal cord and peripheral nerves. Arch Intern Med 44:576-603, 1929.

11. Mirsky IA, Futterman P, Brohkahn RH: The quantitative measurement of vibratory perception in subjects with and without diabetes mellitus. J Lab Clin Med 41:221-235, 1953.

12. Gordon I: The sensation of vibration with special reference to its clinical significance. J Neurol Psychopathol 17:107-134, 1936.

13. Cosh JA: Studies on the nature of vibration sense. Clin Sci 12:131-151, 1953.

14. Pearson GHJ: Effect of age in vibratory sensibility. Arch Neurol Psychiatry 20:482-496, 1928.

15. Rosenberg G: Effect of age on peripheral vibratory perception. J Am Geriatr Soc 6:471-481, 1958.

16. Minor L: Uber die Localisation used klinische Bedeutung der sog. "Knochensensibilitat" oder das "Vibrationsgefuhls". Neurol Centralbl 23:146-199, 1904.

17. Gilmer B von H: A study of the regeneration of vibratory sensitivity. J Gen Psychol 14:461-462, 1936.

18. McQuillan WM: Sensory recovery after nerve repair. Hand 2:7-9, 1970.

19. McQuillan WM, Neilson JMM, Boardman AK, et al: Sensory evaluation after median nerve repair. Hand 3:101-111, 1971.

20. Dellon AL, Curtis RM, Edgerton MT: Evaluating recovery of sensation in the hand following nerve injury. Johns Hopkins Med J 130:235-243, 1972.

21. Dellon AL, Curtis RM, Edgerton MT: Re-education of sensation in the hand following nerve injury and repair. Plast Reconstr Surg 53:297-305, 1974.

22. Jabaley ME, Burns JE, Oratt BS, et al: Comparison of histologic and functional recovery after peripheral nerve repair. J Hand Surg 1:119-129, 1976.

23. Lindblom V, Meyerson BA: Influence on touch, vibration and cutaneous pain of dorsal column stimulation in man. Pain 1:257-270, 1975.

24. Dellon AL: Clinical use of vibratory stimuli to evaluate peripheral nerve injury and compression neuropathy. Plast Reconstr Surg 65:466-476, 1980.

25. Valentin G: Ueber die Dauer der Tasteindrucke. Arch Physiol Heilk 11:438-478, 587-621, 1852.

26. von Frey M: Physiologische versuche uber das Vibrationsgefuhl. Z Biol 65:417-427, 1915.

27. Fox JC, Klemperer WW: Vibratory sensibility. Arch Neurol Psychiatry 48:622-645, 1942.

28. Rumpf J: Ueber exinem Fall von Syringomjlie nebst Beitragen zur Untersuchung der Sensibilitat. Neurol Certralbl 8: 183-190, 222-230, 1890.

29. Gradenigo G: A new optical method of acoumetrie. J Laryngol Rhin Otol 14:583-585, 1899.

30. Symns JLM: A method of estimating the vibratory sensation, with some notes on its application in diseases of the central and peripheral nervous system. Lancet 1:217-218, 1918.

31. Egger M: De la sensibilité osseuse. J Physiol (Paris) 1:511-520, 1899.

32. Rydel A, Seifer W: Untersuchungen ueber das Vibrationsgefuhl oder die sogenannte Knochensensibilitat (Pallasthesie), Arch Psychiatr Nervenkr 37: 488-536, 1903.

33. Tomson WB: The general appreciation of vibration as a sense extraordinary. Lancet 2:1299, 1890.

34. Treitel L: Arch Psychol Bd, 29:633, 1897. Cited by Merzenich MM: Some observations on the encoding of somesthetic stimuli by receptor populations in the hairy skin of primates, doctoral dissertation. Baltimore: Johns Hopkins Univ (Physiol), 1968, pp 145-179.

35. Geldard FA: The perception of mechanical vibration: IV. Is there a separate "Vibratory Sense"? J Gen Psychol 22:291-308, 1940.

36. Head H: *Studies in Neurology.* Cited by Fox JC, Klemperer WW: Vibratory sensibility. Arch Neurol Psychiatry 48:623-645, 1942.

37. Grandis V: Sur la mesure de l'acuite auditive au moyen de valeurs physiques entre elles. Arch Ital Biol 37:358-376, 1902.

38. Tilney F: A comparisive sensory analysis of Helen Keller and Laura Bridgman: Mechanisms underlying sensorium. Arch Neurol Psychiatry 21:1227-1269, 1929.

39. Gray RC: Quantitative study of vibration sense in normal and pernicious anemia. Minn Med 15:674-680, 1932.

40. Cohen LH, Lindley SR: Studies in vibratory sensibility. Am J Psychol 51:44-51, 1938.

41. Daniel CR, Bower JD, Pearson JE, et al: Vibrometry and neuropathy. J Miss State Med Assoc 18:30-34, 1977.

42. Dellon AL: The vibrometer, in press 1981.

43. Moberg E: Fingers were made before forks. Hand 4: 201-206, 1972.

44. Moberg E: Reconstructive hand surgery in tetraplegia, stroke and cerebral palsy: Some basic concepts of physiology and neurology. J Hand Surg 1:29-34, 1976.

45. Grigg P, Finerman GA, Riley LH: Joint-position sense after total hip replacement. J Bone Joint Surg 55A:1016-1025, 1973.

46. Gelfan S, Carter S: Muscle sense in man. Exp Neurol 18:469-473, 1967.

47. Clark FJ, Burgess PR: Slowly-adapting receptors in

cat knee joint: Can they signal joint angel? J Neurophysiol 38:1448–1463, 1975.

48. Grigg P, Greenspan BJ: Response of primate joint afferent neurons to mechanical stimulation of knee joint. J Neurophysiol 40:1–8, 1977.

49. Newman HW, Corbin KB: Quantitative determination of vibratory sensibility. Proc Soc Exp Biol 35: 273–276, 1936.

50. Clark FJ, Horch KW, Bach SM, et al: Contributions of cutaneous and joint receptors to static knee-position sense in man. J Neurophysiol 42:877–888, 1979.

51. Hulliger M, Nordh E, Thelin AE, et al: The response of afferent fibers from the glabrous skin of the hand during voluntary finger movements in man. J Physiol 291:233–249, 1979.

52. Honner R, Fragiadakis FG, Lamb DW: An investigation of the factors affecting the results of digital nerve division. Hand 2:21–30, 1970.

53. Wallace WA, Coupland RE: Variations in the nerves of the thumb and index finger. J Bone Joint Surg 57B:491–494, 1975.

54. Weckesser EC: The repair of nerves in the palm and the fingers. Clin Orthop 19:200–207, 1961.

55. Poppen NK, McCarroll HR Jr, Doyle JR, et al: Recovery of sensibility after suture of digital nerves. J Hand Surg 4:212–221, 1979.

56. Wallace WA: The damaged digital nerve. Hand 7: 139–144, 1975.

57. Posch JL, Marcotte DR: Carpal tunnel syndrome: An analysis of 1,201 cases. Orthop Rev 5:25–35, 1976.

58. Woltman HW: Neuritis associated with acromegaly. Arch Neurol Psychiatry 45:680–682, 1941.

59. Torebjork HE, Hallin RG: Perceptual changes accompanying controlled preferential blocking of A and C fiber responses in intact human skin nerves. Exp Brain Res 16:321–332, 1973.

60. Lewis T, Pickering GW, Rothschild P: Centripetal parapysis arising out of arrested bloodflow to the limbs. Heart 61:1, 1931.

61. Weddell G, Sinclare DC: "Pins and Needles": Observation on some of the sensations aroused on a limb by the application of pressure. J Neurol Neu-

rosurg Psychiatry 10:26–46, 1947.

62. Landau W, Bishop GH: Pain from dermal, periosteal and fascial endings and from inflammations. Arch Neurol Psychiatry 51:1–26, 1944.

63. Denny-Brown O, Brenner C: Paralysis of nerve induced by direct pressure and by tourniquet. Arch Neurol Psychiatry 51:1–26, 1944.

64. Lunborg G: Structure and function of the intraneural microvessels as related to trauma, edema formation and nerve function. J Bone Joint Surg 57A:938–948, 1975.

65. Spinner M: Carpal tunnel syndrome, in: *Injuries to the Major Branches of the Peripheral Nerves of the Forearms*, ed 2. Philadelphia: WB Saunders, 1978, pp 198–202.

66. Spinner M: Cubital tunnel, in: *Injuries to the Major Branches of the Peripheral Nerves of the Forearms*, ed 2. Philadelphia: WB Saunders, 1978, pp 232–234.

67. Salisbury RE, Taylor JW, Levine NS: Evaluation of digital escarotomy in burned hands. Plast Reconstr Surg 58:440–443, 1976.

68. Whitesides TE, Haney TC, Harado H, et al: A simple method for tissue pressure determination. Arch Surg 110:1311–1313, 1975.

69. Matsen FA, Mayo KA, Kriegmire RB Jr, et al: A model compartmental syndrome in man with particular reference to the quantification of nerve function. J Bone Joint Surg 59A:648–653, 1977.

70. Rorabeck CH, Clarke KM: The pathophysiology of the anterior tibial compartment syndrome: An experimental investigation. J Trauma 18:229–304, 1978.

71. Murabeck SJ, Owen CA, Hargen AR, et al: Acute compartment syndromes: Diagnosis and treatment with the aid of a wick catheter. J Bone Joint Surg 60A:1091–1095, 1978.

72. Kingsley NW, Stein JM, Levenson SM: Measuring tissue pressure to assess the severity of burn induced ischemia. Plast Reconstr Surg 63:404–408, 1979.

73. Matsen FA, Wenquist RA, Krugmire RB: Diagnosis and management of compartment syndromes. J Bone Joint Surg 62A:286–291, 1980.

74. Lindsay WK: Hand injuries in children. Clin Plast Surg 3:65–75, 1976.

Chapter 10

EVALUATION OF SENSIBILITY IN THE HAND

INTRODUCTION
TESTING FUNCTIONAL SENSATION
EVALUATION

I am quite convinced that physiology alone, unaided by clinical observation, would be very slow in unraveling the mysterious functions of the nervous system.

M. von Frey, *1906*[1]

INTRODUCTION

Many tests have been described to evaluate sensibility in the hand (Table 10.1). On what basis should we select the tests to use? I suggest that our goal is to evaluate hand sensibility within the framework of rehabilitation of the hand. Our goal is not to localize a lesion within the central nervous system. The main distinction here is that tests must be chosen that have a neurophysiologic basis and that have been demonstrated to correlate with hand function (Table 10.2).

The results of testing for the perception of pain or for the perception of temperature indicate whether protective sensation is present and whether the spinothalamic tracts are intact. Testing for perception of pain and for perception of temperature does not correlate with ability to perform hand functions such as sewing on a button or winding a watch. Tests of pain and temperature are, therefore, "academic" and do not measure functional sensation. Tests of sudomotor function also do not correlate with hand function. If a nerve is divided, all sensory submodalities are effected. If a nerve is repaired with even a small

degree of accuracy, sweating and perception of pain and temperature virtually always recover.[2, 3] I suggest, therefore, that evaluation of sensibility of the hand, within the framework of hand rehabilitation, need not include tests of sudomotor function, pain or temperature perception.

I suggest that evaluation of sensibility of the hand, when the goal is: (1) diagnosis of a peripheral nerve injury or compression neuropathy, (2) evaluating recovery following nerve repair, (3) initiating sensory re-education, or (4) determining functional impairment, may be defined as evaluation of the fiber/receptor systems that mediate the perception of touch. The approach to be outlined below is highly efficient in terms of testing time and valid in terms of its neurophysiologic basis and functional correlation.

To put this approach into perspective, one need only review the most recent four attempts to detail evaluation of hand function.[4-7] There is some attempt to orient hand evaluation by ultimate goal. For example, the approach by Swanson et al.[5] is comprehensive, yet clearly oriented toward the motor aspects of hand function. One of their 19

Table 10.1
Evolution of Clinical Tests of Hand Sensibility [a]

...	Unknown	Pin stick, hot/cold, sweating, finger stroking, cotton wool, paper strips, blunt/sharp
1835	Weber	Two-point discrimination
1852	Valentin	Cogwheel
1894	von Frey	Tactile hairs, pain hairs
1909	Trotter, Davies	Localization [b]
1915	Tinel	"Tingling"
1915	von Frey	"Vibratory hairs"
1928	Minor	Starch iodine [c]
1929	Henney	Pallesthesiometer
1943	Seddon	Digit writing [d]
1945	Seddon	Coin test (after Ridoch)
1956	Dawson	Sensory nerve conduction velocity
1958	Moberg	Pick-up test, tactile gnosis
		Ninhydrin
		Paper clip
1960	Semmes-Weinstein	Monofilaments
1966	Parry	Timed recognition test
1966	Porter	Letter test
1969	Renfrew	Depth-sense aesthesiometer (Poppen's "plastic ridge", 1979)
1972	Dellon	Constant-touch, moving-touch, tuning forks, 30 and 256 cps
1973	O'Rian	Palmar skin wrinkling
1978	Dellon	Moving two-point discrimination

[a] All references for these tests other than those specified may be found in their appropriate book chapter through the index and in the combined bibliography.
[b] Reference 35.
[c] Reference 36.
[d] Reference 37.

Table 10.2
Neurophysiologic Basis of Sensation

Sensation	Clinical Test	Neurophysiologic Correlate	Peripheral Receptor	Nerve Fiber Property
Constant-touch	Fingertip touch	Stimulus	Merkel cell-neurite complex	Slowly-adapting
Pressure	von Frey hair	Threshold		
Tactile gnosis (static)	Classic two-point discrimination	Innervation density		
Moving-touch Flutter	Fingertip stroking 30-cps tuning fork, vibrometer	Stimulus Threshold	Meissner corpuscle	Quickly-adapting
Tactile gnosis (moving)	Moving two-point discrimination	Innervation density		
Moving-touch Vibration	Fingertip stroking 256-cps tuning fork, vibrometer	Stimulus Threshold	Pacinian corpuscle	Quickly-adapting
Tactile-gnosis (movement)	Moving two-point discrimination	Innervation density		

items of clinical information pertains to sensibility, and this item subdivides into the pick-up, two-point, and ninhydrin test (Fig. 10.1). These tests are described in two paragraphs of a 38-page chapter and described under the heading of "neurologic examination." Furthermore, the definition of sensory impairment is "complete loss of palmar sensation." This implies that presence of just protective sensation, that is absence of tactile gnosis, would not be evaluated as impairment of sensation. Fess et al.[6] present a beautifully outlined, balanced approach to evaluating hand function, in which sensibility is given detailed consideration. Their hand charts (Fig. 10.2) require evaluation of classic two-point discrimination, moving-touch, con-

stant-touch, 30-cps and 256-cps vibratory stimuli, Tinel's sign, von Frey hairs, pain and temperature perception, proprioception, hypersensitivity, and the Moberg pick-up test. This comprehensive program is similar to one utilized to evaluate the nerve-injured servicemen recovering from war wounds and reported by Omer.[4] Omer reported 26,900 separate tests! These were performed as a matrix of 12 tests repeated every 6 weeks in the initial phase of sensory recovery. Critical to Omer's approach was the determination of cutaneous pressure thresholds with Semmes-Weinstein monofilaments and classic two-point discrimination with a Boley gauge or eye caliper.[8]* Judith Bell, who also relies heavily on Omer's schema, conceptualized the problem well.[7] She wrote, "What is desired is a simple test that can be easily and reliably performed in a variety of clinical settings. Many are the tests that have been described ... Each test gives us a picture of the elusive perception we call (sensation) ... It may be wise to trade the idea of a simple test for that of thorough testing." Her approach to evaluating sensibility combines exhaustive Semmes-Weinstein monofilament and Weber two-point discrimination testing of the hand supplemented by electrodiagnostic testing. This approach approximates ours in that it emphasizes a quantitative evaluation of the touch submodality but differs from ours in two critical ways: (1) it is limited to the slowly-adapting fiber/receptor system, the smallest subpopulation of the touch spectrum; and (2) it stresses determinations of threshold values in preference to innervation density (Fig. 10.3).

Testing Functional Sensation

Given a choice of just one test of sensibility with which to evaluate a hand and predict the ability of that hand to *function*, which test should be chosen? To answer this question, a study must both evaluate sensibility

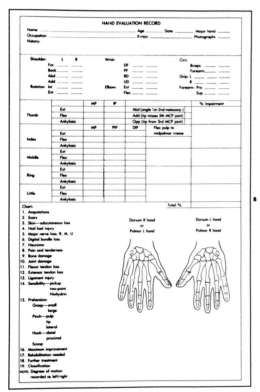

Figure 10.1.   A comprehensive approach for evaluating hand function. Evaluation of sensibility is dominated here by the emphasis on motor function. (Reproduced with permission from A. B. Swanson et al: *Rehabilitation of the Hand*, Hunter JM et al (eds). Saint Louis: CV Mosby, 1978.[5])

* It was in this paper that the numerical values of these Semmes-Weinstein monofilaments (these values are really the $\log_{10}$ [force in milligrams]) were reported erroneously in milligrams (see Chapter 6).

and correlate these test results with a measure of actual hand function.

Throughout the past 2 decades, virtually all studies reporting the results of nerve repair, the quality of sensation in various flaps and grafts, and degrees of sensory impairment in nerve compression and neuropathy have reported their end results in millimeters of classic two-point discrimination. The credit for this universal concurrence belongs to Erik Moberg, who, with almost evangelistic zeal, converted pointed caliphers to blunted tips. Moberg resurrected the paper clip from rusting ruin to the Keys of the Kingdom. His clinical investigation, upon which so much of the present-day approach to sensory testing is based, was the first to correlate clinical tests with tests of hand function. Moberg defined hand function in terms of sensory grips. Good hand function implied the presence of tactile gnosis. This meant that with eyes blindfolded, the patient would still "see" with his fingertips. This was measured by his pick-up test. The only test that Moberg found that correlated with the results of this pick-up test was the Weber two-point discrimination test. Moberg studied 10 patients who had median nerve injuries and who, at the time of evaluation had good motor function (Table 10.3).[2] Of these 10 patients, only three had two-point discrimination less than 15 mm. These patients had precision sensory grip and could perform the pick-up test. Five patients had two-point discrimination between 15 and 40 mm. These patients had gross grip, but could not perform the pick-up test. Two patients with two-point discrimination greater than 40 mm could not even perform gross grips. The von Frey measurements did not correlate with hand function. For example, a threshold of 1.0 gm was associated with two-point discrimination values ranging from 5 mm to greater than 40 mm, with corresponding hand functions ranging from precision grip with pick-up test ability to gross grip without pick-up test ability.

On the basis of Moberg's study, a two-point discrimination of less than 12 or 15 mm has been accepted widely as being required for tactile gnosis (precision-sensory grip and the ability to perform the pick-up test). However carefully this group of patients was stud-

ied, I must emphasize that there were just three patients reported in that group of patients having good recovery of functional sensation. Furthermore, the standard for hand function was chosen to be a static grip and a (nontimed, nonrecognition) pick-up test.

Three studies reported at that same time attempted similar correlations of tests of sensibility with tests of hand function (tactile gnosis). These studies have never been quoted at this point, as far as I am aware, probably because the emphasis of these reports was end-results of nerve repair. Flynn and Flynn's findings[9] confirmed Moberg's (Table 10.4). Precision sensory grip was present with classic two-point discrimination less than 15 mm. McEwan's data.[10] however, suggested that tactile gnosis, as measured by a blindfolded pick up test, could be even in patients with poor classic two-point discrimination. Onne's comments[3] that the blindfolded pick-up test was normal with a classic two-point discrimination of less than 7, and abnormal if 16 to 22 mm, agree with Moberg.

Among earlier studies, I can find only two case reports correlating tactile gnosis and the Weber test (Table 10.4). Oester and Davis[11] detailed the 10 best results following median nerve repair at the wrist. Case 4452 had classic two-point discrimination greater than 25 mm but could button his shirt and pick-up a pin blindfolded. Case 4266 had a classic two-point discrimination of 4 mm (thumb) and 12 mm (index) and could pull the correct coins from his pocket. Although the latter case supports Moberg's position, the first case and the results of McEwan's[10] suggest that the Weber test may be missing something, that there may be more to functional sensation than static grip.

Porter[12] studied fingertips resurfaced with flaps and grafts, comparing sensibility tests with hand function. He found the results of his letter test correlated better with ability to perform Moberg's pick-up test than did classic two-point discrimination testing. The average letter test score for those passing the pick-up test was 2.3 compared to 0.9 for those who failed the test. The mean two-point discrimination for those passing the pick-up test was 7.8 mm versus 9.4 for those who failed. No tests of statistical significance were of-

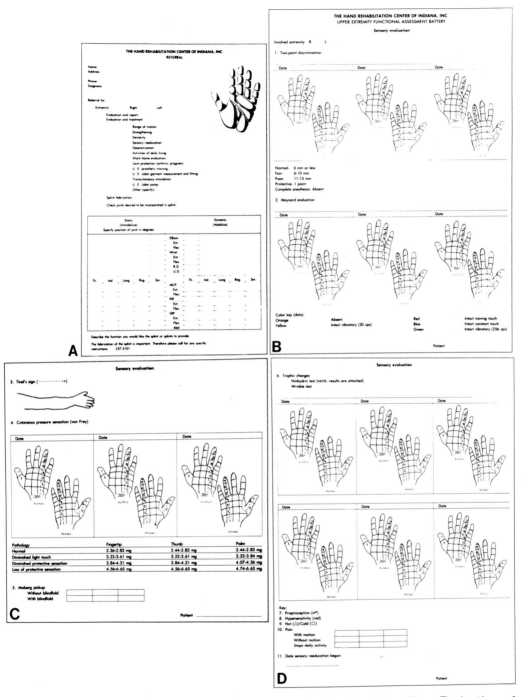

Figure 10.2. A comprehensive approach for evaluating hand function. Evaluation of sensibility plays a prominent role in this balanced approach. (Reproduced with permission from E. E. Fess et al: *Rehabilitation of the Hand*, Hunter JM et al (eds). Saint Louis: CV Mosby, 1978.[6])

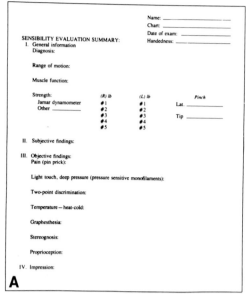

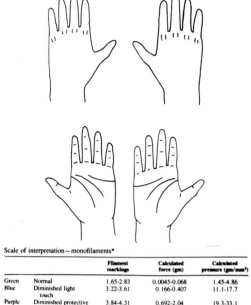

Scale of interpretation — monofilaments*

		Filament markings	Calculated force (gm)	Calculated pressure (gm/mm²)
Green	Normal	1.65-2.83	0.0045-0.068	1.45-4.86
Blue	Diminished light touch	3.22-3.61	0.166-0.407	11.1-17.7
Purple	Diminished protective sensation	3.84-4.31	0.692-2.04	19.3-33.1
Red	Loss of protective sensation	4.56-6.65	3.63-447	47.3-439
Red-lined	Untestable	Greater than 6.65	Greater than 447	Greater than 439

*From Levin, S., Pearsall, G., and Ruderman, R.: J. Hand Surg. 3(3):211, 1978.

B

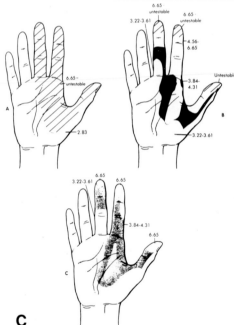

C

Figure 10.3. A comprehensive approach for evaluating hand function. This approach (*A* and *B*), in fact, emphasizes primarily the determination of pressure thresholds (*C*). (Reproduced with permission from J. A. Bell: *Rehabilitation of the Hand*, Hunter JM et al (eds). Saint Louis CV Mosby, 1978.[7])

fered. In another correlation of sensibility tests and hand functions done on patients with flaps (neurovascular island flaps), Krag and Rasmussen[13] noted that patients had the ability to perform the pick-up test yet had poor two-point discrimination.

There has been a recent study on end-results after nerve injury that also attempted to relate sensibility testing to hand function.[14]

In this study, a Vietnam serviceman's nine object recognition test was scored and the results correlated with the Weber test during the course of his sensory recovery (Table 10.5). Although with a Weber test of 16 mm or less, he identified most of the objects correctly, he could also identify some objects when he had effectively no classic two-point discrimination.

Table 10.3
Correlation of Sensibility Testing with Hand Function [a]

Case	von Frey (gm)		Weber test (mm)		Grip Function		Pick-up Test
	Index	Thumb	Index	Thumb	Gross	Precision	
1	1	1	8	5	+	+	+
2	1	0.5	20	15	+	−	−
3	0.5	0.5	15	12	+	+	+
4	1	0.5	12	12	+	(+)	(+)
5	1.5	1	>20	>20	+	−	−
6	1.5	1	>40	>40	+	−	−
7	2.5	1	>60	15	+	−	−
8	2.5	1.5	>40	>40	−	−	−
9	2.5	2.5	>60	>40	−	−	−
10	2.5	1.5	>40	>40	+	−	−

[a] Adapted from E. Moberg.[2]

Table 10.4
Correlation of Tactile Gnosis and Weber Test after Nerve Repair [a]

Age at Injury (yr)	Follow-up (mo)	Grip Function		Weber Test (mm)		
		Gross	Precision	Thumb	Index	Middle
3	84	++	++	3	3	4
10	24	++	++	6	8	8
23	96	+	+	12	14	16
26	84	+	+	14	12	14
24	72	−	+	12	12	12
16	96	−	−	26	26	26
52	132	−	−	40	40	40
16	24		−	26	26	22

[a] Adapted from J. E. Flynn and W. F. Flynn.[9]

Table 10.5
Correlation of Tactile Gnosis and Weber Test after Nerve Repair [a]

Time after Repair (mo)	Classic Two-Point Discrimination (mm)	Object Recognition No. Correct/No. Tried
5	>45	2/9
6	>45	3/9
7	>45	5/9
→[b]		
10	20	6/9
11	16	7/9
12	6	9/9

[a] Patient is 25 years old, with median nerve repair at wrist. (Reproduced with permission from R. L. Reid et al: *Am Soc Surg Hand Newsletter* 15, 1977.
[b] Sensory re-education was begun 8 months after the primary nerve repair.

These types of observations, as discussed in Chapter 8, were part of the stimulus that led me to develop the moving two-point discrimination test.[15] In that study, hand function was related to moving two-point discrimination only in terms of the patients' return to work or to the preinjury level of activity. Specific tests of hand function were not evaluated.

A recent comprehensive report evaluated sensibility after digital nerve suture.[16] Although this study makes conclusions regarding tactile gnosis, it in fact failed to test hand functions. The study did graphically contrast results of von Frey hairs (Semmes-Weinstein monofilaments) with results of the classic Weber two-point discrimination. There was no correlation between these two tests of sensibility (see Chapter 5). For a von Frey range of less than 1.0 gm (their normal threshold value), two-point discrimination ranged from 3 to 32 mm (normal being less than 6 mm). Furthermore, for two-point discrimination values in the 6- to 12-mm range, in which, according to Moberg, tactile gnosis should still be possible, there were many patients with abnormal von Frey values.

Onne's data[3] also demonstrated no correlation between results of the Weber test and von Frey test (Table 10.6).

Poppen et al.[16] used a modified Renfrew depth-sense esthesiometer for evaluating sensibility. This "plastic ridge device" gave values which correlated with neither von Frey hair nor Weber test results. I have explained[17] these findings in light of the neurophysiologic principles discussed in Chapter 3. The Plastic Ridge Device is testing the quickly-adapting while von Frey and Weber test the slowly-adapting fiber/receptor populations. The importance of the Poppen et al.[16] study does not lie in their presentation of a "new test" of sensibility. As discussed in Chapter 8, the Ridge Device is not only based on inappropriate philosophical speculation (there is no somatic sense of space or choraesthesia), but also is poorly calibrated, has a wide range of normal, is difficult to use, and, so far, is difficult to obtain. They failed to correlate Ridge results with either the pick-up or object identification test, so they cannot make a valid correlation of Ridge results with tactile gnosis. The importance of their work is the further confirmation that tests of threshold (von Frey) do not necessarily correlate with tests of innervation density.

In a given test area the threshold for perception of constant-touch/pressure can be normal if just one slowly-adapting fiber reinnervates the appropriate Merkel cell-neurite complex and this has had time to "mature" prior to testing. In an adjacent area this reinnervation may not have occurred, and the threshold would be abnormal (higher). In such a situation, there would be a low peripheral innervation density, a poor (high) two-point discrimination, but in certain areas

Table 10.6
Absent Correlation Between Weber and von Frey Testing[a]

Nerve	Von Frey (gm)	Weber Range (mm)
Digital	0.3	2–18
	1.0	7–25
Median	0.3	2–27
	1.0	6–30

[a] Adapted from L. Onne.[3]

of the fingertip, normal threshold values. Onne's data[3] are also explained by this hypothesis (Fig. 10.4). I believe the slowly-adapting fiber/receptor system is predisposed for this to occur following nerve repair for three reasons: (1) The Merkel cell-neurite complex degenerates more rapidly than its quickly-adapting fiber/receptor system counterpart (see Chapter 4). Therefore, there will be less Merkel cells in an optimal state for reinnervation by the regenerating axon; (2) The ratio of axon to corpuscle in this system is less than one (Merkel cell-neurite complex: <1, Pacinian corpuscle: 1, Meissner corpuscle >1, see Fig. 7.5). Therefore, the chances of a Merkel cell being reinnervated by a regenerating axon is the least likely of the sensory corpuscular endings; and, 3) The slowly-adapting fibers comprise only about one-third of the group A beta fibers (see Chapter 3). Therefore, if only a fraction of the proximal axons re-enter distal endoneurial sheaths, and if only a fraction of these are correctly redirected, i.e., to the correct distal locations and to the correct sensory receptor, the actual number of regenerating slowly-adapting axons is more likely to be below the critical number required to give a peripheral innervation density capable of tactile discrimination. To restate this thesis: regeneration favors recovery in the quickly-adapting Meissner afferent system, the system for movement detection.

Moberg recognized that we needed a new test of functional sensation. Delivering the first Sterling Bunnell Memorial Lecture before the American Society for Surgery of the Hand in 1964, he said[18] "The tools are still crude and must be improved." These concerns have been echoed in 1978 by Narakas,[19] whose sensory evaluation in patients recovering from brachial plexus injuries has demonstrated that "achieved tactile gnosis is not parallel to the clinical tests we have. Good results in the laboratory (clinical examination) can be useless in life and vice versa." The moving two-point discrimination test was presented to the American Society for Surgery of the Hand in 1978, as a quantitative test which answered the criticisms outlined above and in Chapter 6 of the static Weber test. "Every time we conceive and express

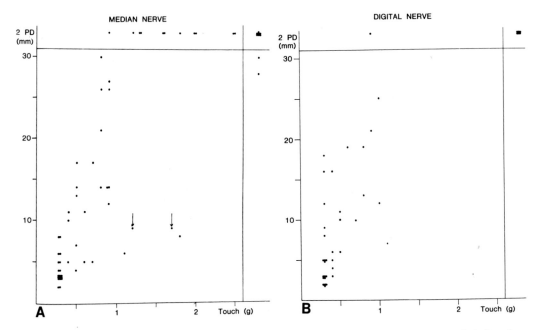

Figure 10.4. Lack of correlation between von Frey hairs and classic two-point discrimination. These data from Onne's work[3] demonstrate a wide range of two-point discrimination values possible for any given pressure threshold under 1.0 gm. For example, for a threshold of 0.3 gm in a fingertip following digital nerve repair, the Weber test result might range from 3 mm (S4 normal) to 18 mm (S3, only gross grip possible). (Reproduced with permission from L. Onne: *Acta Chir Scand [Suppl]* 300:5–9, 1962.[3])

quality as quantity, our knowledge increases and along with it our powers of thinking and acting correctly."[20]

This focus on movement has been emphasized most recently (1980) in a review of thumb replantation from Louisville.[21] A comparison was made between results of classic two-point discrimination (sensibility) and the patient's subjective assessment of his sensory recovery (sensation). Patients listed decreased thumb motion highest as the cause of decreased usefulness of their replanted thumb (Table 10.7). The authors concluded "that greater than 10 mm of two-point discrimination is compatible with good sensation" and that these findings indicate that "motion, as well as sensibility, is important in the replanted thumb." The static thumb cannot use its movement detection system.

The moving two-point discrimination test was validated as a test of tactile gnosis by correlating its results with a test of hand function.[22] In this recent study, patients with

Table 10.7
Correlation between Sensibility and Sensation[a]

Sensibility (Weber Test)	Sensation[b]			
	Poor	Fair	Good	Excellent
<10 mm	0	1	5	3
>10 mm	3	4	4	0

[a] Adapted from J. D. Schlenker et al.[21]
[b] Values indicate number of patients making objective assessment. Ability to move thumb, making moving-touch possible, was more critical to patient assessment than presence of a >10-mm Weber test result.

abnormal sensation following injury to the median nerve, but with normal thenar and ulnar motor function (Moberg's criteria[2]), had a comprehensive evaluation of hand sensibility. This evaluation included moving- and constant-touch, 30- and 256-cps vibratory stimuli, classic and moving two-point discrimination, vibratory (Biothesiometer) and cutaneous pressure (Semmes-Weinstein monofilaments) thresholds, and a timed pick-up (sighted) and object recognition (blind-folded) test. The results demonstrated that tactile gnosis begins to recover when the moving two-point discrimination is less than 7 mm, a time during recovery from nerve repair when classic two-point discrimination is usually greater than 15 mm (see Table 10.8).

This study[22] demonstrated for the first time the functional difference between a recovered peripheral innervation density of the group A beta fiber subpopulations. Among the patients studied were those following nerve repair who had recovered to the point where they could perceive constant-touch, had wide ranging cutaneous pressure thresholds, and two-point discrimination greater than 15 mm. By Moberg's criteria, these patients should have no tactile gnosis. I found that these patients could not perceive an object between their thumb and index finger if they held it with a static grip, nor could they identify the object using a static grip. They could perceive

moving-touch, had near normal vibratory threshold at 120 cps, and moving two-point discrimination between 4 and 6 mm. I found that they could easily identify objects placed between their thumb and index finger if they *moved* the object between their fingers (Table 10.8). As moving two-point discrimination improved below 6 mm, the patients could identify objects more quickly and could identify smaller and more closely related objects. Certainly these patients without classic two-point discrimination had tactile gnosis.

Several patients in the study[22] permitted a fingertip biopsy in an area of carefully evaluated pulp (Fig. 10.5). For example, light and electron microscopy (Figs. 10.6 and 10.7) demonstrated absent Merkel cell-neurite complexes in an area, correlating with the absence of perception of constant-touch, unobtainable cutaneous pressure threshold and absent two-point discrimination. A pattern of reinnervated Meissner corpuscles was present (Fig. 10.8), in an area with perception of 30-cps vibratory stimuli, an elevated vibratory threshold, and moving two-point dis-

Table 10.8
Correlation of Sensibility Testing with Hand Function [a]

Patient, Age	Pressure Threshold (Semmes-Weinstein Markings)			Vibratory Threshold (Vibrometer in microns)			Two-Point Discrimination (mm)				Tactile Gnosis	
							Classic		Moving		No. of Objects Recognized of 12	Mean Recognition Time per Object (sec)
	Control	Thumb	Index	Control	Thumb	Index	Thumb	Index	Thumb	Index		
Nerve repair												
L. F., 27	2.44	5.18	5.18	0.09	0.36	0.66	35	40	12	11	4	12.5
B. K., 22	3.84	4.31	4.56	0.09	0.09	0.09	13	25	7	10	6	4.5
K. L., 29	2.83	4.93	4.93	0.25	1.00	2.60	19	22	7	7	8	4.8
C. E., 24	2.83	4.74	4.93	0.09	0.36	0.66	50	50	10	10	8	7.5
O. O., 30	2.44	4.56	4.31	0.09	0.36	0.16	18	16	8	5	9	7.3
L. T., 30	3.84	5.80	6.10	0.16	0.36	0.50	40	40	6	6	11	17.0
E. L., 60	3.22	4.74	6.45	0.12	0.50	0.36	40	40	6	4	12	9.9
J. C., 34	3.84	4.93	5.18	0.25	1.00	1.00	40	40	4	4	12	9.8
C. H., 18	2.83	4.08	3.84	0.09	0.16	0.09	13	12	5	3	12	2.0
R. O., 23	3.61	3.61	3.84	0.09	0.09	0.66	9	12	2	4	12	5.7
J. M., 32	2.36	3.61	4.17	0.12	0.16	0.16	6	7	3	4	12	3.3
Nerve compression												
P. D., 37	3.61	5.46	5.46	0.25	0.66	0.66	40	40	10	8	10	9.9
D. C., 47	3.61	4.74	6.45	0.16	0.36	3.30	3	13	3	8	12	2.8
M. H., 47	2.83	3.84	3.84	0.25	0.66	0.66	4	7	3	3	12	2.6

[a] Adapted from A. L. Dellon and B. Munger.[22]

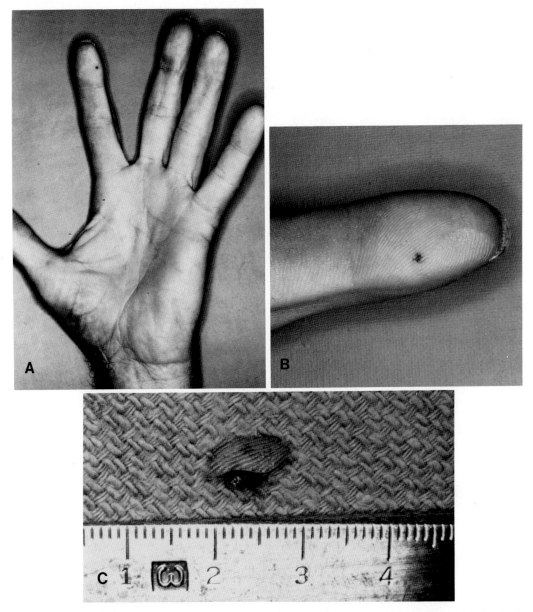

Figure 10.5. Correlation of sensibility tests, functional tests and histology. *A*, Hand of 62-year-old man 1 year after median nerve repair at wrist. *B*, Dot on index fingertip is center of area of high pressure threshold and absent two-point discrimination. *C*, Biopsy of this area in which vibratory threshold was near normal and moving two-point discrimination was present. (Reproduced with permission from A. L. Dellon and B. Munger, in press 1981.[22])

crimination of 10 mm. An innervated Pacinian corpuscle was present in this area, which correlated with the perception of the 256-cps vibratory stimulus.

Would electrodiagnostic techniques provide an alternative method or important adjunct to the evaluation of functional sensation? Should they be obtained routinely? It

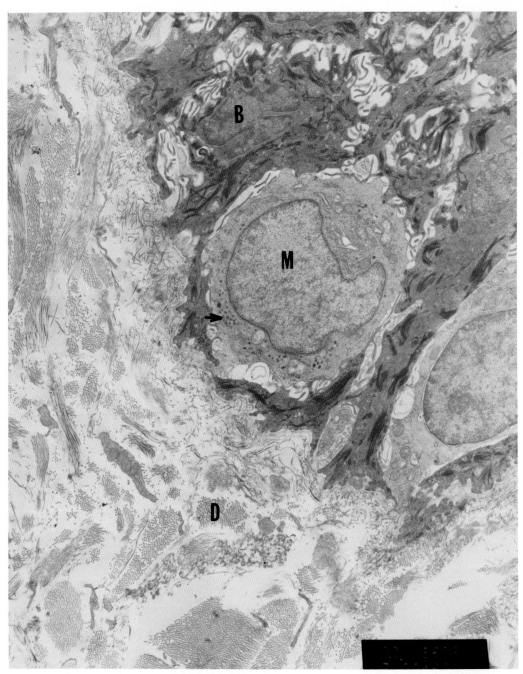

Figure 10.6. Correlation of sensibility tests, functional tests and histology. Electron micrograph (×4600) demonstrating a noninnervated Merkel cell from directly beneath blue dot seen in Fig. 10.5. Merkel cell identification by irregularity of nucleus (*M*) in cell at base of intermediate epidermal ridge with granular cytoplasm. Note absence of axon terminals around the Merkel cell. This was the only Merkel cell in the serial sections of the specimen except for that in Fig. 10.7. *D*, dermal papilla; *B*, nucleus of cell in basalar layer of epidermis. (Reproduced with permission from A. L. Dellon and B. Munger, in press 1981.[22])

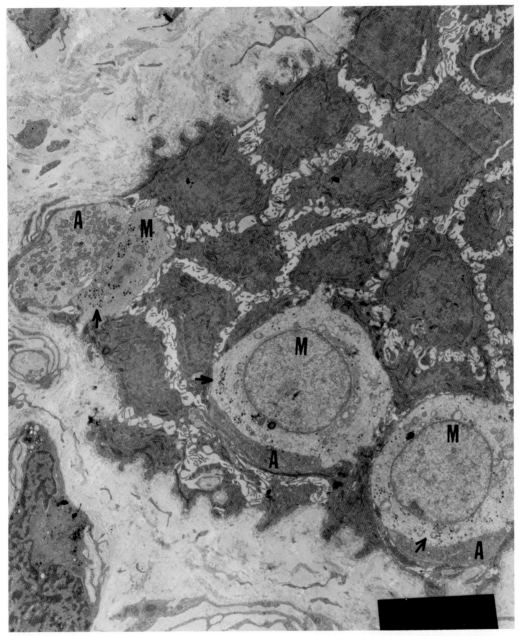

Figure 10.7.   Correlation of sensibility tests, functional tests and histology. Electron micrograph (×2750) demonstrating an innervated Merkel cell (Merkel cell-neurite complex) from the most proximal end of the biopsy specimen in Fig. 10.4. These were the only other Merkel cells in the entire specimen. *M*, Merkel cell nucleus. Note axon terminals (*A*) forming "disc" below the Merkel cell and increased density of the granules in these innervated cells' cytoplasm. The presence of three Merkel cells in this one field is abnormal and represents a reinnervation pattern. (Reproduced with permission from A. L. Dellon and B. Munger, in press 1981.[22])

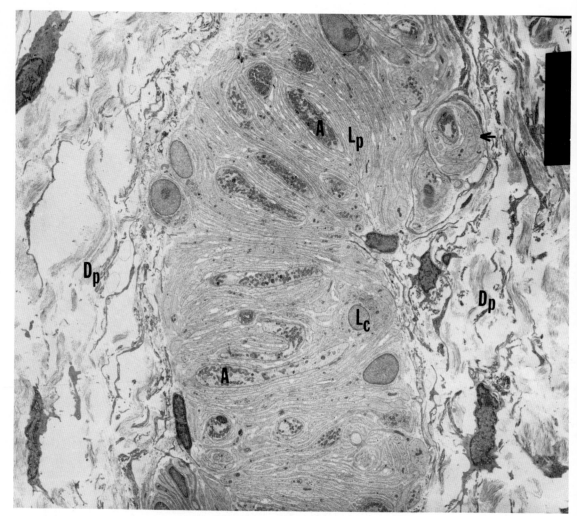

Figure 10.8. Correlation of sensibility tests, functional tests and histology. Electron micrograph (×1650) demonstrating an innervated Meissner corpuscle from the specimen in Fig. 10.4. Note lobulated appearance, multiple axon terminals (*A*) ensheathed by lamellar cell processes (*L_p*). Lamellar cell nuclei (*L_c*) are present at periphery of corpuscle which lies in a dermal papillae (*D_p*). Fully and partially reinnervated Meissner corpuscles were abundantly present throughout specimen. (Reproduced with permission from A. L. Dellon and B. Munger, in press 1981.[21])

has been only relatively recently that sensory nerve conduction velocities have been measured by Dawson[23] in both antidromic and orthodiomic directions (1956). Melvin et al.[24] have demonstrated that the sensory latency becomes prolonged sooner than motor latency in peripherial compression neuropathy. My preliminary data on correlating a comprehensive clinical evaluation with electro-

diagnostic studies in the carpal tunnel syndrome[25] suggested that the tuning fork examination and moving two-point discrimination tests become abnormal earlier than the electrodiagnostic studies. These findings were supported by a later study including 80 extremities with nerve compression.[26] Bell noted that "when a loss of sensibility was measured by the monofilaments, so also was there a delayed or untestable sensory nerve conduction . . . However it is true that nerve conduction can sometimes show indications of a decreased latency before it can be measured by the monofilaments." In 1970, Almquist and Eeg-Olofsson[27] reported nerve conduction-velocity in 19 patients who were at least 5 years after median and/or ulnar nerve suture at the wrist. There was no correlation between either conduction velocity or stimulus threshold and the degree of sensory recovery as evaluated by the classic two-point discrimination (Fig. 10.9). Of potential interest is the recent work of Conomy et al.[28] with cutaneous electrical threshold testing. They are able to detect an abnormal threshold for detection of a 200-msec train of rectangular pulses at 20 Hz in children and adults. This, however, would seem to have little applicability to patients following nerve repair. I conclude that the results of electrodiagnostic studies now available do not correlate with functional sensation in the hand.

In summary, critical review demonstrates inadequacies in the correlation of tactile gnosis with classic two-point discrimination testing. These inadequacies are intrinsic to the test which measures the innervation density of only the slowly-adapting fiber/receptor system. These inadequacies are overcome by the moving two-point discrimination test. The results of moving two-point discrimination test correlate precisely with tactile gnosis throughout the period of recovery of sensation.

EVALUATION

The clinician attempting to evaluate hand sensibility must have at his disposal reliable and valid tests, a knowledge of the regional anatomy and the realization that his sensory examination must vary depending upon the clinical setting. In the setting of acute trauma, the goal of the examination is to determine the integrity of the involved nerves. In the setting of nerve compression, the goal of the examination usually is to determine the presence of early or subtle changes in sensibility. With more advanced cases of nerve compression, the goal is to determine the presence of intraneural fibrosis and, thereby, guide the therapeutic approach to include an internal neurolysis. In the setting of recovery following nerve repair, the goal of the examination is first to determine if axonal regeneration is occurring at all. If regeneration is occurring, then the goal becomes to determine the sequence of recovery of sensory submodalities as a guide to instituting sensory re-education. Once sensory recovery has progressed, the goal of the examination changes again to determining the final status of sensibility in a way that reflects hand function. The sensibility evaluation charts in Fig. 10.10 are helpful.

Fig. 10.9. Correlation of electrodiagnostic studies with Weber test. There was no correlation between nerve conduction velocity and Weber test results in patients studied 5 years after nerve repair. If there had been a correlation, line would have sloped from upper left to lower right. (Reproduced with permission from E. Almquist and O. Eeg-Olofsson: *J Bone Joint Surg* 52A:791–796, 1970.[27])

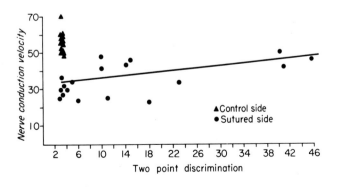

Patient's name : _____

Examination date: _____

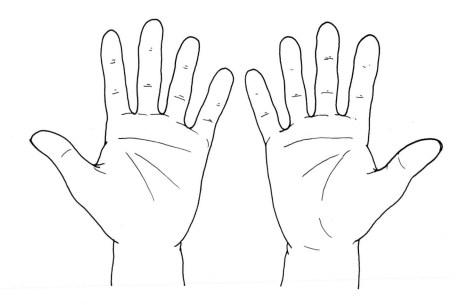

Left		Right
	Tinel's	
	Wrist	
	Elbow	
	Phalen's	
	Extrinsics	
	FDP$_L$	
	FPL	
	Intrinsics	
	AbP	
	OpP	
	AbDM	
	IDI	

Ulnar vs. radial dorsal sensation

Left				Right		
Th	In	Li	sensory	Th	In	Li
			30 cps			
			256 cps			
			2PD			
			m2PD			
			misc.			

∗	Tinel's	
⋯⋯	30 cps	
ooooo	256 cps	
∿∿∿	Moving touch	
—	Constant touch	

Figure 10.10. Chart I use to record sensibility evaluation.

Trauma

When evaluating the acute injury, the nerves at risk for potential crush or division are suggested immediately by the location of the injury. Knowledge of the regional anatomy should guide the examination to the thumb, index, middle, and ring fingers for potential median nerve injury at the wrist, the little finger for a potential injury to the ulnar nerve at the wrist, and to the radial dorsal or ulnar dorsal aspects of the hand if injury may have occurred to the dorsal sensory branch of the radial or ulnar nerves, respectively. With an injury in the palm, the common volar digital nerves are, of course, at risk, and the adjacent volar surfaces of the fingers on both sides of the web space must be examined. More distal injuries of course, may involve just a single digital nerve.

The examiner must be suspicious of puncture wounds. These are especially common in the palm and more often than not cause injury to the common volar digital nerves, usually the one to the ring/little finger web space.

The examiner must be suspicious of partial nerve division. These are most likely to occur to the median nerve at the wrist. Because of the ulnar nerve overlap in the ring and sometimes the middle finger, these injuries may be initially unnoticed by both patient and examiner.

In the acute setting in the emergency room, with the patient apprehensive and in pain, the environment loud and threatening, and the hand bandaged and often bleeding, the circumstances are clearly not ideal for comprehensive evaluation of sensibility. Furthermore, the patient is likely to be uncooperative, often being a child or an intoxicated adult. The diagnostic test must be one that is readily available, quick, reliable, valid and nonthreatening. My choice is the tuning fork.[25] I never use a needle. The tuning fork is demonstrated to the patient on his noninjured hand. Usually the examiner is not the first person to see the patient, and in that case if the fingertips are exposed, the bandage is not removed again. The use of the tuning fork is discussed in detail in Chapter 9. In brief, the prong end of the tuning fork (usually a 256-cps tuning fork is available, but

any one can be used in this situation) is touched to each finger and the patient asked if he can perceive the stimulus. If he says yes, he is then asked where he felt it, to be sure he is localizing it to the fingertip and not to the palm or proximal dorsal finger skin. He is then tested in this area again and asked if that stimulus feels the same as the stimulus applied to an adjacent finger, the contralateral finger, or the other digital nerve autonomous zone on the same finger, depending upon which nerve the examiner thinks is at risk for injury.

A diminished vibratory perception means there is loss of neural conduction in the nerve tested, and this loss is almost always due to nerve division. Occasionally, it has been found associated with a traction injury or a nerve contusion.[25] With careful testing, that is, being sure that the patient's perception is not from a more proximal level or from an uninjured adjacent nerve territory, I have not yet had a false negative or false positive with this test.

With a puncture wound or missile injury, if a diminished vibratory perception is present, the possibility of a reversible nerve lesion, a neuropraxia, exists. If the wound would not otherwise require exploration, I suggest the patient be observed and serial sensory evaluations conducted. If by 4 to 6 weeks the vibratory perception remains abnormal, and local wound conditions permit, exploration is indicated.

In the acute situation, if time, the wound, and the patient permit, additional evaluations of sensibility can be carried out, either to "confirm" for the examiner or the patient the results of the tuning fork test or for the sake of "completeness" or "thoroughness." I emphasize that the tuning fork exam in this setting is reliable and valid. What other sensory testing might meaningfully be done? For all the reasons discussed earlier in this chapter, the only other test that might prove useful, as a baseline or diagnostic study is the moving two-point discrimination test.[15] This is performed exactly like the classic two-point discrimination test (see Chapter 8) except that the two prongs are moved only in a longitudinal direction, from proximal to distal and at a perceptible pressure. Values of 4 mm or greater are abnormal and suggest nerve compression, single digital nerve injury or partial division of a more proximal major nerve. Absent moving two-point discrimination in a fingertip indicates complete conduction block (usually nerve transection) proximal to the common volar digital nerve level.

Nerve Compression

The sensory examination of the patient with a potential nerve compression is usually performed under more ideal circumstances than the examination on the trauma patient. The patient's history and his complaints are most frequently sufficient to make the diagnosis of a peripheral nerve compression and often to suggest which nerve is compressed. However, to localize the level or the site of the compression, and the degree or the presence of intraneural fibrosis, evaluation of sensibility is a must.

The two indispensible tests are the tuning fork test[25] and the moving two-point discrimination test.[15] The only clinical tests of median nerve compression at the wrist to be evident earlier than abnormal vibratory perception in the thumb, are the provocative tests such as Phalen's and Tinel's sign.[25,26] We have found abnormal vibratory perception in the presence of a normal Phalen's and Tinel's sign, and sometimes, in the rheumatoid, or after wrist fractures, Phalen's sign is not possible to test.

In the early nerve compression, a hyperesthesia occurs and the patient may perceive the tuning fork to be more, not less, intense.

Abnormal vibratory perception means the presence of a peripheral nerve conduction block but does not indicate the degree or severity of the block. This is assessed with the moving two-point discrimination test.[15] A value of 4 mm or more is abnormal and correlates with intraneural fibrosis.[29] The patient's history at this point usually is positive for a persistent sensory disturbance, and I suggest that nerve decompression should be accompanied by internal neurolysis to give the best chance of complete recovery of sensation.[29]

With sensory disturbance related to the thumb, index, and middle finger, and abnormal vibratory perception in the thumb and index in contrast to the little finger or contra-

lateral fingers, the diagnosis of median nerve entrapment is made. Weakness of the abductor pollicis brevis or opponens pollicis may be present (rarely) ahead of sensory change. Muscle wasting without diminished tactile discrimination is also an indication for internal neurolysis.[30]

With sensory disturbance related to the ring and little fingers, and abnormal vibratory perception in the little finger in contrast to the thumb and contralateral finger, the diagnosis of ulnar nerve compression is secure. However, at which level? Motor evaluation of the ulnar innervated intrinsics will confirm an ulnar nerve compression, but will not resolve the question, "At which level is compression occurring, wrist or elbow?" I have found the sensory examination of the dorsum of the hand to be critical. Often there will still be strength in the flexor profundus to the little finger, especially if the ulnar nerve compression at the elbow is in the dominant upper extremity. Almost invariably there will be diminished vibratory perception over the dorsal ulnar skin surface, in contrast to the ipsilateral dorsal radial and contralateral dorsal ulnar skin surface with ulnar nerve compression at the elbow. This indicates entrapment above the wrist. This, perhaps neurologically "soft sign" can be confirmed by gently stroking the dorsal skin with the examiner's finger longitudinally, and moving these strokes successively from the radial to the ulnar half. Ask the patient to tell you when the sensation begins to change, or if it begins to change in quality.

A positive Tinel's sign at the elbow over the cubital tunnel or just proximal to it is common throughout the population, especially if the person spends much time on the phone or working at a desk (elbows flexed). Thus, this sign, unless "four plus" is more confirmatory than pathognomonic. I have found, however, a positive Tinel's sign just distal along the course of the ulnar nerve at the point where it goes between the two heads of the flexor capri ulnaris is highly diagnostic of ulnar nerve compression by Osborne's band.[31] In the clinical setting of ulnar nerve entrapment, with abnormal dorsal sensory examination, a tender area distal to the cubital tunnel has correlated invariably, in my experience, with the presence of a fibrous band at this point.

Nerve compression is commonly a bilateral problem, and both median and ulnar nerve compression can occur in the same extremity. In these cases, tuning fork evaluation may not appear to be altered because the comparison area also has abnormal innervation.[26] For this reason, a quantitative test of sensibility is of value in all cases of suspected peripheral nerve compression. I favor the moving two-point discrimination test.[15] Although the classic two-point discrimination test becomes abnormal with advanced nerve compression, the relatively wider range of normal usually given, i.e., 2 to 6 mm, makes the test inherently less sensitive than the moving two-point discrimination test. For example, if perception of the tuning fork were equal in the thumb, index, and little finger, the classic two-point discrimination was 6 mm in each of these fingers and the moving two-point discrimination was 4 mm in each of these fingers, I would suspect compression of both the median and ulnar nerve in that extremity and proceed to very carefully compare both extremities again. I have operated upon four patients so far with bilateral nerve compression of the median, at the wrist, and ulnar, at the elbow. In these difficult bilateral cases, a quantitative measurement of vibratory threshold (vibrometer)[32] or cutaneous pressure threshold (Semmes-Weinstein monofilaments) can be helpful, but remember that these "absolute" values vary, for example, with age.

Nerve Repair

The sensory examination of a patient following nerve repair must be considered as a series of observations along the time continuum of recovery. If we accept the average rate of regeneration of a peripheral nerve in the distal end of the extremity to be 1 mm per day, or 1 inch per month (see Chapter 7), then it should take about 6 months after nerve repair for the regenerating axons to reach the fingertip following suture at wrist level.

During the first 2 to 4 months following suture, axon sprouts of all sensory submodalities are regenerating and are entering the palm. Most axons are destined for the fingertips and will not reinnervate the palm. The axon sprouts from the smaller diameter fibers are in advance of the larger diameter fibers. At this stage, the evaluation of sensibility can be limited simply to following the Tinel's sign progressing distally.[33,34] As reinnervation occurs, there will be the development of a state of "hypersensitivity," "dysethesia" or "paresthesia." Recovery of moving- and constant-touch and the perception of vibratory stimuli occurs next and these are often poorly localized. The goal of the evaluation at this point is to establish within 4 months whether regeneration is proceeding satisfactorily, which is to say at a pace commensurate with the patient's age, the type of injury and its repair, skill of the surgeon, etc. If regeneration is not proceeding as expected, then, as discussed in Chapter 4, surgical intervention is justified before the sensory corpuscle population suffers irreversible degenerative changes. For "satisfactory regeneration", I require: (1) an advancing Tinel's sign and (2) the orderly distal progression across the palm of the expected pattern of sensory recovery (see Chapter 7). During this period it is useless and a waste of time to measure two-point discrimination or thresholds, as it is simply too early for them to have recovered in the palm and impossible for them to be present in the fingertips. The qualitative tests give the desired information.

From 4 to 6 months following nerve suture at the wrist, the axon sprouts are entering the fingers. The goal of sensibility evaluation now is to guide rehabilitation. Moving-touch, constant-touch, 30- and 256-cps vibratory stimuli are used exclusively until all have been recovered to the fingertips. Because of variability in peripheral nerve innervation patterns, the middle and ring fingers are not tested nor are the dorsal aspects of the fingers. (The thumb, however, is carefully assessed during this time to ascertain the degree, if any, of anomalous radial nerve innervation of the thumb pulp.) Once each of these four sensory tests can be perceived at the fingertip it is not repeated at subsequent examinations.

Moving two-point discrimination is not tested until moving-touch is perceived at the fingertip. Moving-touch is then no longer individually tested. The tuning forks serve both as the earliest tests of recovery of the touch submodality and as an important guide to the institution of sensory re-education. However, once perception of moving-touch has recovered in the fingertip, the only test required thereafter in the routine evaluation of sensibility is the moving two-point discrimination test.[15]

The vibratory threshold is not evaluated routinely.[32] It may be of value in checking occasionally, as its progressive return towards normal can be recorded and demonstrated to the patient as a means of reassurance, helping him to endure the first postoperative year. The cutaneous pressure threshold (Semmes-Weinstein, von Frey) is not evaluated at all. I evaluated cutaneous pressure thresholds in the comprehensive study correlating sensibility tests with function and found these not to correlate.[22] There is a progressive change in cutaneous pressure threshold over time, but as this change can be shown with the vibrometer[32] and the vibrometer is quicker and easier to use (no log conversion scale or calibration problem), I prefer, in those rare cases where it is needed, the vibrometer (see Chapter 9). Furthermore, by its very nature, the cutaneous pressure threshold must be done for multiple spots on a fingertip, using the series of different filaments at each spot. The vibrometer, since it employs a traveling wave as its stimulus, is more efficient. It can be tested on just one "spot," the fingertip, giving an "average threshold" for the whole area. The patient, after all, feels with the fingertip, not a small spot somewhere on its tip.

The classic two-point discrimination is not tested until perception of constant-touch has been recovered at the fingertip. At present, I am still recording both the moving and classic two-point discrimination in each patient. Theoretically, this is not necessary. It has been shown that the curve of classic two-point discrimination recovery over time parallels that for moving two-point discrimination, but is, in every instance, slower to recover (delayed, on the average, 6 months) and is in every instance, a higher value (demonstrating a poorer degree of recovery, a poorer result).[15] I continue to record it for

three reasons: (1) At present, it remains the standard of comparison throughout the world; (2) it serves as a link between today's evaluation and those classic studies of the past; and, (3) although the moving two-point discrimination test does test the slowly-adapting fiber/receptor population, in addition to its measurement of the quickly-adapting fiber/receptor population, the classic two-point discrimination test permits a separate quantitation of the system that mediates perception of constant-touch and pressure. This later information is worth knowing functionally and is discussed below.

End Results of Nerve Repair

The goal of evaluating the end result of a nerve repair is to determine the functional capacity of the hand. What type of work is the hand capable of performing? What is the permanent partial impairment? How does the technique of nerve repair or sensory re-education compare with some other techniques? How good a job did the surgeon do? What can the patient expect?

The first question is not "how should the evaluation be done? but, "when should the evaluation be done?" Much of the past lack of understanding of sensory recovery came from the view that "sensory recovery continues throughout the fifth postoperative year." A sense of frustration and complacency permeated the field. Once the repair was done, there seemed to be little to do except sit back, check the patient at yearly intervals, reassure them, and after 5 years record their "final check." Of course, somewhere between 6 months and 1 year postinjury, or whenever motor function seems to return, or whenever the workmen's compensation insurance carrier or the lawyer needed a disability rating, a detailed sensory examination could always be done!

A program of sensory re-education (see Chapter 12) must be an integral part of the care of every patient with a nerve injury if the patient is to maximize the full sensory potential given to him by the nerve repair in the shortest possible time. Clearly then, frequent and early evaluation of sensibility must be done both by the therapist and the surgeon. If the evaluation of sensibility program outlined immediately above is employed, these evaluation sessions are brief because only those tests appropriate for the given degree of neurophysiologic recovery are used. An entire "battery" of sensibility testing is not ritually repeated every time the patient is seen. Sensory testing does not become a half hour chore.

At 1 year following repair of the median nerve at the wrist, even in the adult, an excellent approximation to the traditional 5-year result can be found if the patient has been in a program of sensory re-education. By 1 year, virtually all nerve fibers that are ever going to regenerate to the fingertips have done so. Threshold values, which reflect fiber/receptor maturation (the trophic influence of the regenerated corpuscular component) will continue to improve beyond 1 year. Tactile gnosis, which reflects the totality of axonal regeneration, maturation, and re-education, will continue to improve beyond 1 year, and require continuing education or practice to be maintained. We have seen this 1 year mark delayed by intercurrent problems, such as pregnancy, where peripheral edema clearly slowed the recovery process. But, as a general statement, a good approximation of the 5-year end result and an accurate prognosis can be made at 1 year following nerve repair in a patient receiving postoperative sensory rehabilitation.

Given only one test instrument to carry out the evaluation of sensibility in this end result type of examination, the paper clip should be chosen. Given only one test to carry out the evaluation of sensibility in this end result type of examination the moving two-point discrimination test should be done. Only the moving two-point discrimination test correlates with the hand function defined as tactile gnosis when the fingertips are allowed to move.[22] Movement is the way of life. The questing, working, active hand is most always a moving hand. The proof of this is that thumb, index and middle finger, with no "measurable useful" classic two-point discrimination (greater than 15 to 20 mm) can readily identify objects placed within their grasp by manipulating these objects.[22]

The classic two-point discrimination tests underestimates hand function greatly. It lags behind recovery of useful moving two-point discrimination by 6 months, usually never recovers to the same level as moving two-point discrimination, and accurately reflects only those hand functions for which a static precision sensory grip is employed. However, it provides one critical piece of information required for the comprehensive evaluation of sensibility. In the blindfolded patient, the hand with 5 mm of moving two-point discrimination and 15 mm of classic two-point discrimination can identify small objects placed within its grasp, but when the fingers stop moving, they become unaware that the objects are still within their grasp. The afferent information required to know how tightly to hold the object is not sufficient. Classic two-point discrimination testing is still recommended, therefore, to provide this information.

References

1. von Frey M: The distribution of afferent nerves in the skin. JAMA 47:645–648, 1906.
2. Moberg E: Criticism and study of methods for examining sensibility of the hand. Neurology (Minneap) 12:8–9, 1962.
3. Onne L: Recovery of sensibility and sudomotor activity in the hand after nerve suture. Acta Chir Scand [Suppl] 300:5–9, 1962.
4. Omer GE: Injuries to nerves of the upper extremity. J Bone Joint Surg 56A:1615–1624, 1974.
5. Swanson, AB, Goran-Hagert C, Swanson GD: Evaluations of impairment of hand functions, in Hunter JM, Schneider LH, Mackin EJ, et al (eds): *Rehabilitation of the Hand*. Saint Louis: CV Mosby, 1978, Ch 4.
6. Fess EE, Harmon KS, Strickland JW, et al: Evaluation of the hand by objective measurement, in Hunter JM, Schneider LH, Mackin EJ, et al (eds): *Rehabilitation of the Hand*. Saint Louis: CV Mosby, 1978, Ch. 5.
7. Bell JA: Sensibility evaluation, in Hunter JM, Schneider LH, Mackin EJ, et al (eds): *Rehabilitation of the Hand*. Saint Louis: CV Mosby, 1978.
8. Werner JL, Omer GE Jr: Evaluating cutaneous pressure sensation of the hand. Am J Occup Ther 24:347–356, 1970.
9. Flynn JE, Flynn WF: Median and ulnar nerve injuries. Ann Surg 156:1002–1009, 1962.
10. McEwan LE: Median and ulnar nerve injuries. Aust NZ J Surg 32:89–104, 1962.
11. Oester VT, Davis L: Recovery of sensory function, in Woodhall B, Beebee GW (eds): *Peripheral Nerve Regeneration*. Washington DC: US Gov Print Office, 1956, Ch 5.
12. Porter RW: New test for fingertip sensation. Br Med J 2:927–928, 1966.
13. Krag K, Rasmussen KB: The neurovascular island flap for defective sensibility of the thumb. J Bone Joint Surg [Br] 57B:495–499, 1975.

14. Reid RL, Werner J, Sunstrum C: Preliminary results of sensibility re-education following repair of the median nerve. Am Soc Surg Hand Newsletter 15, 1977.
15. Dellon AL: The moving two-point discrimination test: Clinical evaluation of the quickly-adapting fiber/receptor system. J Hand Surg 3:494–481, 1978.
16. Poppen NK, McCarroll HR Jr, Doyle JR, et al: Recovery of sensibility after suture of digital nerves. J Hand Surg 4:212–226, 1979.
17. Dellon AL: The plastic ridge device and moving two-point discrimination. (Letter to the Editor). J Hand Surgery 5:92–93, 1980.
18. Moberg E: Aspects of sensation in reconstructive surgery of the upper extremity. J Bone Joint Surg 46A:817–825, 1964.
19. Narakas A: Brachial plexus injuries. Clin Orthop 133:71–90, 1978.
20. Tsatsos C: Address by His Excellency, President of the Hellenic Republic, to the Institute of Management Science, Athens, Greece, July 1977, quoted by Conomy JP, Barnes KL, Cruse RP: Quantitative cutaneous sensory testing in children and adolescents. Cleve Clin Q 45:197–206, 1978.
21. Schlenker JD, Kleinert HE, Tsai T: Methods and results of replantation following traumatic amputation of the thumb in sixty-four patients. J Hand Surg 5:63–70, 1980.
22. Dellon AL, Munger B: Correlation of sensibility evaluation, hand function and histology, in press 1981.
23. Dawson GD: The relative excitability and conduction velocity of sensory and motor nerve fibres in man. J Physiol 131:436–451, 1956.
24. Melvin JL, Harris DH, Johnson EW: Sensory and motor conduction velocities in the ulnar and median nerves. Arch Phys Med Rehabil 47:511–519, 1966
25. Dellon AL: Clinical use of vibratory stimuli to evaluate peripheral nerve injury and compression neuropathy. Plast Reconstr Surg 65:466–476, 1980.
26. Spindler H, Dellon AL: Results of electrodiagnostic studies in a well-defined population of peripheral compression neuropathies, in press 1981.
27. Almquist E, Eeg-Olofsson O: Sensory nerve-conduction velocity and two-point discrimination in sutured nerves. J Bone Joint Surg 52A:791–796, 1970.
28. Conomy JP, Barnes KL, Cruse RP: Quantitative cutaneous sensory testing in children and adolescents. Cleve Clin Q 45:197–206, 1978.
29. Dellon AL: Internal neurolysis, in press 1981.
30. Curtis RM, Eversmann WW: Internal neurolysis as an adjunct to the treatment of the carpal tunnel syndrome. J Bone Joint Surg 55A:733–740, 1973.
31. Osborne G: The surgical treatment of tardy ulnar neuritis (abstr). J Bone Joint Surg 39B:782, 1957.
32. Dellon AL: The vibrometer, in press 1981.
33. Henderson WR: Clinical assessment of peripheral nerve injuries: Tinel's test. Lancet 2:801–805, 1948.
34. Napier JR: The significance of Tinel's sign in peripheral nerve injuries. Brain 72:63–82, 1949.
35. Trotter WB, Davies HM: Experimental studies in the innervation of the skin. J Physiol 38:134–246, 1909.
36. Minor V: Ein neues Verfahren zu der klinischen Untersuchung der Schweissabsonderung. Deutsch Z Nervenheilk 101:302, 1928.
37. Seddon HJ, Medawar PB, Smith H: Rate of regeneration of peripheral nerves in man. J Physiol 102:191–215, 1943.

SECTION 3

Re-Education of Sensation

Chapter 11

RESULTS OF NERVE REPAIR IN THE HAND

MEDIAN NERVE
ULNAR NERVE
DIGITAL NERVE
CONCLUSIONS

The proliferation of published symposia and monographs on upper extremity peripheral nerve problems in the last decade[1-13] attests to the continued general interest, numerous basic investigations, clinical work and FRUSTRATION in this field. Following World War II, debate turned (although unresolved) from the superiority of primary versus secondary nerve repair to three brightly glowing areas on the horizon: microsurgery,[14-16] nerve repair techniques,[17-27] and nerve grafting.[28-34] The hand surgeon today, with superior training, technical skill, instrumentation, and a versatile eclectic approach to the injured nerve, nevertheless, still is reporting end results of nerve repair that cannot be shown statistically to be superior to those reported 2 decades ago.

The purpose of this chapter is to tabulate the past results of nerve repair to serve as an historic baseline for future comparison. We feel that part of the failure of recent reports to document the desired improved end result following the recent technical advances in nerve repair is less a failure of the technique than a failure of our ability to quantitate those end results. Furthermore, we feel that the observed failure to improve end results is less a failure of the technique than a failure of the patient to achieve the full potential inherent in the nerve repair. The first "fail-ure" can be overcome, we suggest, by an improved measurement of end results of sensory recovery, the moving two-point discrimination test (see Chapter 8).[35] The second "failure" can be overcome, we suggest, with a regular program of sensory re-education, instituted at the appropriate time in the recovery process (see Chapter 12).

The studies included in this chapter are all those published since the end of World War II that contain sufficient information to permit their inclusion as baseline data. Because the majority of these studies have reported their end results according to the modification by Zachary and Holmes[36] of Highet's scheme, we have also presented the results in that format (see Tables 11.1 and 11.2). This scheme does not define a "good" or "bad" result, but rather permits the author to consider, for example, "useful median nerve recovery as M3 and S2+, useful ulnar nerve recovery as M2+ and S2+."[29]

The diversity of criteria for judging end results by this scheme may be seen from the following. Nicholson and Seddon[43] regarded useful recovery as M4, S3+. Some authors have a different criteria depending upon which nerve is being discussed. For example, McEwan[46] regarded "useful" ulnar nerve as M2+, and "useful" median nerve as M3. For the median nerve, Sakellarides[47] regarded

Table 11.1
Classification of Sensory Recovery

Grade	Recovery of Sensibility
S0	No recovery of sensibility in the autonomous zone of the nerve
S1	Recovery of deep cutaneous pain sensibility with the autonomous zone of the nerve
S1+	Recovery of superficial pain sensibility
S2	Recovery of superficial pain and some touch sensibility
S2+	As in S2, but with over-response
S3	Recovery of pain and touch sensibility with disappearance of over-response[a]
S3+	As in S3, but localization of the stimulus is good and there is imperfect recovery of two-point discrimination[a]
S4	Complete recovery[a]

[a] These classifications were modified to include classical two-point discrimination ranges as follows: S3 has 2PD greater than 15 mm, S3+ includes 7- to 15-mm range, S4 includes 2- to 6-mm range.

Table 11.2
Classification of Motor Recovery

Grade	Motor Recovery
M0	No contraction
M1	Return of perceptible contraction in the proximal muscles
M2	Return of perceptible contraction in both proximal and distal muscles
M3	Return of function in both proximal and distal muscles to such a degree that all important muscles are sufficiently powerful to act against gravity
M4	All muscles act against strong resistance and some independent movements are possible
M5	Full recovery in all muscles

"good" as M3, S2+ and S3, and "excellent" as M4, S3+. For the ulnar nerve, Sakellarides[47] regarded "good" as M2+ and M3, S2+ and S3, and "excellent" as M4, S3+. Most recent use of the scheme[53] considered "good" for both median and ulnar nerves to be M3, S2+ and "excellent" to be M4, S3+. It is thus evident that "normal", M5, S4 is a level to be approximated, a level rarely, if ever, reached.

As discussed fully in Chapter 10, "useful" recovery must be considered functional recovery, and functional recovery must be measured in terms of the presence of two-point discrimination. None of the studies included here were published after the description of the moving two-point discrimination test,[35] and so, this end result cannot be used for retrospective comparison. In the tables to follow, category S3+ includes patients with "some" recovery of two-point discrimination, while category S4 is "normal." Based on Moberg's work,[37, 38] we assigned patients with two point discrimination of 7 to 15 mm to the S3+ group and those with less than 6 mm to the S4 group. Those with two point discrimination greater than 15 mm are in the S3 group. All the studies reported have been redefined in these terms and listed in the tables to follow (Tables 11.3 through 11.10).

MEDIAN NERVE

Low Repair

In the war injuries, of the 864 patients reported, just one patient recovered to S4 and less than 20% to S3+. About 40% recovered to M4. These results were not better after Vietnam than after World War II.[52] In the civilian adult injuries treated with nerve repair, of the 465 patients reported, just two patients recovered to S4 and 33% to S3+. Less than 5% recovered to M5 and 40% to M4 (within this M4 group, studies ranged from 11%[47] to 65%[44]). Among these 158 patients who recovered good to excellent sensory function were probably the 48 children included in these studies, but it is impossible to separate them from these "adult" results. It is quite possible that no adults recovered to S4 and that just 24% recovered to S3+ when evaluated at an average of 5 years after their nerve repair (see Table 11.3).

High repair

In the war injuries, 0% recovered S4, 3% recovered S3+, and 5% recovered M5, 20% recovered M4, and 17% recovered M3. In the civilian injuries, 0% recovered S4, 17% recovered to S3+, and 0% recovered M5, 30% recovered M4, and 44% recovered to M3.

These reports included no children (see Table 11.4).

Nerve Graft

Taken as a whole, the nerve graft patients had 2% recover to S4, 24% to S3+ and 20% to M5, 13% to M4 (see Table 11.5).

ULNAR NERVE

Low Repair

In the war injuries, of the 1098 reported patients, none recovered to S4, and less than 15% to S3+ and 40% to M4. The results were not better after Vietnam than they were after World War II.[52] In the civilian adult injuries treated with nerve repair, of the 466 patients reported, just three patients recovered to S4 and 34% to S3+. Thirty-two percent recovered to M4 (within this M4 group, reports ranged from 3[47] to 67%[46]). Among the 146 patients who recovered good to excellent sensory function were probably the 49 children included in these studies, but it is impossible to separate them from these "adult" results. It is quite possible that no adults recovered

Table 11.3
Results of Median Nerve Repair—Low

Reference, Date	Type of Trauma	Repair Timing	No. of Cases	Age	% Children	Follow-up (yr)	Motor Recovery (%)				Sensory Recovery (%)				
							M2	M3	M4	M5	S2	S2+	S3	S3+	S4
39, 1949	War	All	235	Adults	0	2	67				27		73		
40, 1954	War	Secondary	290	Adults	0	5	31	14	18	0	47	15	30	9	0.2
41, 42, 1956	War	Secondary	244	Adults	0	4	11	23	29	31	17	28	14	18	
43, 1957	Civilian	Secondary	52		16	5	21	27	39	0	21	15	40	25	0
44, 1958	Civilian	Primary	54		16	1–7	35	0	65	0	3	0	26	71	0
44, 1958	Civilian	Secondary	24		16	1–7	50	0	50	0					
45, 1961	Civilian	All	46			2–24									9
46, 1962	Civilian	All	27	<14	100	"Long"	0	0	27	65	4	0	4	7	86
46, 1962	Civilian	All	16	>14	0	"Long"	13	20	27	13	17	0	17	61	0
47, 1962	Civilian	Primary	38	3–81	26	2–31	13	37	11	0	15	33	13	5	0
47, 1962	Civilian	Secondary	20	3–81	26	2–31	25	35	25	0	20	29	32	4	0
48, 1962	Civilian	Primary	40			1–12	25	38	15	7	50	0	7	10	3
49, 1962	Civilian	Primary	15	<14	100	4–11	20	13	40	27	0	0	0	27	73
49, 1962	Civilian	Primary	17	>14	0	4–11	30	23	18	29	22	18	18	41	0
50, 1964	Civilian	All	10	5–58	33	1–3	30		70			30		70	
51, 1965	Civilian	All	26		35	1	0				0		88	8	4
2, 1972	Civilian	Secondary	110			5	5	47		44	4	5	47	44	0
52, 1974	War	Secondary	95[a]	Adults	0	1	61		39	0	61		39		0
53, 1980	Civilian	Primary	14		6	2–11	0	43	57	0	7	7	29	57	0

[a] Value includes ulnar nerve cases too.

Table 11.4
Results of Median Nerve Repair—High

Reference, Date	Type of Trauma	Repair Timing	No. of Cases	Age	% Children	Follow-up (yr)	Motor Recovery (%)				Sensory Recovery (%)				
							M2	M3	M4	M5	S2	S2+	S3	S3+	S4
39, 1949	War	All		Adult	0	<2					37		47		
40, 1954	War	Secondary	95	Adult		5	42	13	6	0	47	23	25	6	0
41, 42, 1956	War	Secondary	124	Adult	0	>4	17	25	30	13					
43, 1957	Civilian	Secondary	6	Adult		5	33	0	50	0	50	0	34	16	0
44, 1958	Civilian	Primary	14			1–7	0	14	36	0		8	50	42	0
47, 1962	Civilian	All	7	Adult		2–31	42	14	0	0	42	0	14	0	0
2, 1972	Civilian	Secondary	100			>5	6	61		30	3	6	61	30	
52, 1974	War	Secondary	48[a]	Adult	0	>1	7	3	27	0	7	3	27	0	0
53, 1980	Civilian	Primary	12	Adult	0	2–11	16	60	8	0	8	8	60	17	0

[a] Value includes ulnar nerve cases too.

to S4, and that just 20% recovered to S3+ when evaluated at an average of 5 years after their nerve repair (see Table 11.6).

High Repair

In the war injuries, 0% recovered to S4 or S3+, while 6% recovered to M5 and 23% to M4. In the civilian injuries, 0% recovered to S4, 20% to S3+ and 0% to M5, 17% to M4 (see Table 11.7).

Nerve Graft

Taken as a whole, the nerve graft patients had 7% recover to S4, 14% to S3+ and 23% to M5, 20% to M4 (see Table 11.8).

DIGITAL NERVE

Nerve Repair

In the civilian adult injuries treated with nerve repair, of the 381 patients reported, 11% recovered to S4 and 48% to S3+. Among these 221 patients who recovered good to excellent sensory function, were probably the 47 children included in these studies, but it is impossible to separate them from these "adult" results. In the two studies in which children were separated from adults,[49, 56] when the results are pooled and averaged, 60% of children and 12% of adults recovered to S4, while 16% of the children and 30% of the adults recovered to S3+ when evaluated

Table 11.5
Results of Median Nerve Graft

Reference, Date	Type of Trauma	Gap Grafted	No. of Cases	Age	% Children	Follow-up (yr)	Motor Recovery (%)				Sensory Recovery (%)				
							M2	M3	M4	M5	S2	S2+	S3	S3+	S4
59, 1939	Civilian	3–15 cm	32ᵃ			1–15									3
60, 1947	War	5–15 cm	11	Adult		2–3	0	36	18	0	10	18	45	18	0
61, 1955	Civilian	>7 cm	33			>5	0	69	0	0	21	0	69	0	0
31, 32, 1976	Civilian	2–20 cm	38	8–62	3	5–11	7	21	14	46	3	0	60	34	3
63, 1977	Civilian	5–10 cm	8	17–38	0	1.5–2.5	12	0	50	0	13	0	12	63	12
64, 1978	Civilian	4–15 cm	6			1.5–2.5		33	16	33				33	
34, 1980	Civilian	>2 cm	8	15–57	0	1–5		0	0	0	0	37	38	25	0

ᵃ Value includes ulnar and digital nerves too.

Table 11.6
Results of Ulnar Nerve Repair—Low

Reference, Date	Type of Trauma	Repair Timing	No. of Cases	Age	% Children	Follow-up (yr)	Motor Recovery (%)				Sensory Recovery (%)				
							M2	M3	M4	M5	S2	S2+	S3	S3+	S4
39, 1949	War	All	158	Adults	0	<2					0	31	69	0	0
40, 1954	War	Secondary	384	Adults	0	>5	72	14	5	0	54	15	28	3	0
41, 42, 1956	War	Secondary	441	Adults	0	>4	5	34	38	16	16	24	19	13	0
43, 1957	Civilian	Secondary	60		16	>5	32	32	35	0	18	14	47	21	0
44, 1958	Civilian	All	62		16	1–7	63	0	37	0	4	0	33	63	0
45, 1961	Civilian	All	32			2–24									3
46, 1962	Civilian	All	23	<14	100	"Long"	4	25	67	4	0	0	5	23	72
46, 1962	Civilian	All	23	>14	0	"Long"	32	36	23	0	8	0	24	48	12
47, 1962	Civilian	Primary	39	3–81	26	2–31	30	6	0	0	25	15	23	5	0
47, 1962	Civilian	Secondary	29	3–81	26	2–31	20	7	3	0	30	13	27	13	0
48, 1962	Civilian	Primary	40			1–12	57	15	18	0	50	0	13	7	0
49, 1962	Civilian	Primary	10	<14	100	5–10	8	30	30	32	0	0	10	30	60
49, 1962	Civilian	Primary	7	>14	0	5–10					0	0	57	43	0
50, 1964	Civilian	All	16	5–58	33	1–3	30	70			38		62		
51, 1965	Civilian	All	19		35	1					4		76	20	0
2, 1972	Civilian	Secondary	119			>5	10	43		45	2	10	43	45	0
52, 1974	War	Secondary	95ᵃ	Adults	0	>1	61	39	0		61		39		0
53, 1980	Civilian	Primary	20		6	2–11	55	30	10	0	50	0	10	30	0

ᵃ Value includes median nerve cases too.

Table 11.7
Results of Ulnar Nerve Repair—High

Reference, Date	Type of Trauma	Repair Timing	No. of Cases	Age	% Children	Follow-up (yr)	Motor Recovery (%)				Sensory Recovery (%)				
							M2	M3	M4	M5	S2	S2+	S3	S3+	S4
40, 1954	War	Secondary	105	Adult		5	23	5	1	0	53	24	23	0	0
41, 1956	War	Secondary	240	Adult	0	>4	9	38	32	10					
43, 1957	Civilian	Secondary	9	Adult		3	33	22	22	0	33	11	44	11	0
44, 1958	Civilian	Primary	18			1–7	0	0	0	0	0	16	44	44	0
47, 1962	Civilian	All	18	Adult		2–31	56	11	0	0	40	22	11	0	0
2, 1972	Civilian	Secondary	140			>5	13	61		22	4	13	61	22	0
52, 1974	War	Secondary	48[a]	Adult	0	>1	73		27	0	73		27	0	0
53, 1980	Civilian	Primary	11	Adult	0	2–11	54	18	9	0	27	9	27	0	0

[a] Value includes median nerve cases too.

Table 11.8
Results of Ulnar Nerve Graft

Reference, Date	Type of Trauma	Gap Grafted	No. of Cases	Age	% Children	Follow-up (yr)	Motor Recovery (%)				Sensory Recovery (%)				
							M2	M3	M4	M5	S2	S2+	S3	S3+	S4
59, 1939	Civilian	3–15 cm	32[a]			1–15									0
31, 32, 1976	Civilian	2–20 cm	39	11–69	23	5–11	8	31	18	31	0	15	65	15	5
63, 1977	Civilian	2–6 cm	2	16–50		1.5–2.5	0	50	0	0	50	0	50	0	0
64, 1978	Civilian	3–7 cm	10			1.5–3.5	20	50	30	0	20	20	40	20	0
34, 1980	Civilian	>2 cm	5	15–57		1–5			20		0	0	60	0	40

[a] Value includes median and digital nerves too.

Table 11.9
Results of Digital Nerve Repair

Reference, Date	Type of Trauma	Repair Timing	No. of Cases	Age	% Children	Follow-up (yr)	Nerve Block	Sensory Recovery (%)				
								S2	S2+	S3	S3+	S4
54, 1927	Civilian	All	105				No					
44, 1958	Civilian	All	142		16	1–7	No	7	0	29	64	0
55, 1961	Civilian	Primary	12	7–55	8		No	0	0	16	42	25
55, 1961	Civilian	Secondary	12	7–48	8		No	0	16	16	21	63
49, 1962	Civilian	Primary	8	<14	100	4–15	Yes	0	0	0	0	100
49, 1962	Civilian	Primary	14	>14	0	4–15	Yes	28	0	29	43	0
56, 1970	Civilian	Primary	24	<19	100	2–6	Yes	12	0	20	20	48
56, 1970	Civilian	Primary	50	>19	0	2–6	Yes	28	0	28	28	16
57, 1972	Civilian	All	18	6–51	5		No	0	0	22	28	50
58, 1979	Civilian	Primary	62	6–67	22	5–15	Yes	0	10	16	55	19
53, 1980	Civilian	Primary	71		6	2–11	No	20	0	32	48	0

at an average of 5 years after the repair (see Table 11.9).

Nerve Graft

Taken as a whole, the nerve graft patients had 9% recover to S4 and 20% recover to S3+ (see Table 11.10).

CONCLUSIONS

Seddon began his chapter on "Results of Repair of Nerve"[2] without such a review of the literature on end results. He wrote, "Earlier series of results of nerve suture have been reported, but even to summarize them would be a fruitless exercise, largely because there have been no universally agreed criteria for assessment." As indicated in the introduction to this chapter, the main purpose of this review is to serve as the "historic control" for the chapter to follow, which will include the effect of a sensory re-education program on the results of nerve repair. But this chapter's

Table 11.10
Results of Digital Nerve Graft

Reference, Date	Type of Trauma	Gap Grafted	No. of Cases	Age	% Children	Follow-up (yr)	Nerve Block	Sensory Recovery (%)				
								S2	S2+	S3	S3+	S4
60, 1947	War	3–8 cm	15	Adults		2–4	No	46	12	24	6	12
61, 1955	Civilian	>2 cm	17			>5	No	18	0	47	0	0
62, 1976	Civilian	1.5–3.5 cm	13	20–59		0.75–2	No	0	15	39	46	0
34, 1980	Civilian	>2 cm	27	15–57		0.5–5	Yes	0	0	60	25	15

review of 27 studies, precisely because it does highlight the deficiencies of previous end result reports, hopefully will be fruitful in providing a stimulus for the appropriate design of future studies.

What can be concluded from the studies reviewed? All who addressed the question of the effect of age on results of nerve repair agreed that children obtain better results than adults.[4] The few studies that subdivided their patient population into children (usually less than age 14 or 16) versus adults[4] demonstrated this conclusively for sensory recovery in distal, median and ulnar nerve[46, 49] and digital nerve repairs.[49, 56] The results are not as clear with respect to motor recovery[49] (see Table 11.11). However, even with these studies, we can criticize their basic design. McEwan's study[46] included both primary and secondary repairs, while the study of Onne[49] has very small numbers. I feel, however, that it is probably the most valid conclusion of all to state that the patient's age at the time of nerve repair directly affects the degree of sensation recovered. Seddon's[2] data effectively demonstrates this (Table 11.12), and this was one of the basic conclusions of Onne's study of "ideal" nerve repairs.[49]

When the S4 and S3+ columns of Tables 11.3 through 11.10 are examined for each paper with respect to the children included in each study, and when each author's text is carefully examined, it appears that the vast majority of those patients reported to have achieved excellent sensory recovery are children. This age-related effect is so critical to end result analysis that Moberg[4] suggests all future reports be tabulated so as to relate patient age and recovered (classical) two-point discrimination.

A second area about which all studies agree is the effect of the level of nerve repair, in terms of proximal (high) versus distal (low). For the median nerve (Table 11.3 versus 11.4) and the ulnar nerve (Table 11.6 versus 11.7), it is clear that the more distal the nerve repair, the better is the degree of both motor and sensory recovery (see Table 11.11). Even when the most distal nerve repairs are subdivided (Table 11.13), the results of sensory recovery can be related to the level of repair.

Most disturbing, perhaps, is that after 3 decades of analyzing results of nerve repairs, we are still unable to say with certainty whether primary versus secondary or nerve repair versus nerve graft gives the better results. Why haven't we been able to answer these questions? Studies haven't been designed correctly. For example, those that subdivided their cases into primary versus secondary didn't further subdivide into children versus adult[44, 47, 55] and had very small groups of patients.[55] It is not appropriate to compare the reports of primary[48, 49, 53, 56–58] to those of secondary[2, 40, 43, 52] repair because left uncontrolled would be mechanism of injury (war versus civilian), surgical technique, and patient age. Of course those studies that lumped all nerve repairs together are useless in this regard.[39, 44–46, 50,51] These same criticisms apply to the question of nerve repair versus nerve graft. A nerve graft procedure implies a secondary repair, and usually a mechanism of injury less favorable than that in the patient group for whom primary repair was possible. Thus, it is probably never correct from a statistician's point of view to compare these two groups of patients. However, given all these caveats, it is interesting to note that for civilian injuries, the best nerve graft results[31, 32] (Tables 11.5, 11.8) compare quite favorably (if not better) than the best primary nerve repair results[48, 49, 53] (Tables 11.3, 11.6) and even to the best secondary nerve repair

Table 11.11
Results Summary

	No. in Group	Degree of Recovery			
		M4 (%)	M5 (%)	S3+ (%)	S4 (%)
Median					
Low repair					
War injury	864	40	0	20	0.1
Civilian injury[a]	465	40	5	33	0.5
Children	42	31	51	14	83
High repair					
War injury	266	20	5	3	0
Civilian injury	139	30	0	17	0
Graft					
Civilian injury	104	13	20	24	2
Ulnar					
Low repair					
War injury	1098	40	0	15	0
Civilian injury[b]	466	32	0	34	0.7
Children	33	55	12	24	70
High repair					
War injury	393	23	6	0	0
Civilian injury	196	17	0	20	0
Graft					
Civilian injury	56	20	23	14	7
Digital					
Civilian injury[c]	381			48	11
Children	32			16	60
Graft	72			20	9
Total	4607				

[a] Group includes 48 children.
[b] Group includes 49 children.
[c] Group includes 47 children.

Table 11.12
Influence of Age on End Results of Nerve Repair[a]

Age Group	n	Good (M4, S3+)	Fair (M3, S3)	Poor (M2, S2)	Bad (M1, M0, S1, S0)
0–10	35	71	29		
11–15	47	58	32	4	6
16–20	106	33	46	9	12
21–30	231	25	59	9	8
31–40	109	30	46	16	8
41–50	32	31	50	19	
51	24	20	58	13	8
Total	584				

[a] Adapted from H. J. Seddon,[2] includes median and ulnar nerves, all levels of repair.

results[2] (Tables 11.3, 11.6) in adults for both median and ulnar nerves (see also Table 11.11).

If the "odds" are stacked against the nerve graft, how can the results of Millesi[65] be comparable to or better than nerve repairs? Certainly his emphasis on a tension-free repair, meticulous preparations of the nerve stumps, microsurgical techniques, and interfascicular grafting are critical. Millesi's patients also, however, receive significant postoperative sensory rehabilitation. The nerve grafting results being reported from the Saint Louis group[34] are also comparable to or better than the results of nerve repair (see Table 11.11). Although these patients did not uni-

Table 11.13
Effect of Level of Repair on Outcome of Digital Nerve Repair[a]

Level of Repair	Recovery of S3+ (%)
Proximal palm	25
Mid-palm	50
Metacarpal	50
Proximal interphalangeal joint	48
Distal interphalangeal joint	75

[a] Adapted from J. L. Posch and F. de la Cruz-Saddul.[53]

formly go through a sensory re-education program,[66] they were in a hand center that is well aware of our approach of applying specific sensory exercises at the appropriate times in the recovery process.[9] These patients must have received frequent postoperative sensory testing. This postoperative attention, similar to that now devoted to the postoperative care of replant patients, I believe, places these patients into a separate category, a category that bridges the gulf between the nerve repair patient, who in the past has received little if any organized sensory rehabilitation, and the nerve repair patient of today, who has available the benefits of a formal program of Sensory Re-education (see Chapter 12).

References

1. Cramer LM, Chase RA: *Symposium on the Hand.* St. Louis: CV Mosby, 1971.
2. Seddon HJ: *Surgical Disorders of the Peripheral Nerves.* Baltimore: Williams & Wilkins, 1972.
3. Weckesser EC: *Treatment of Hand Injuries.* Chicago: Western Reserve Press, 1974.
4. Michon J, Moberg E: *Traumatic Nerve Lesions of the Upper Extremity.* London: Churchill Livingstone, 1975.
5. Ito T: *Surgery of the Peripheral Nerve.* Tokyo: Igaku Shoin, 1977.
6. Sunderland S: *Nerves and Nerve Injuries,* ed 2. London: Churchill Livingstone 1978.
7. Fredricks S, Brody GS: *Symposium on the Neurologic Aspects of Plastic Surgery.* St. Louis: CV Mosby, 1978.
8. Hunter JM, Schneider LH, Mackin EJ, et al: *Rehabilitation of the Hand.* St. Louis: CV Mosby, 1978.
9. Weeks PM, Wray RC: *Management of Acute Hand Injuries; A Biological Approach,* ed 2. St. Louis: CV Mosby, 1978.
10. Spinner M: *Injuries to the Major Branches of Peripheral Nerves of the Forearm,* ed 2. Philadelphia: WB Saunders, 1978.
11. Jewett DL, McCarroll HR Jr: *Nerve Repair and Regeneration.* St. Louis: CV Mosby, 1980.
12. Omer GE, Spinner M: *Management of Peripheral Nerve Problems.* Philadelphia: WB Saunders, 1980.
13. Green D (ed): *Operative Treatment of Nerve Problems.* Edinburgh: Churchill Livingstone, 1981.
14. Smith J: Microsurgery of peripheral nerves. Plast Reconstr Surg 33:317–329, 1964.
15. Daniel RK: Microsurgery: Through the looking glass. N Engl J Med 300:1251–1257, 1979.
16. Jabaley ME, Wallace WH, Heckler FR: Internal topography of major nerves of the forearm and hand: A current review. J Hand Surg 5:1–18, 1980.
17. Sunderland S: Funicular suture and funicular exclusion in repair of several nerves. Br J Surg 40:580–587, 1953.
18. Edshage S: Peripheral nerve suture. Acta Chir Scand [Suppl] 331:1–101 (99 references), 1964.
19. Bora FW Jr: Peripheral nerve repair in cats: The fasicular stitch. J Bone Joint Surg 49A:659–666, 1967.
20. Hakistian RW: Funicular orientation by direct stimulation; an aid to peripheral nerve repair. J Bone Joint Surg 50A:1178–1186, 1968.
21. Grabb WC, Bement SC, Koepke G: Comparison of methods of peripheral nerve suturing in monkeys. Plast Reconstr Surg 46:31–38, 1970.
22. Gruber H, Zenker V: Acetylcholinesterase: Histological differentiation between motor and sensory nerve fibers. Brain Res 51:207–214, 1973.
23. Cabaud HE, Rodkey WG, McCarroll HR Jr, et al: Epineural and perineural fascicular nerve repair: A critical comparison. J Hand Surg 1:131–137, 1976.
24. Bora FW Jr, Pleasure DE, Didizan NA: A study of nerve regeneration and neuroma formation after nerve suture by various techniques. J Hand Surg 1:138–143, 1976.
25. Orgel MG, Terzis JK: Epineurial vs. perineurial repair: An ultrastructural and electrophysiologic study of nerve regeneration. Plast Reconstr Surg 60:80–91, 1977.
26. Rosen JM, Kaplan EN, Jewett DL, et al: Fascicular sutureless and suture repair of the peripheral nerves: A comparison study in laboratory animals. Orthop Rev 8:85–92, 1979.
27. Sunderland S: The pros and cons of funicular nerve repair. J Hand Surg 4:201–211, 1979.
28. Holmes W: Histologic observations on the repair of nerves by autografts. Br J Surg 35:167–173, 1947.
29. Sanders FK: Histopathology of nerve grafts, in Seddon HJ (ed): *Peripheral Nerve Injuries.* London: Her Majesty's Printing Office, 1954, pp 134–155.
30. Seddon HJ: Nerve grafting and other unusual forms of nerve repair, in Seddon HJ (ed): *Peripheral Nerve Injuries.* London: Her Majesty's Printing Office, 1954, pp 389–417.
31. Millesi H, Meisse G, Berger A: The interfascicular nerve-grafting of the median and ulnar nerves. J Bon Joint Surg 54A:727–750, 1972.
32. Millesi H, Meisse G, Berger A: Further experience with interfascicular grafting of the median, ulnar and radial nerves. J Bone Joint Surg 58A:209–218, 1976.
33. Mayamoto Y: Experimental study of results of nerve suture under tension vs. nerve grafting. Plast Reconstr Surg 64:540–549, 1979.
34. Young VL, Wray CR, Weeks PM: The results of

nerve grafting in the wrist and hand. Ann Plast Surg 5:212–215, 1980.

35. Dellon AL: The moving two-point discrimination test: Clinical evaluation of the quickly-adapting fiber receptor system. J Hand Surg 3:474–481, 1978.

36. Zachary RB, Holmes W: Primary suture of nerves. Surg Gynecol Obstet 82:632–651, 1946.

37. Moberg E: Objective methods for determining the functional value of sensibility in the skin. J Bone Joint Surg [Br] 40B:454–476, 1958.

38. Moberg E: Criticism and study of methods for examining sensibility in the hand. Neurology (Minneap) 12:8–19, 1962.

39. Kirklin JW, Murphy F, Berkson J: Suture of peripheral nerves: factors affecting prognosis. Surg Gynecol Obstet 88:719–730, 1949.

40. Zachary RB: Results of nerve suture, in Seddon HJ (ed): *Peripheral Nerve Injuries*. London: Her Majesty's Stationery Office, 1954, Ch 8, pp 34–388.

41. Yahr MD, Beebe GW: Recovery of motor function, in Seddon HJ (ed): *Peripheral Nerve Regeneration*. Washington DC: US Gov Printing Office, 1956, Ch III, pp 71–202.

42. Oester VT, Davis L: Recovery of sensory functions, in Woodhall B, Beebe GW (eds): *Peripheral Nerve Regeneration*. Washington DC: US Gov Printing Office, 1956, Ch V, pp 241–310.

43. Nicholson OR, Seddon HJ: Nerve repair in civil practice. Br Med J 2:1065–1071, 1957.

44. Lansen RD, Posch JL: Nerve injuries in the upper extremity. Arch Surg 77:469–482, 1958.

45. Stromberg WB, McFarlane RM, Bell LL, et al: Injury of the median and ulnar nerves. J Bone Joint Surg 43A:717–730, 1961.

46. McEwan LE: Median and ulnar nerve injuries. Aust NZ J Surg 32:89–104, 1962.

47. Sakellarides H: A follow-up study of 173 peripheral nerve injuries in the upper extremity of civilians. J Bone Joint Surg 44A:140–148, 1962.

48. Flynn JE, Flynn WF: Median and ulnar nerve injuries. Ann Surg 156:1002–1009, 1962.

49. Onne L: Recovery of sensibility and sudomotor activity in the hand after nerve suture. Acta Chir Scand [Suppl] 300:1–70, 1962 (135 references).

50. Nielsen JB, Torup D: Nerve injuries in the upper extremities. Dan Med Bull 11:92–95, 1964.

51. Boswick JA, Schneewind J, Stromberg W: Evaluation of peripheral nerve repairs below the elbow. Arch Surg 90:50–51, 1965.

52. Omer G: Injuries to nerves of the upper extremities. J Bone Joint Surg 56A:1615–1624, 1974.

53. Posch JL, dela Cruz-Saddul F: Nerve repair in trauma surgery: A ten-year study of 231 peripheral injuries. Orthop Rev 9:35–45, 1980.

54. Bunnell S: Surgery of the nerves of the hand. Surg Gynecol Obstet 44:145–152, 1927.

55. Weckesser EC: The repair of nerves in the palm and the fingers. Clin Orthop 19:200–207, 1961.

56. Honner R, Fragiadakis FG, Lamb DW: An investigation of factors affecting the results of digital nerve division. Hand 2:21–31, 1970.

57. Buncke HJ: Digital nerve repairs. Surg Clin North Am 52:1267–1285, 1972.

58. Poppen NK, McCarroll HR Jr, Doyle JR, et al: Recovery of sensibility after suture of digital nerves. J Hand Surg 4:212–226, 1979.

59. Bunnell S, Boyes JH: Nerve grafts. Am J Surg 44:64–75, 1939.

60. Seddon HJ: The use of autogenous grafts for repair of large gaps in peripheral nerves. Br J Surg 35:151–167, 1947.

61. Brooks D: The place of nerve grafting in orthopedic surgery. J Bone Joint Surg 37A:299–326, 1955.

62. McFarlane RM, Moyer JR: Digital nerve grafts with the lateral antebrachial cutaneous nerve. J Hand Surg 1:169–173, 1976.

63. Walton R, Finseth F: Nerve grafting in the repair of complicated peripheral nerve trauma. J Trauma 17:793–796, 1977.

64. Tallas R, Staniforth P, Fisher TR: Neurophysiological studies of autogenous nerve grafts. J Neurol Neurosurg Psychiatry 41:677–683, 1978.

65. Millesi H: Personal communication, 1980.

66. Wray C: Personal communication, 1980.

Chapter 12

RE-EDUCATION OF SENSATION

ROOTS OF SENSORY RE-EDUCATION
TECHNIQUES OF SENSORY RE-EDUCATION
RESULTS OF SENSORY RE-EDUCATION AFTER NERVE REPAIR
OTHER APPLICATIONS OF SENSORY RE-EDUCATION

Without sensation, a worker can scarcely pick up a small object, and he constantly drops things from his grasp. The so-called eyes of his fingers are blind.

S. Bunnell, 1927[1]

My interest in evaluating sensibility grew from the experiences of the summer of 1968. During the preceding Spring quarter, as a sophomore medical student at Johns Hopkins, I had taken a research elective with Doctor John E. Hoopes in the Division of Plastic Surgery. We worked on cleft palate speech problems. There was a bimonthly Hand Surgery Conference, attended by both Doctor Milton T. Edgerton, Chief of the Division, and Doctor Raymond M. Curtis, Hand Consultant. The conferences were stimulating. That summer, while continuing work with lateral view, sound cineradiography to evaluate cleft palate speech, I received per-

mission to observe Doctor Curtis in surgery at the Children's Hospital on Tuesdays. One day, after witnessing a meticulous nerve repair, I asked Doctor Curtis, "What are the results of nerve repair?" "Very few people recover normal sensation," he said.

The apparent gap between technical expertise in the operating room and functional recovery in the examining room was disturbing to me. In the hand, especially, structure and function were so intimately related, so clearly evident. Yet with a nerve, precise fascicular realignment seemingly failed to result in a correspondingly good functional result. In the Fall of 1968, during my clinical rotations, I began to review Doctor Vernon B. Mountcastle's neurophysiology course from my freshman year of medical school. The basic neurophysiologic concepts which had been revealed by his laboratory, and reviewed in his textbook[2] quite suddenly seemed immediately relevant to the clinical paradox of sensibility! As outlined earlier (see Chapter 3), the definitions of subpopulations of the group A beta fibers, based upon their properties of adaptation, could be translated clinically into a subdivision of touch as moving-touch and constant-touch. The subdivision of the quickly-adapting group A beta fibers, based upon their tuning curves, could be translated clinically into a 30-cps and a 256-cps tuning fork examination. I obtained permission to study a group of patients recovering from nerve injury. This approach to evaluating sensibility in the hand was begun in the Department of Rehabilitation Medicine, where Janice Maynard, M.A.O.T., O.T.R, was in charge of Occupational Therapy.

During my Junior year in medical school I continued to attend the Hand Conferences. When a patient recovering from a nerve injury was presented, I observed that after the patient would respond to pinprick, light fingertip stroking and pressure, he was still unable when "blindfolded" to pick out correctly a nickel from a quarter held in the examiner's palm. Leaving the conference room with the patients, I would meet them in the hall and ask to examine their hand again. It seemed to me that the necessary sensory submodalities had recovered but, perhaps because of "incomplete recovery" or fiber misdirection, the patient was simply confused by what he was feeling. I would place the nickel in the patient's hand and then the quarter, asking him "Can you feel these?" The answer would be "Yes." Then with his eyes shut and after feeling each again, I would ask him "Do these two feel different from each other?" The answer would be "Yes." Then, "Do they feel like a nickel and quarter used to feel?" The answer, "No." Clearly there was sufficient sensory information being perceived to permit a distinction by the patient between the two objects but the question "Is that a nickel?" was ambiguous. Upon

reflection I realized it was really two questions. One, "Do you feel something in your hand?" and two, "What is it?" The patient was passing the object perception question but failing the object recognition question. His sensibility had recovered but his attempted matching of the new, altered profile of impulses with past association cortex profiles always read "mismatch." Now, giving the nickel back, I'd say, "Shut your eyes. This is a nickel. It doesn't feel the way a nickel used to feel, but you must now call whatever you are feeling a nickel." The same was repeated with the quarter. Then, upon retesting, the patient could correctly, "blindfolded," choose the nickel or the quarter from my palm. Within a few minutes he had re-learned the names of common objects, his sensation had been re-educated.

This approach to evaluating sensibility in the hand and the results of the first series of patients we re-educated were presented to the Johns Hopkins Medical Society in May of 1970, just prior to my graduation from medical school. This work was presented to the American Society for Surgery of the Hand at their 1971 meeting in San Francisco, during my internship. The abstract of that presentation was published in the *Journal of Bone and Joint Surgery* in 1971.[3] The full manuscript, rejected by the Journal, ultimately was published. It had to be divided into a part on evaluating recovery of sensation, which was published in the *Johns Hopkins Medical Journal* in 1972,[4] and a part on re-education, published in *Plastic and Reconstructive Surgery* in 1974![5]

ROOTS OF SENSORY RE-EDUCATION

We see a little farther ahead because we are standing on the shoulders of those who came before.[6]

Sir Isaac Newton, 1675

As I reviewed the literature in preparing this monograph, it has become very clear that examples of sensory re-education have been documented previously, although they were unrecognized as such. One category of observations that may be explained on the basis of sensory re-education is the universal finding that sensory recovery continues to improve slowly for many years after nerve repair. Hakstian[7] calls this phenomenon "the drop-off in recovery toward completion of regeneration that characterizes all peripheral nerve sutures." An example of this phenomenon is supplied from the Nicholson and Seddon[8] data. In a group of ulnar nerve repairs, 5% of patients had achieved sensory grade of 3+ by 1 year following repair. By 3 years following the repair, this sensory grade had been achieved by 15% of the group and at 5 years by 21% of the group. Moberg[9] also seems to favor a prolonged course of nerve regeneration as an explanation for this. His "working hypothesis" is that "the larger fibers for tactile gnosis regenerate slower than the small fibers for sudomotor functions. Two-point discrimination is not regained for five years." I believe this hypothesis is untenable in view of the known capacity of axons to regenerate at about 1 mm per day in the distal upper extremity[10-11] (see Chapter 3). Even at 1 mm per day (1 inch per month), in the average sized adult, with the distance from the wrist to the fingertips being about 6 inches, regenerating axons of the thinnest diameter should arrive no later than 6 months, and probably by 1 year all axons have regenerated to the fingertip. I suggest that the further continued improvement in sensation is in part due to maturation of the newly re-united fiber/receptor systems, but primarily to the subliminal re-education that attends the daily, though guarded, use of the injured hand.

Sensory re-education allows the patient to achieve the potential for functional recovery provided by the nerve repair. Implicit in this statement is the assumption of use of the injured hand, if not in a formal sensory re-education program, then in an intrinsically motivated setting. I believe Davis[12] reported essentially this in 1949. Davis was working with Bowden on the staff of the Medical Research Council in London and was a Lecturer in psychopathology at the University of Cambridge. He studied 82 patients who had been treated in the Peripheral Nerve Units during the war. He related their "relative academic and functional recovery" to their

degree of disability, present and previous employment, and job satisfaction. He concluded that functional recovery was favored by exercise and that recovery was better where the tendency to use the limb was stronger and where use was begun earlier. More recent, but parallel, observations by Honner, Fragiadakis, and Lamb[13] support this general hypothesis. They found that "the best results (of nerve repair) were obtained in skilled or dexterous workers, compared with semi-skilled, or heavy manual labourers, clerical workers or housewives."

The ultimate capacity for tactile discrimination in the normal hand remains to be defined. Observations that may be interpreted as demonstrating sensory re-education in the noninjured hand are available in the control groups in Onne's series[14] and in my own series.[5] In establishing normal values for the two-point discrimination test, Onne tested a series of controls on two separate occasions. One patient's two-point discrimination decreased by 6 mm between trials. In our initial group of patients having sensory re-education, we tested two-point discrimination in the normal hand at each testing session. In four patients, the initial value decreased from 6 to 3.5 mm, 4 to 2 mm, 3 to 2.5 mm, and 4 to 2 mm as the program progressed. This sensory re-education in the normal hand is emphasized by the capacity of formerly sighted (blind) individuals to read braille. Heinricks and Moorehouse[15] evaluated two-point discrimination in nondiabetic blind people. Whereas the normal value in their control group was 3 to 5 mm, the blind braille readers had a two-point discrimination of 1.5 mm. These findings have been supported by the independent study of Almquist.[16]

The results of nerve repair in children have been found consistently superior to those in adults (see also Chapter 11).[12, 14, 17] The usual "explanation" for these better results is a presumed superior ability of their central nervous system to compensate for misdirected axons. However, Bach-y-Rita's extensive experience in retraining blind people with the tacile visual substitution system,[18-19] and his experience with recovery from brain lesions, i.e., strokes,[20, 21] has demonstrated that the young adult and the senior citizen also possess a remarkable capacity for cerebral reorganization. "However, training has been found crucial in adaptation to the tactile visual substitution system, even as it is in obtaining functional recovery from experimental or clinical brain lesions. The cerebral reorganization revealed by such functional recovery may have features in common with the reorganization necessitated by processing information received through the skin in visual terms."[20] Retraining has been found to enable monkeys to recover precision tactile activities after parietal lobe lesions, too.[22] I wonder, therefore, if the success of children in recovering their functional sensations after nerve injury is not at least partially due to their continual curious investigation of their environment with their hands.

Another set of observations that may be interpreted to demonstrate sensory re-education is derived from the relationship between the Meissner corpuscles and moving-touch. In Chapters 3 and 10, the neurophysiologic basis for designating the Meissner corpuscle as the receptor for the low frequency quickly-adapting fiber/receptor system, and the function of the system in mediating the perception of moving-touch was outlined. It has been demonstrated that the absolute number of Meissner corpuscles diminished with age (Fig. 12.1).[23] It would seem natural therefore if Meissner corpuscle function diminished with age, that when a specific test of this sensibility, such as receptor threshold, is studied by means of vibration of varying amplitude, an age-related effect is found. Vibratory thresholds, indeed, do increase with increasing age (Fig. 12.2).[24] However, the normal values for the moving two-point discrimination test show little change with increasing age (Fig. 12.3).[25] Moving two-point discrimination is a test of the innervation density of the quickly-adapting fiber/

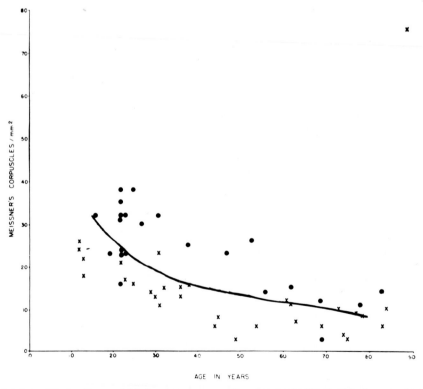

Figure 12.1. Diminution of Meissner corpuscle concentration with increasing age in the fingertip of man. (Reproduced with permission from C. F. Bolton et al.: *Neurology* 16: 1–9, 1966[23])

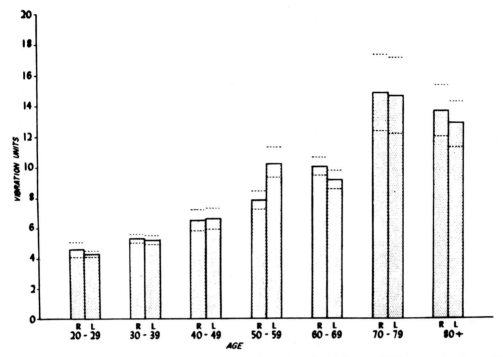

Figure 12.2. Increase in vibratory perception threshold for a 125-cps stimulus with increasing age. (Reproduced with permission from G. Rosenberg: *J Am Geriatr Soc* 6: 471–481, 1958.[24])

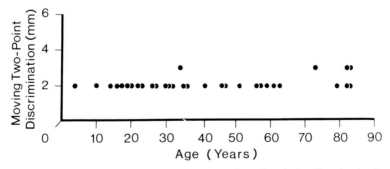

Figure 12.3. Normal value of the moving two-point discrimination test, demonstrating little, if any, increase in the limen with increasing age. (Reproduced with permission from A. L. Dellon: *J Hand Surg* 3:474–481, 1978.[25])

receptor systems and might be expected to show, therefore, more variation with age. However, this test requires conscious discrimination of tactile patterns. I suggest that the component of central learning can be invoked to "override" a physiologic peripheral loss, and thus there is little change in moving two-point discrimination with age. I suggest that if the fingers are kept active, then despite advancing chronologic age, the biologic capacity for tactile discrimination will not be diminished. Constant activity is the sensory re-education that provides a physiologic face-lift to the wrinkled hand.

Another example that demonstrates re-education is that a transplant assumes the sensory characteristics of its recipient site. In the classic study of Hutchinson, Tough, and Wynburn,[26] from 1949, classic two-point discrimination was measured in human abdominal skin grafted to the face or fingertips. The two-point discrimination of the normal abdominal skin was 20 to 25 mm. When tested 2 to 18 years later, there were examples of recovered two-point discrimination of 4 mm on the face and 6 mm on the fingertip. Sturman and Duran[27] reported similar results, including donar sites of forearm skin, dorsal, palmar, and abdominal flaps.

Transferring toe pulp to the fingertip offers another demonstration of sensory re-education having occurred. The plantar tissue has been found to have an average classic two-point discrimination of 11.3 mm for the great toe (range, 7 to 18 mm), and an average of 16.4 mm for the second toe (10 to 25 mm)[28] In 1974, Maquieric reported transferring a plantar nerve innervated pulp graft to the fingertip in eight patients. Six of the eight recovered a classic two-point discrimination of less that 6 mm! With the advent of microvascular transfer of tissue, the great toe-to-thumb[30] and the second toe-to-thumb[31] reconstructions have also reported recovery of classic two-point discrimination that is better than it was in the toe prior to transfer.[32] Similar gains in tactile discrimination have been reported for microvascular transfer of dorsal first-second toe web space to the hand[33, 34] with improvement of from 15 mm for the donor to 3 mm for the recipient. These results can only be interpreted as demonstrating fulfillment of unrealized sensory potential in the transplanted tissue brought about by sensory re-education during and after nerve regeneration.

What is the origin of the term "sensory re-education?" In August of 1971 Doctor Curtis sent me a copy of a letter he had received from Group Captain C. B. Wynn Parry, Consultant Adviser in "Physical Medicine, Royal Air Force, Chessington, Surrey, England." The letter began:

I was sorry not to be at the meeting of the Society for Surgery of the Hand when you gave your Presidential address. I am particularly sorry as I read in the *Journal of Bone and Joint Surgery* of June, 1971 your experience with Doctor Dellon

and Doctor Edgerton in sensory re-education. I would be most grateful for any published materials you have on this as to my knowledge you are the only other team to have worked in this field. I do not know whether you are aware that I have a fairly extended treatment of the importance of sensory re-education which I published in my book "Rehabilitation of the Hand," Butterworth, 1966 ... I hope you may find time to look through the relevant pages in my book as I would be very glad to know how our techniques compare.

In fact, Doctor Curtis had known of Wynn Parry's work, and once I had begun to discuss the project with him, he referred me to Wynn Parry's monograph.[35] My notation on my copy of that book indicates I bought it in June of 1969. Wynn Parry, to the best of my knowledge, was the first to utilize sensory re-education for patients with nerve repair in a formal program of rehabilitation. He wrote:

Although it has been accepted for many years that re-education of motor function is most important in the management of peripheral nerve injuries, little or no attention seems to have been paid to the problem of re-education of sensation after nerve suture. It is widely felt that the quality of sensation after median nerve suture is poor. At the most, protective sensation can be expected, and in very rare cases is there an expectation of perfect two-point discrimination or stereognosis. In our experience over the last twelve years, in patients with combined median and ulnar nerve sutures who have had full-time treatment, function is remarkably good. Our studies of such patients suggested that they were instinctively retraining themselves to learn to use their abnormal sensation for function. We therefore decided to apply sensory re-education techniques in a more formal manner in the Physiotherapy Department.[35]

Rehabilitation centers, however, had been applying the sensory retraining techniques for the decade prior to Wynn Parry's monograph. His techniques appear to be linear descendents from these. In 1955, the neurology section of the Minneapolis Veteran's Administration Hospital evaluated sensibility in 35 postcerebrovascular accident hemiplegics. Eighty percent had impaired sensation. Their length of hospital stay and ultimate recovery were found directly related to their recovery of sensation. In the rehabilitation unit, though, no definite sensory retraining program was used. The patient's sensibility was retested weekly. The authors concluded "retraining may play a significant role in return of function."[36] Forster and Shields,[37] from the Neurology and Rehabilitation Departments at Georgetown University, reported in 1959 the first specific program for sensory retraining in hemiplegics. The technique was one of conditioning, with the patient alternately observing and blinded to his hand's activity. Activities included positioning of the digits, pinprick localization, weight discrimination with sandbags and attempted recognition of large objects of differing shapes and textures. In 1962, Vinograd et al.[38] utilized a modification of Forster and Shields' technique to retrain sensation in the hemiplegic hand. This group, from the Rehabilitation Department of the Wilmington, Delaware Veteran's Administration Hospital, used common household objects, like a ball, can opener, and keys for their object recognition. Patients were trained and retested daily for an average of 7 weeks. Results encouraged the authors to recommend sensory retraining "as an adjunct in the management of suitable patients."

The roots of re-education go back farther, however. In the Medical Research Council 1954 monograph on peripheral nerve injuries, for which Seddon was the editor, Ruth E. M. Bowden wrote an extensive chapter (54 pages) on "Factors Influencing Functional Recovery." Her final segment is subtitled "Reeducation after Nerve Injuries." She wrote, "The aim of re-education of patients with nerve injuries is to aid the restoration of function in the damaged limb and facilitate the adjustment of the individual to his disability." She goes on, however, to discuss essentially only motor function rehabilitation and expresses almost pessimism over the potential of its sensory counterpart. "On the whole, there is no definite evidence to suggest the existence of compensatory adjustments in the central nervous system to faulty peripheral connections. However, there is an indication that constant usage may lead to greater manual dexterity even in the presence of such abnormalities."[39]

Possibly, the first to demonstrate that hemiplegics could be retrained were Ruch et al.[40] in 1938. They reviewed their work in sub-human primates demonstrating that removal of the parietal lobe resulted in astereognosis. Then in the monkeys, and in humans following cortical loss, they demonstrated that sensory retraining or reconditioning resulted in some recovered function. This suggested the potential that led to the sensory retraining programs of Forster and Shields.

The roots of re-education go back even further. Just recently I was referred to an article by John S. B. Stopford[41] written in 1926. The reference to this article, and the only time I've ever seen it referred to, was in a recent paper by Horch.[42] The Stopford reference does not appear in the extensive bibliographies of Winkelmann, Sunderland or Seddon. Stopford was an ardent supporter of Henry Head's theories. The purpose of Stopford's paper was to provide an explanation for the two-stage recovery of sensation. Stopford noted, "We find the elements of sensation ... which recover late and which most frequently show imperfect recovery ... are those (epicritic) which Head has shown to have cortical representation." The protopathic sensations Stopford attributed to the thalamus. He went on:

> If the thalamus and sensory cortex provide a reason for the two stages of recovery, it is possible to understand why a longer period must elapse before the fibres subserving the cortical forms of sensation function correctly ... a very much more complex readjustment and *re-education* (emphasis mine) must occur after regeneration of the fibres ... In consequence of the inevitable disturbance of the intraneural pattern after suture, chance plays a considerable part in the success of the result, since a variable number of regenerating fibres must grow down the endoneural, perineural, or epineural connective tissues and be functionally lost, whilst others grew down heterogeneous peripheral fibres ... Fibres previously concerned with transmission of impulses excited by pain may grow down ... "localization" paths ... It is conceivable that after the lapse of time, a capable patient would by *re-education* overcome this and localize the stimulus more or less accurately. Such a period of *re-education* would explain the occurrence of an interval between the recovery of the crude forms (protopathic) and the higher forms (epicritic) of sensation ... It seems possible that by *re-education* some recovery may follow at a later date.

With that amazing quote, I will leave the "roots" of re-education to a future "gardener" who may wish to dig deeper.

TECHNIQUES OF SENSORY RE-EDUCATION

This section is entitled technique*s*. There is no one technique of sensory re-education.

Sensory re-education is a method or combination of techniques that help the patient with a sensory impairment learn to re-interpret the altered profile of neural impulses reaching his conscious level after his injured hand has been stimulated.

In the normal state, stimulation of the hand by contact with the external environment stimulates the sensory receptors, a profile of neural impulses is elicited, these impact upon the sensory cortex, associate with previous memory or experiences, and ultimately become consciousness, a perception. After a nerve division and nerve repair, the same contact with the external world, the same stimulus, now elicits a different or an altered profile of neural impulses. When these reach the sensory cortex, they may find no match in the association cortex. Thus, the sensation is new, cannot be named, and may even pass unnoticed (Fig. 12.4).

Despite any future refinement in technical skill with nerve repair, altered peripheral sensibility is statistically inevitable (Fig. 12.5). With microsurgical fascicular repair, hopefully, the "majority" of regenerating axons will cross the suture, enter their own or a closure cousin's endoneurial tube, and distally reinnervate the correct type of sensory

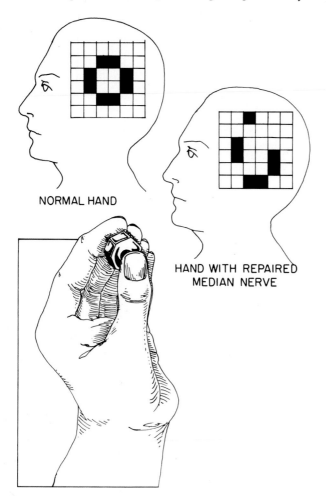

NORMAL HAND

HAND WITH REPAIRED MEDIAN NERVE

Figure 12.4. In the normal hand, a stimulus, such as this gripped bolt, elicits a profile of neural impulses which reaches the sensory cortex, and ultimately is perceived, as represented by the checkerboard pattern. After a nerve repair, the same stimulus elicits an altered profile of impulses, which reaches the sensory cortex. The new perception, the altered checkerboard pattern, may be so different from the previous one, that object recognition is at first impossible.

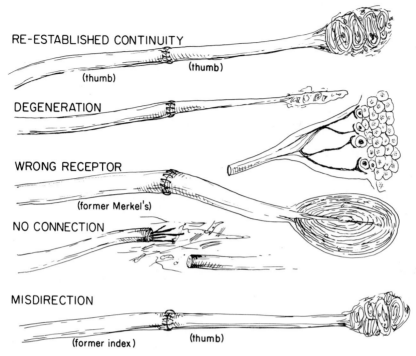

Figure 12.5. The inevitable altered profile of impulses. The majority of regenerating axons will re-establish continuity with the appropriate end organ in the appropriate digital area. However, some axons will arrive to find an irreversibly degenerated end organ, others will arrive at the correct digital area, but reinnervate the wrong end organ, while others will either never re-enter a distal endoneurial sheath or be misdirected to the wrong finger. Thus, a stimulus gives rise to a different profile of nerve impulses than this stimulus elicited prior to nerve repair.

end organ. Some regenerating axons will arrive distally to find their former home destroyed, degenerated beyond salvage. Some regenerating axons will arrive distally to the correct locale but find themselves in the wrong home. A former index fingertip Pacinian afferent may return to the index fingertip but reinnervate a Merkel cell-neurite complex, or a former index fingertip resident may find himself in the thumb. Then there will be the group of axons that either never cross the suture line and grow out of the epineurium to form a neuroma, or grow distally into the epi-, peri- or endoneurial connective tissue. These possibilities create the following potential alterations: (1) an absolute decrease in the number of normally functioning peripheral receptive fields; (2) a new set of abnormal peripheral receptive fields (wrong fiber/receptor combinations, one fiber reinnervating multiple receptive fields); (3) a new set of misdirected peripheral receptive fields (index referred to thumb, proximal referred to distal, etc.); (4) dysesthetia (axons trapped in scar at repair site) (Fig. 12.5).

Refinements in surgical technique should be giving patients an increasing potential for sensory recovery. It is my belief that the present failure to demonstrate improved end results following nerve repair is less a failure of the surgeon to achieve fascicular alignment as it is a failure of the patient to realize the potential given to him at surgery. The goal of sensory re-education is to help the patient achieve the full potential for functional sensory recovery given to him by his nerve repair (Fig. 12.6).

The first published formal program of sen-

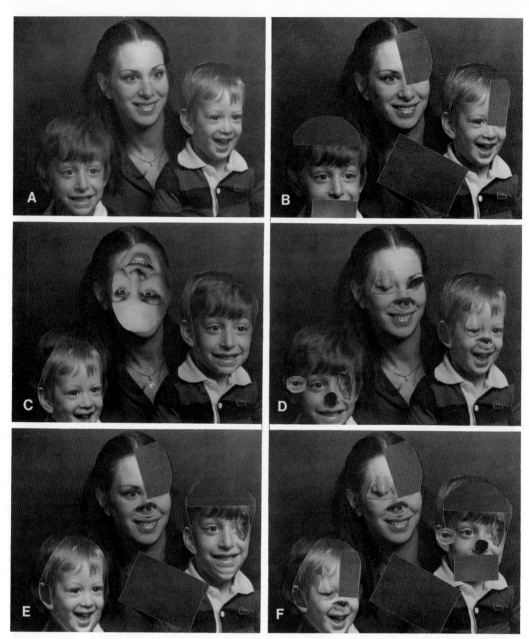

Figure 12.6. Conceptual basis for altered profile of neural impulses after nerve repair. *A*, The three people here are seen by stimulation of sensory receptors in the eye, causing neural impulses to be received in the visual cortex of the brain. These impulses are associated with previous visual memory patterns and given a name, e.g., Evan (*left*), Marge (*center*), Glenn (*right*). The analogous series of events occurs normally in the hand, e.g. tactile gnosis. After a nerve repair, a number of axons never regenerate causing discrete loss of impulses from the previous pattern (*B*). After a nerve repair, a number of axons will regenerate to the wrong topographic area, i.e., index to thumb, or Evan to Glenn (*C*). After a nerve repair, a number of axons will reinnervate an inappropriate sensory end organ, creating unnatural combinations, of unknown potential, e.g., eye for nose, eye for an ear (*D*). Even in the microsurgical repair, all of these combinations occur to a degree (*E*) and in some repairs the resulting combinations (*F*) may create impulse patterns that are impossible to recognize. Sensory re-education can overcome much of this distortion, and allow recovery of tactile gnosis.

sory re-education following nerve repair is that of Wynn Parry.[35, 43] In essence, blindfolded patients are given a series of familiar, large, household objects to identify. The time required for object identification is recorded and used as a basis of comparison during subsequent testing and training sessions. Tasks are increased in complexity as the patient improves. They are begun on coins, erasers, paper clips, keys, cards, etc. If they can't recognize an object in 60 seconds they go on to the next, for 10 objects. Failing these, they begin with large wood blocks of varying weight, shape, and size, covered with different textured materials. If they still cannot identify the object, they are permitted to open their eyes, "study the object carefully and then feel it again with their eyes shut, thus trying to combine the mental with the visual picture. The patient carries out the same procedure with the unaffected hand so that he may compare the sensation on the two sides." Training is given daily or patients are asked to get someone to help them at home daily.

Following the appearance in the *Journal of Bone and Joint Surgery* of the abstract of my presentation on sensory re-education at the 1971 meeting of The American Society for Surgery of the Hand, I received many requests from hand surgeons and therapists for a copy of my "program." As mentioned earlier, the *Journal of Bone and Joint Surgery* had rejected our manuscript. Their letter of August 17, 1971 said in part, "All of us thought the study was pertinent to the practical concerns of a good number of our Journal's readers, but many of us thought that . . . the experimental plans did not sufficiently take into account one possible source of error—bias on the part of both subject and observer." The letter concluded, "We think your method and experience with it should first be shown to be acceptable to the physiologists and should appear in their literature as a valid study." I was undoubtedly biased. I was also in the midst of my surgical residency. I wrote up our program and sent off xeroxed copies to all who requested them. Interestingly, in 1978 I was shown a book available through Sammon, Inc. which included this program as a chapter on sensory re-education.[44] They never asked our permis-

sion to publish it, but I thank them now for distributing it!

My program consists of a series of specific sensory exercises instituted at the appropriate time in the recovery process. One can't run before he can walk. The pattern of sensory recovery outlined in Chapter 7 may be thought of as the timetable on which to base the introduction of sensory exercises. Initiating an exercise before the appropriate fiber/receptor system has reunited can only lead to frustration and failure. Instituting the appropriate exercises at the appropriate time speeds patient recovery, builds patient confidence, and facilitates recovery of maximal function in the minimal time.

Early Phase Sensory Re-education

The pattern of sensory recovery is charted by evaluating sensibility (see Chapter 10) with the 30-cps tuning fork, moving-touch, constant-touch and the 256-cps tuning fork. The perception of these stimuli will recover in this same time sequence, i.e., 30 cps first, 256 cps last. When 30 cps and moving-touch have returned to an area, for example, the palm, early phase re-education may be begun. It is most critical to begin by the time recovery has reached the proximal phalanges. The goal at this stage is (1) to re-educate submodality-specific perceptions, movement versus constant-touch and pressure and (2) to re-educate misdirection or incorrect localization. The exercise simply is for the patient to use a soft instrument like a pencil's eraser, or someone else may use their fingertip to stroke up and down the length of the area being re-educated. The patient observes what is happening, shuts his eyes and concentrates on what he is perceiving, and then opens his eyes to confirm again what is really happening (Fig. 12.7). He should verbalize to himself what he is perceiving as specifically as he can, i.e., I feel something moving up (down) my index finger near the palm.

When the patient can perceive constant-touch, the same type of Early Phase Re-education is done for this touch submodality, i.e., the eraser is pressed down into one spot on the palm or finger within the area of recovered constant-touch perception, and the

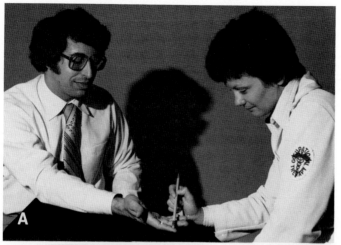

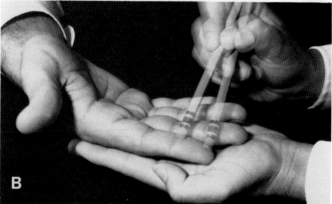

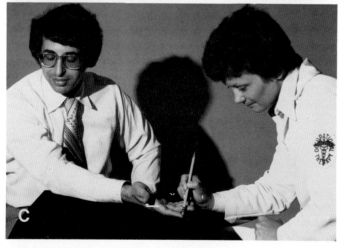

Figure 12.7.   Early Phase Sensory Re-education. The perception of moving-touch is returning to the finger. The patient (*A*) directly observes the stimulus (*B*), a moving pencil eraser, on his fingertip, then (*C*) shuts his eyes (emphasized here by also turning the head), and concentrates again on the stimulus. At this point he should be telling himself, "I feel something moving on my index finger." This is repeated several times in each area recovering sensation. Goal is to (1) re-educate touch submodalities and (2) re-educate mislocalization.

patient first directly observes what is occurring, then shuts his eyes and repeats the stimulus, verbalizes to himself what he is perceiving, opens his eyes and reaffirms the stimulus/perception. Again, he should be saying "I feel something pressing (soft, hard) on my index finger near my palm."

How hard should the stimulus be pressed into the finger? Remember that the newly reunited fiber/receptor system is "immature," its threshold is therefore high, and early in the recovery of sensation more stimulus intensity must be used for perception to occur (see Fig. 7.3). Press the moving or still eraser as hard as necessary for the patient to perceive constant-touch or movement. However, stimulus intensity should never be such as to evoke the perception of pain. We are not re-educating pain perception.

The patient should not stimulate one hand directly with the other. The patient's right index finger should not be used to stroke or press upon the patient's left palm or left thumb. If this were to occur, the patient would be receiving two sets of sensory information, one from each hand. At this early point in re-education, this only confuses the distorted sensory picture.

Who does Early Phase Re-education? We all do, the entire hand rehabilitation team. The surgeon, whenever he examines the patient, will be doing these exercises to ascertain for his own records the degree of recovery. This may be about once a month and should re-enforce the whole motivational/emotional system and the need for re-education. The hand therapist should be doing sensory re-education concomitant with motor re-education, range of motion, strength exercises, and massage. If there is dichotomy in the rehabilitation department with specific skills being assigned to physical and occupational therapy, a good workable arrangement we have found is for the physical therapist to do the motor re-education, including range of motion, strength, massage, whirlpool, ultrasound, etc., and for the occupational therapist to do the sensory re-education program. Certainly, any interested therapist or individual (mother, sister, boyfriend, visiting nurse) can be shown the sensory re-education technique and be "pressed" into service. The therapist should be seeing the patient at least once a week, if possible, for just 10 to 15 minutes to reinforce the goals, check the progress, provide reassurance, and establish that individual one-to-one contact that often makes the difference in the marginally motivated patient. The patient, himself, should be encouraged to practice Early Phase Sensory Re-education four times a day, even if just for 5 minutes a day.

The environment in which re-education is done is important. Janice Maynard, the therapist with whom our first sensory re-education work was done, has emphasized this.[45] A quiet room is essential. A soundproof room in the Hand Center is ideal. A bustling, noisy area is to be avoided. The patient is trying to concentrate on early, altered sensory perceptions. During this phase, if hyperesthesia or dysesthesia develops, specific desensitization should be begun concomitant with Early Phase Re-education.[45] Specific re-education exercises occasionally may need to be discontinued until a period of extreme "over-response" passes or is worked through. But, the exercises being used for desensitization, gentle stroking with different fabrics, gentle tapping, etc., can be re-educational in themselves, and, conversely, the Early Phase Re-education exercises can help desensitize the mild case of hyperesthesia.

You may find a patient who recovers the perception of 30 cps at the fingertip while the perception of moving-touch remains in the palm. Or you may find the patient who recovers both 30 cps and 256 cps at the fingertip while perception of constant-touch remains in the palm and perception of moving-touch is in the proximal phalanx. The patient has re-established the requisite fiber/receptor system for perception of moving-touch at the fingertip in the former, and for both moving- and constant-touch in the latter case. A "potential" gap exists. Within 2 to 3 weeks of intensive Early Phase Re-education, this gap can be overcome (see Fig. 12.8).[5] In these situations, the tuning fork is your guide to instituting the specific sensory exercises. Once the perception of 30 cps has reached the fingertip, you need not wait to institute the movement exercises to the distal phalanx. Once the 256 cps has reached the fingertip, you need not wait to institute the constant-touch/pressure exercises to the distal phalanx. Early Phase Re-education should be introduced to the fingertip 4 to 6 months following a median or ulnar nerve repair at the wrist level.

Late Phase Sensory Re-education

Late Phase Sensory Re-education should be begun as soon as moving-touch and constant-touch can be perceived definitely and unambiguously at the fingertip with good

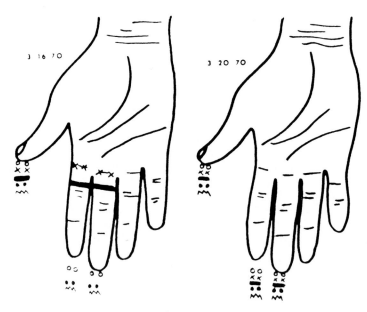

Figure 12.8. Early Phase Sensory Re-education. When perception of vibratory stimuli can be perceived at the fingertip and touch stimuli cannot (see text), a potential gap exists that can be filled quickly with specific re-education exercises. Legend (for this figure only) •••, 30 cps; ○○○, 256 cps; ∿, pain; ×××, constant-touch; ▬, moving-touch. (Reproduced with permission from A. L. Dellon et al: *Plast Reconstr Surg* 53: 297–305, 1974.[5])

localization. In our experience, this often can be as early as 6 to 8 months after median or ulnar nerve repair at the wrist.

It is never too late to begin Late Phase Sensory Re-education.

Beginning it too early leads to inevitable patient failure at the recognition tasks and heightens patient/therapist frustration. It is important to tell the patient at the beginning of this phase that he will continue slow improvement in his ability to recognize objects. He simply will not be physiologically ready to differentiate the smallest objects until 10 to 12 months after nerve repair at the wrist if he is "young" and has a good repair. It is critical to give the patient a timeframe for improvement so his expectations can be realistic.

The goal of Late Phase Sensory Re-education is to guide the patient to recovery of tactile gnosis, nothing less. If we expect less, we'll get less.

Sensory re-education cannot induce axonal regeneration. Sensory re-education can only help the patient achieve the fullest potential provided by the nerve repair. However, we do not know the consequences of improper fiber/receptor connections. For example, it is entirely possible, indeed probable, that a quickly-adapting, former Pacinian afferent can reinnervate a Meissner corpuscle (which is, of course, the transducer for the other

quickly-adapting fiber/receptor system) and form a functional unit. But, what happens if a quickly-adapting fiber enters a previous Merkel cell-neurite complex, or a slowly-adapting fiber enters a Meissner corpuscle? These may give rise to cortical level confusion, such as the type shown by Paul, et al. (Fig. 12.9)[46] or dorsal horn confusion, such as the type recently shown by Brushart and Terzis.[47] Furthermore, a regenerating axon, by virtue of its multiple axonal sprouts, may reinnervate receptors in two different areas, thereby having one fiber innervate two separate peripheral receptive fields. Such an occurrence has been demonstrated recently by Horch[42] and by Dykes and Terzis.[49] Horch demonstrated a slowly-adapting fiber reinnervating more than one Merkel cell-neurite peripheral receptive field. Dykes and Terzis demonstrated a quickly-adapting fiber reinnervating two different Meissner afferent receptive fields, and another fiber reinnervating both a quickly-adapting and slowly-adapting peripheral receptive field (Fig. 12.10). The possibilities here for altered patterns of neural profiles are obvious, and create situations requiring Late Phase Sensory Re-education.

Re-education may enable central reorganization. Groups of fiber/receptors which otherwise would have been totally lost to meaningful perception, if not groups that

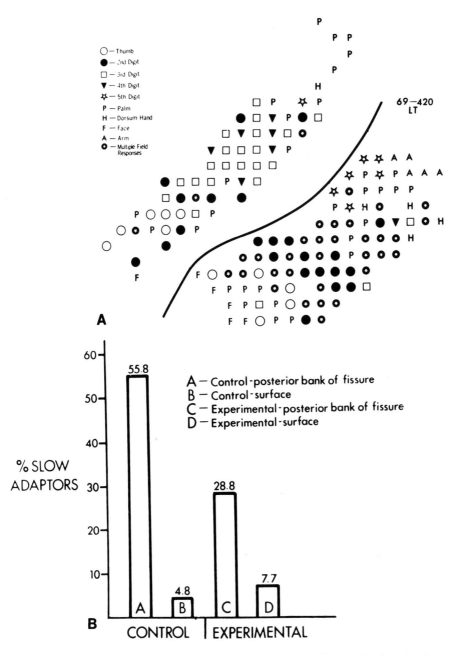

Figure 12.9. Cortical alterations following nerve repair. *A*, Example of evoked response recordings from postcentral gyrus of monkey after nerve repair demonstrating a large number of MFR (multiple field responses) in Brodmann's area 1 (to right) and fewer number in area 3 (to left). The MFR represents a cortical neuron now representing more than one peripheral receptive field. *B*, Demonstrates the average change in percentage of submodality-specific cortical neurons after nerve repair for bars A and C (area 3) and B and D (area 1). (Reproduced with permission from R. L. Paul et al: *Brain Res* 39:1–19, 1972.[46])

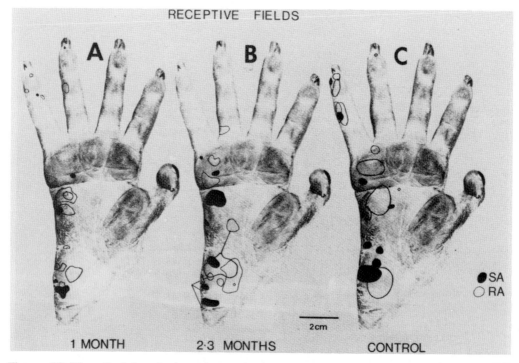

RECEPTIVE FIELDS

A   B   C

● SA
○ RA

2cm

1 MONTH   2·3 MONTHS   CONTROL

Figure 12.10. Peripheral alterations following nerve repair. The center hand has a single fiber reinnervating two rapidly-adapting peripheral receptive fields and another fiber reinnervating both rapidly-adapting and slowly-adapting peripheral receptive fields. (Reproduced with permission from R. W. Dykes and J. K. Terzis: *J Neurophysiol* 42: 1461–1478, 1979.[48])

would have interfered with meaningful perception, may be recruited, retrained, and provide meaningful sensory input. If re-education can achieve such "central reorganization"[21] of these types of peripheral fiber/receptor misconnections, then re-education conceivably could help the patient enhance or even exceed the potential given by the nerve repair.

Since the goal of Late Phase Sensory Re-education is recovery of functional sensations, the specific exercises should involve object identification. Tactile discrimination recovers progressively over time as measured by both classic and moving two-point discrimination.[25] Since, at any given time in the recovery process, moving two-point discrimination has recovered to a greater degree than classic two-point discrimination,[25] the object recognition tasks should incorporate movement. The tasks or exercises should be graded, beginning with the discrimination of

larger objects, with greater differences among them in size, shape, and texture, if possible, and progressing to finer and more subtle differences. Although it was generally accepted that tactile gnosis could not be present unless the classic two-point discrimination was less than 12 to 15 mm, I have demonstrated recently[49] (see Chapter 10), that even in the absence of classic two-point discrimination (>25 mm) if moving two-point discrimination is less than 7 mm, a patient can identify objects by manipulating them between his thumb and index finger.

Late Phase Sensory Re-education is begun with a set of familiar household objects, differing widely in shape, size, and texture (Fig. 12.11, top). Again, the sequence of object grasp with eyes open, eyes shut with concentration on perception, eyes open for reinforcement is utilized. After the patient has practiced with the objects, the therapist may test him and record either the number of

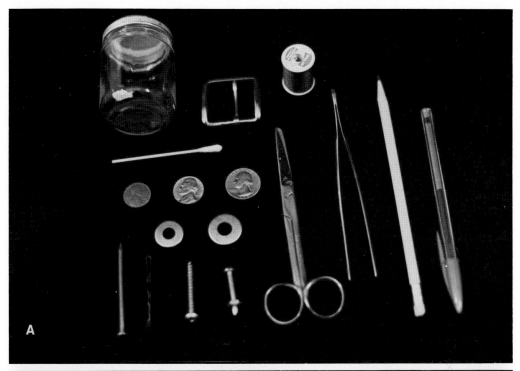

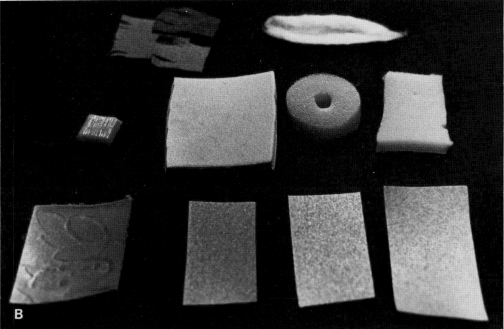

Figure 12.11. Late Phase Sensory Re-education. As moving two-point discrimination begins to return, and before classic two-point discrimination returns, movement must be incorporated into the object identification exercises. *A,* Familiar household objects, differing markedly in shape, size, and texture are used, progressing to *B,* objects differing, for example, primarily in texture, such as felts, polyethelene, plastic, leather, and grades of sandpaper.

objects identified correctly or the time required (in seconds with a stop watch) for object identification. A record such as this provides evidence to the patient, therapist, and referring physician that progress is occurring. It gives the patient a goal "to beat" next time. It assists patient motivation. A chart, such as the one used for our standard timed object recognition test (Fig. 6.7), can be prepared for the set of household items, mimeographed, and be available to fill out and place into the patient's chart.

Late Phase Sensory Re-education is continued by progressing to objects differing largely in texture (Fig. 12.11, bottom) and then to objects that are smaller, differing in size and shape but not in texture, and requiring subtle discrimination (Fig. 12.12). At this stage, the patient will be clinically recovering classic two-point discrimination, and moving two-point discrimination will be less than 7 mm. As moving two-point discrimination drops below 5 mm, patients will be able to identify the smallest objects correctly, although the objects may fall from the patient's grasp because the slowly-adapting fiber/re-

ceptor system has not regenerated and matured sufficiently. (It may never do so.)

It should be obvious that Late Phase Sensory Re-education also provides motor re-education (Fig. 12.13).

For the patient who worked before his injury, as soon as possible in Late Phase Re-education, activities that duplicate or incorporate work motions or activities should be included. To this end, a workshop within the Hand Center is ideal. A therapist with a background in industrial arts can design a program of workshop activities that coincide in sensory requirements with the degree of sensory recovery actually present. A Work Simulator, such as that recently designed by John Engalitcheff for the Raymond M. Curtis Hand Center at the Union Memorial Hospital in Baltimore, is ideal to practice a specific sensory grip before the patient is ready to try the actual tool at work (Fig. 12.14).

Who performs Late Phase Sensory Re-education? The entire hand team should participate. The hand surgeon during the office examination should test moving and constant two-point discrimination and object recog-

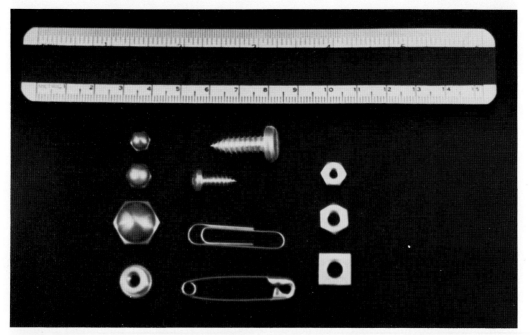

Figure 12.12. Late Phase Sensory Re-education. As moving two-point discrimination begins to return, smaller objects requiring more subtle discrimination in size and shape, but not texture, are used for object identification.

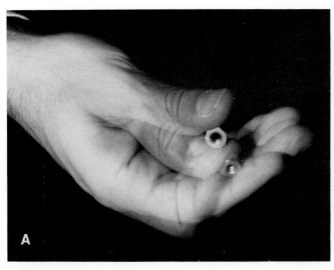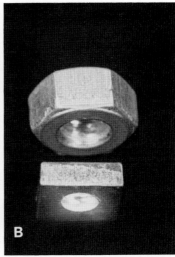

Figure 12.13.   Median nerve-injured patients are re-educated with exercises involving manipulating the object for recognition between the thumb and index and/or middle finger (*A*). For final stages of re-education, patient attempts discrimination between the square and hex nut (*B*).

nition. In so doing, praise, reinforcement, reassurance, and motivation are provided to sustain the patient and back-up what the therapist has been doing. At this point, the surgeon should be seeing the patient every 3 months. The therapist should be seeing the patient weekly, progressing to bi-weekly and perhaps monthly between the start of the Late Phase (6 to 9 months postrepair) and the patient's return to work. The therapist should be working through the Late Phase exercises, testing and recording the results of object recognition, encouraging and reinforcing the patient. At each session both classic and moving two-point discrimination are recorded. The patient should be practicing at home three to four times a day, 5 to 10 minutes each time. Frequent short sessions are more productive than longer, less frequent sessions. When the patient reaches the Fig. 12.12 stage, he is encouraged to carry the smaller objects in his pocket, or she in her purse, and to practice identifying them and picking them out during the day.

Late Phase exercises can be modified depending on the nerve involved. For the median nerve, all of the tests described above are applicable and essentially involve three-point pinch or gripping of the object between thumb, index, and middle fingers, and manipulating the object (Fig. 12.13). For ulnar or digital nerve injuries, a second person's presence during exercise is helpful (Fig. 12.15). That person can place the object for recognition onto the surface of the fingertip being re-educated. Less precise but still helpful is for the patient to manipulate the object between the thumb and the fingertip being re-educated. Here the patient must try to concentrate upon the perceptions being transmitted via the injured finger instead of those coming from the thumb.

Other Techniques

At the outset, it was noted that there is no one technique. If it works for you and your patient, use it. Mansat and Delprat,[50] from Toulouse, France, employ a program of sensory re-education modeled after ours. In addition to techniques discussed above, they show a patient receiving vibratory stimuli and placing geometric-shaped pegs into geometric-shaped slots. The success in training blind people to read braille was the inspiration behind Millesi's program of sensory re-education.[51] This program employs metal plates with standardized prominences, like braille, arranged in straight and wavy lines in

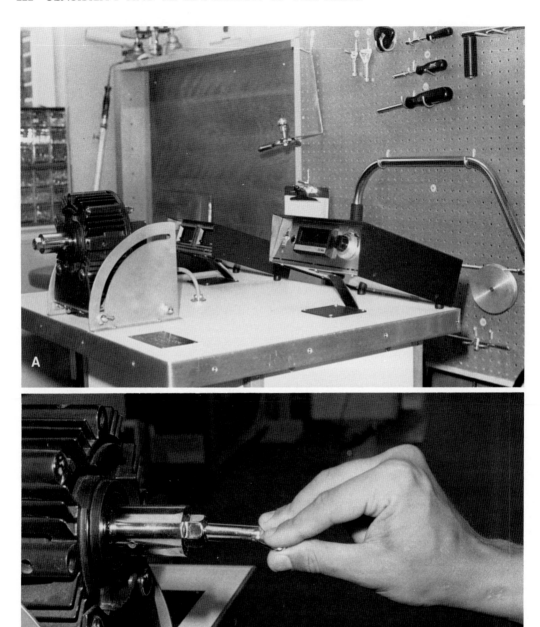

Figure 12.14. The Work Simulator (*A*). This rehabilitation machine was designed, and a prototype built by John Engalitcheff to fulfill the need of the Hand Surgeon and Hand Therapist as outlined by Raymond M. Curtis, M.D. Multiple attachments are available that connect to a calibrated resistance device. This permits a wide range of gross and precision sensory grips to be utilized with increasing strength (*B*). The patient's sensory re-education program can thus include actual work-simulated activities.[118]

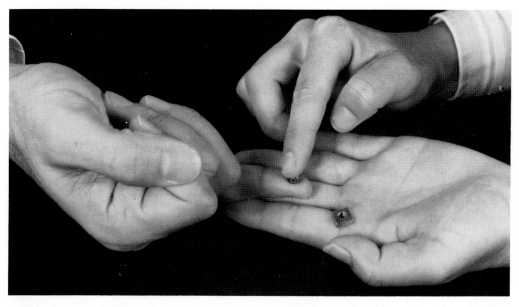

Figure 12.15.   Ulnar or digital nerve-injured patients are re-educated with exercises requiring object recognition, and this requires another person; e.g., a friend, placing the object upon the fingertip to be re-educated.

a circle, square, and triangle. There are also plates with rows of irregularly spaced dots. The patients practice *moving* their fingers along the figures and learning to identify them. The most recent sensory program of which we are aware is that described by Pegge Carter.[52] In addition to our program as outlined above, she adds "sensory bombardment" and the recognition of objects out of the visual field hidden in a sand or bean media (Fig. 12.16).

If sensory re-education were being done on an investigational level, a technique that allowed comparisons would be important. When I did my first small series of patients in 1969, I allowed them to plateau in their recovery, and then instituted sensory re-education, late phase, with a few small hex and cap nuts in an attempt to standardize our procedure as much as possible.[5] Recently, Colonel Reid and his hand therapists, Janet Werner, O.T.R., and Carl Sunstrum, O.T.R., presented the "preliminary results" of their sensory re-education program.[53] Their goal was to be able to relate the results of their program to the results of nerve repairs done in the past. They knew that classic two-point discrimination results improved with repeat

testing and gave measurable results. Accordingly, their program employed the use of classic two-point discrimination testing, using a Boley gauge, begun at the time 256 cps had progressed to the fingertip. Patients received "twenty minutes of supervision twice a day for six weeks" in the military base hospital (excellent motivation for servicemen). The patients were also encouraged to carry a gauge with them and continue the training "while watching television or other educational endeavors." The results of these programs will be discussed below.

How long should sensory re-education be continued once the patient has recovered functional sensation? The program should be followed for a long time. If the patient returns to active work, or resumes housekeeping or hobbies, or is a child, the re-education is being continued at this level and no formal program is required. However, Wynn Parry[43] and Reid et al.[53] for median nerve repair, and Narakas[54] for brachial plexus repair, as well as I, have noted that if sensory re-education stops and the patient discontinues active daily use of his hand, the effect of the re-education is lost by the time the patient is next tested. Now this is "early on." If re-education is

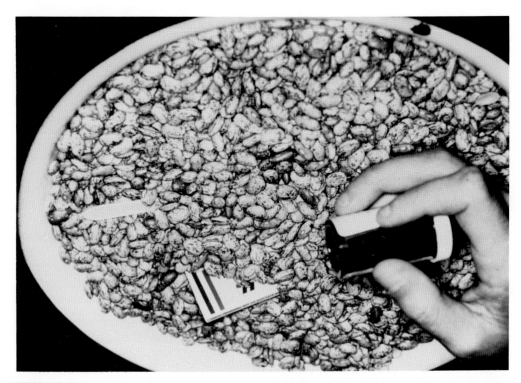

Figure 12.16. Bean media for sensory re-education. Patients, without visual clues, must identify objects within a pile of beans. (Reproduced with permission from M. S. Carter: *Re-education of Sensation.* Presented at the Hand Rehabilitation Symposium, Philadelphia, 1980.[52])

resumed, function is quickly recovered. After recovery has proceeded for "some time," the patient becomes increasingly able to maintain his re-educated status. Obviously, the program must be designed and modified on an individual basis.

RESULTS OF SENSORY RE-EDUCATION AFTER NERVE REPAIR

How may we ever know what is true? What constitutes a significant difference and what a chance observation? In the introduction to his monograph,[55] Seddon addressed this very subject. He wrote that he had the opportunity to conduct a "controlled clinical trial," even with a prospective randomized design. He lamented that so many nerve-injured patients had passed his way, but he had not conducted this "scientific study." The answer to even

"simple" questions like the "primary vs. secondary nerve repair controversy" remained scientifically unanswered. He concluded that studies needed to be conducted properly, and that even "forthright dogmatism was better than arguments based upon shaky statistics."

Moberg[56] attempted to answer the same question. He described the clinical investigator's dilemma:

To progress in this complicated and difficult field, we must pick out almost ideal cases, with clean cuts, little scar tissue, and correct timing of the procedure. We must divide our cases into relatively small age groups ... The level of the lesion must be approximately the same. Loss and recovery must be tested by reliable methods. The precise methods used must be described ... test only one surgical variant at a time. Now where in the world can such an enormous number of nerve lesions be found? ... I believe that our only way of getting ahead in the sensibility problems in this field will be to collect cases from several centres in the world. Then all these results ... could be plotted on a curve corresponding to that of Onne.... If the results are above the "mean for average cases" it should mean "no improvement on present techniques." If the results are below this line, it might mean that the technical variation has contributed an improvement. This will be the way to get precise knowledge.

Moberg is suggesting the comparison of appropriately studied new patients with the historic control. This is an accepted statistical comparison, but it assumes that only the variable studied has been varied over time. The historic control he suggests is "Onne's reported end results."[14] Onne measured classic two-point discrimination in ideal cases of nerve repairs and related these measurements to the patient's age (see Fig. 12.17). Onne reported that in general the classic two-point discrimination value recovered (in millimeters) equaled the patient's age (in years). Thus a graph of two-point discrimination versus age would be a straight line with a slope of 1.0. I will, below, report the results of my own small series of end results after re-education on a graph such as Moberg suggested. Chapter 11 was written to serve as an historic control for comparison of end results of nerve repair previously reported with those of sensory re-education programs. I believe that this use of an historic control is as close as we will ever come to a "scientific comparison" of the effect of sensory re-education upon the results of peripheral nerve repair.

There is, perhaps, one other way we can know if something is "true." Felix Freshwater,[57] in a wonderful chapter on the history of Plastic Surgery, discusses the claim for historic priority. Who should receive the credit for a "discovery," Freshwater writes, the one who first discovers it or the one who makes it known throughout the world (if it happens that they are not both the same individual)? Freshwater quotes Owen[58] as saying: "He becomes the true discoverer who establishes the truth: and the sign of the proof is the general acceptance." I believe that sensory re-education has received "general acceptance." For the past 8 years, Sensory Re-education has appeared on the program of at least one, and usually more than one, nationally publicized hand symposium. For the academic year 1979–80, it

has been on at least five national programs and one international program! Sensory re-education has been described in detail as a chapter in seven books[35, 44, 45, 59–62] (not counting this one), described in brief in nine books,[63–71] and discussed as part of the methodology employed in 12 scientific reports.[5, 25, 50, 51, 53, 72–78] I am aware of active sensory re-education programs in the United States in Baltimore, Carville, Denver, Downey, Durham, Loma Linda, Louisville, New York, Philadelphia, and Saint Louis. I am aware also of active sensory re-education programs in Australia, Austria, Canada, England, France, India, Japan, Sweden, and Switzerland. If, as Owen said, "the sign of the proof is in the general acceptance," then I believe sensory re-education can be said to be of proven value.

The *results of Early-Phase Sensory Re-education* are dramatic. The goal is to correct mislocalization and a lagging of moving- and constant-touch behind 30- and 256-cps perception in reaching the distal phalanx. Early Phase Re-education results in virtually 100% correction of mislocalization (false localization).[5, 56, 72] This can occur after just 3 to 4 weeks, if the patient has not previously been on a re-education program.[5] Once perception of the 256-cps stimulus is present at the fingertips, Early Phase Re-education has been 100% successful in the small group of patients we carefully studied and reported[5] in achieving the "catch-up" of moving- and constant-touch perception to the fingertip. This occurred in less than 1 week of intensive re-education.

There are only two studies that give examples of the end results achieved after nerve repair in patients who have been through a formal program of sensory re-education. Reid et al.[53] presented data to the membership of the American Society for Surgery of the Hand via its Newsletter in 1977. They gave no percentage end results, but did document the course of recovery of sensibility in two patients (Fig. 12.18). These show recovery of normal classic two-point discrimination in less than 2 years in each case! Wynn Parry's results, also discussed below, are given in exact relationship to age for just one median nerve patient,[75] while it is given in this detail for four patients by Reid et al.[53] In Figure

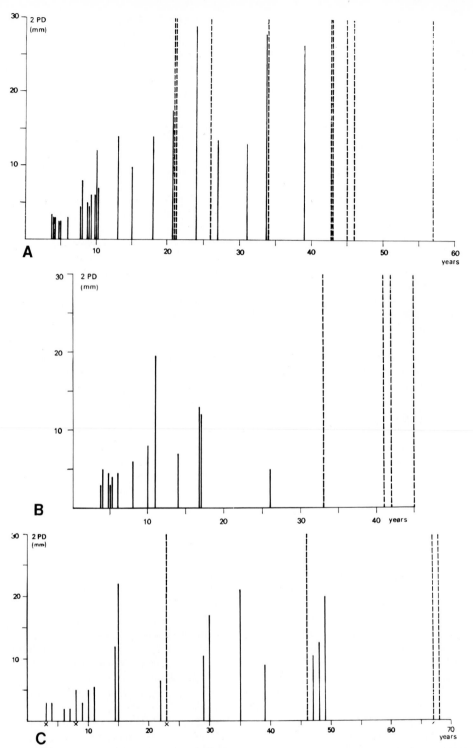

Figure 12.17. Onne's end results of nerve repair in ideal cases related to age (at time of repair) for median (*A*), ulnar (*B*) and digital (*C*) nerve repairs. Each line represents one patient, and dotted lines have 2PD greater than 30 mm. These results have been interpreted as demonstrating that 2PD is recovered in millimeters equal to the patient's age. (Reproduced with permission from L. Onne: *Acta Chir Scand [Suppl]* 300, 1962.[14])

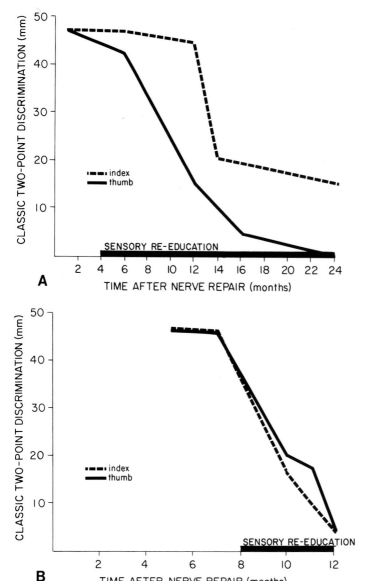

Figure 12.18. Late Phase Sensory Re-education results. *A*, Patient, L.M., 26 years old. *B*, Patient, J.H., 21 years old. Both with primary median nerve repair in distal forearm. Examples of results achieved with formal program of Late Phase Sensory Re-education. (Adapted from R. L. Reid et al.[53])

12.19, these five patients are plotted, as suggested by Moberg,[56] against Onne's results for the ideal nerve repair. All five points fall well below the line, indicating that not only are these results absolutely better in achieving sensory grades S3+ and S4, but they were achieved in 2 years after nerve repair, not 5 years. Since the remaining numbers of patients studied and exact results achieved are not specified in these studies, the overall results cannot be compared to the historic controls of Chapter 11 on a percentage basis.

But note from Table 11.11, that there probably have been no adults previously reported who recovered to the S4 level.

The *results of Late-Phase Sensory Re-education* are also dramatic. Using Chapter 11's historic controls to compare the end results of nerve repair patients who have not had sensory re-education with those who have had sensory re-education, we can make the following comparisons with Wynn Parry's results.[35] Compare Chapter 11's summary table, Table 11.13, with Table 12.1. For the historic control, adult civilian nerve repairs, 33% of median and ulnar nerve repairs recovered S3+. Wynn Parry's patients did too. None of the historic control adults achieved level S4. Wynn Parry reported that 50% of his median and 25% of his ulnar nerve patients recovered near normal sensation. The only other reported Late Phase Sensory Re-education results are those of Wilgis and Maxwell[77] for patients with digital grafts. Again, compare Chapter 11's summary table, Table 11.13, with Table 12.1. Of the historic

controls for digital nerve grafts, 20% recovered to S3+ and 9% to S4. With sensory re-education, Wilgis and Maxwell reported recovering S3+ in 33% and S4 in 67% of their patients!

I have just two criticisms of Wynn Parry's studies. He does not give quantitative data in terms of numbers of patients, or how long it took them to recover. He just reports, "50%," for example. The theoretical basis of his sensory re-education program is pattern theory. He believes the skin is reinnervated at ran-

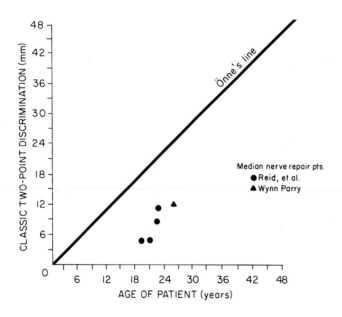

Figure 12.19. Late Phase Sensory Re-education results. Individual cases given as examples of the end results of their sensory re-education program by Wynn Parry[75] and Reid et al,[53] plotted as suggested by Moberg.[56] Diagonal line represents graph of Onne's results of ideal cases of nerve repairs.[14] Patient points falling below the diagonal line are those with results better than expected from repair of the "ideal nerve suture at five years."

Table 12.1
Results of Late Phase Sensory Re-education in Patients Following Nerve Repair

Reference, Date	Type of Trauma	Repair Timing	No. of Cases	Age	% Children	Follow-up (yr)	Motor Recovery (%)				Sensory Recovery (%)				
							M2	M3	M4	M5	S2	S2+	S3	S3+	S4
Median nerve repair															
35, 1966	Civilian	—[a]	—	—	—	2	—	25	50	—	—	—	—	33	50
75, 1976	Civilian	—[a]	23	—	—	3	—	—	—	—	—	—	—	—	—
53, 1977	War	All	150	Adults	—	—	—	—	—	—	—	—	—	—	—
Ulnar nerve repair															
35, 1966	Civilian	—[a]	—	—	—	2	—	—	40	40	—	—	—	50	25
Digital nerve graft		Gap Length					Nerve Block								
77, 1979	Civilian	1–2.5 cm	12	17–54	0	1–2	Yes				0	0	0	33	67

[a] Only examples of individual cases that demonstrated excellent response to re-education were reported. No statistics were reported (see Fig. 12.19).

dom, and that the patient must learn this new pattern. This, as pointed out to me by Julia Terzis,[79] is different from the specificity theory, upon which my entire sensory exam and re-education program are based. That is, reinnervation of specific end organs must occur, as explained earlier in this chapter and in Chapters 3 and 5. Of course, Wynn Parry's conclusion is identical to mine, namely, that patients need sensory re-education after nerve repair. The implementation of our two programs does differ. As per his more nebulous pattern theory, his program is non-specific. My program applies specific sensory exercises at the appropriate time in the recovery process.

Results of Late Phase Sensory Re-education: Personal Series

In this section, I will report the results achieved with 42 patients. These represent all the patients I have re-educated personally since I began in 1969, and who continued in the program for at least 1 year after their nerve repair. Most of these patients went through both early and late phase sensory re-education. These patients include 16 median,

9 ulnar, and 17 digital nerve repairs. The patient's individual data, including age, type of repair or graft, follow-up interval, and tactile discrimination testing are listed in Tables 12.2, 12.3 and 12.4. The median and ulnar nerve repairs were done, to use present terminology, as microsurgical grouped fascicular repairs and the digital nerves by microsurgical epineurial repair (except for median

Table 12.2
Results of Sensory Re-education Median Nerve (Dellon's Series)

Pa-tient	Age at Repair	Type of Re-pair	Follow-up (mo)	Two-Point Discrimination (mm)	
				Moving	Classic
1	28	Primary	16	ND[a]	5
2	49	Primary	18	ND	6
3	20	Primary[b]	36	3	10
4	34	Primary	24	3	9
5	20	Primary	23	2	4
6	37	Primary	14	2	10
7	19	Primary	12	3	5
8	21	Primary	12	3	3
9	10	Primary	12	2	3
10	19	Primary	12	4	8
11	49	Primary	12	3	5
12	60	Primary	18	4	25
13	30	Primary	22	4	13
14	27	Primary	17	4	15
15	29	Primary[c]	12	6	19
16	30	Primary	18	3	5

[a] ND, not done.
[b] Plexus level.
[c] Elbow level.

Table 12.3
Results of Sensory Re-education Ulnar Nerve (Dellon's Series)

Pa-tient	Age at Repair	Type of Re-pair	Follow-up (mo)	Two-Point Discrimination (mm)	
				Moving	Classic
1	18	Primary	18	ND	2
2	20	Primary[a]	36	9	15
3	17	Primary	24	2	7
4	20	Primary	23	2	6
5	16	Primary	15	2	5
6	35	Graft	13	6	20
7	27	Primary	17	2	5
8	29	Primary[b]	12	6	18
9	9	Primary	24	2	4

[a] Plexus level.
[b] Elbow level.

Table 12.4
Results of Sensory Re-education Digital Nerve (Dellon's Series)[a]

Pa-tient	Age at Re-pair	Type of Repair	Follow-up (mo)	Two-Point Discrimination (mm)	
				Moving	Classic
1	47	Primary	18	ND	6
2	57	Secondary	22	5	5
3	24	Graft	12	4	6
4	18	Primary	12	2	4
5	18	Secondary	12	7	11
6a	46	Primary	15	6	10
6b	46	Primary	15	8	18
7	20	Graft	12	4	5
8	21	Graft	14	3	6
9	35	Primary	12	3	6
10	61	Primary	22	2	5
11	49	Graft	12	3	5
12	22	Primary	18	2	2
13	52	Graft	12	3	5
14a	28	Primary	12	3	4
14b	28	Primary	12	3	5
14c	28	Primary	12	3	6

[a] Results after nerve block of intact digital nerve. Block was not done if both digital nerves were repaired.

cases 1 and 2, and ulnar case 1, which were done as microsurgical epineurial repairs). Many of the early cases in the series were done by the Plastic Surgery residents at Johns Hopkins, who were kind enough to allow me to test and re-educate their patients after the nerve repairs. I re-emphasize that this series is a personal series in which patients were seen often monthly, by myself. This kept even those with low intrinsic motivation working (and me too!).

The data in this personal series is first analyzed as suggested by Moberg, against the age line devised by Onne[14] for ideal nerve repair cases as evaluated at 5 years after their nerve repair. However, as seen in Tables 12.2, 12.3 and 12.4, the mean follow-up for the median nerve (at the wrist) patients is 17 months, for the ulnar nerve (at the wrist) patients is 19 months, and for the digital nerve patients is 14 months. As is evident from Figures 12.20, 12.21, and 12.22 for median, ulnar, or digital nerves, respectively, this analysis demonstrates that *all* patients who received sensory re-education did better than the ideal result predicted for their age. Even the two patients with high median and ulnar nerve lesions did far better than the predicted age-matched low lesion!*

The data in this personal series can be analyzed also in comparison with the historical controls for adult civilian peripheral nerve repair, without sensory re-education, as summarized in Table 11.11. Historically 33% of low median and ulnar adult nerve repairs recover to S3+, and 0% to S4 by 5 years after nerve repair. In my total series, 38% of median and 22% of ulnar nerves recovered to S3+ and 50% of median and 56% of the ulnar nerves to S4 (Table 12.5). If just primary adult repairs at the wrist level are considered, then 39% of median and 20% of ulnar nerves recovered to S3+ and 54% of median and 80% of ulnar nerves recovered to S4 in less than 2 years after nerve repair. For the historic control digital nerves, 48% recovered S3+ and 11% recovered S4 (the adult

results for this group are really poorer because 12% of these were children) by 5 years after nerve repair. In my series of adult digital nerve repairs, 12% recovered to S3+ and 82% to S4 by 2 years after nerve repair. These results are far superior to the historic control.†

In summary, the success of sensory re-education in patients recovering from nerve repair has been demonstrated, in general, by the worldwide acceptance of the technique, and in particular, by the results published in the few studies available. The success achieved with sensory recovery is in both the percentage of patients achieving the higher level of recovery (S4) and in the savings in time (1 to 2 years, instead of 5) in which this level is achieved. This is schematically represented in Figure 12.23.

Table 12.5
Results of Sensory Re-education Dellon's Series Summary[a]

	No. in Group	Degree of Recovery		
		S3 (%)	S3+ (%)	S4 (%)
Median				
Total series	16	12	38	50
Adult, wrist level	13	7	39	54
Ulnar				
Total series	9	22	22	56
Adult, wrist level	5	0	20	80
Digital				
Total series	17	6	12	82

[a] Patients are less than 2 years after repair.

OTHER APPLICATIONS OF SENSORY RE-EDUCATION

Replantation

Because of the newness, excitement, and curiosity that surround the replant patient and his replant, more rehabilitation and more home care are usually devoted to these nerve repairs. This intention may be secondary or intended, but I suggest that each replant re-

---

* Although I am biased, I believe that if statistics could be applied to this type of data, I am sure they would demonstrate that sensory re-education made a statistically significant difference.

† I have done a chi-square test on these data although I am sure a statistician would shudder at the assumption that these are all comparable groups. However, I know no other way to compare these data. The value is $p < 0.001$ for each group.

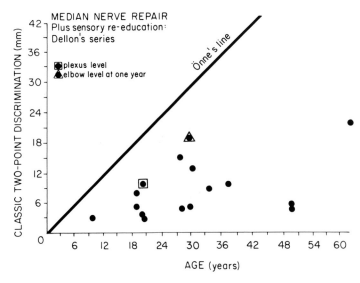

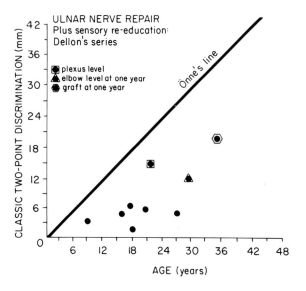

Figure 12.20. Late Phase Sensory Re-education results: median nerve. Patients are charted in relation to Onne's line, which is the 5-year postoperative result of the ideal nerve repair (measured in classic two-point discrimination) plotted against patient age. Patients are from Dellon's personal series. Note that all points are below Onne's line. This means that for each patient, the final result is much better than previously achieved by surgery alone. Sensory re-education permitted these greatly improved results just 1 to 2 years after nerve repair.

Figure 12.21. Late Phase Sensory Re-education results: ulnar nerve. See legend for Figure 12.20.

ceives enough attention to be considered as having received sensory re-education. If they have not received this attention, certainly they should.

There have been three reports published of digital replantation in which the report has gone beyond the concern with replant survival and evaluated sensibility in terms of classic two-point discrimination.[80-82] The Louisville group has stated that their replants do receive formal sensory re-education.[83] The Australian[84] and Duke[85] groups have patients who have been exposed variably to formal sensory re-education, but who, nevertheless, have received the attention, referred to above, that is unique to the replant patient.

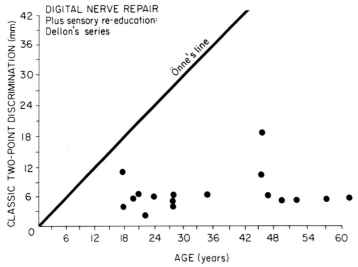

Figure 12.22. Late Phase Sensory Re-education results: digital nerve. See legend for Figure 12.20.

I suggest that the replant patients be considered as having been re-educated. The results of these three studies[80-82] appear in Table 12.6. By comparison with Table 11.11, it may be seen that the replanted digits with sensory re-education are recovering a greater degree of sensation than did the historic control group of digital nerve repairs.

Toe-to-Thumb Transfers

Foucher et al.[78] have reported most recently a series of toe-to-thumb transfers in which a formal program of sensory re-education was incorporated in the postoperative rehabilitation. Four patients were re-educated and followed sufficiently long to evaluate (8 to 15 month range with a mean of 10.5 months). These patients had classic two-point discrimination values of 3, 4, 4, and 7 mm in contrast to the classic two-point discrimination values of 14, 13, 12, and 15 mm in the contralateral toe pulp. Four patients in the series did not receive sensory re-education. Their values were >15, 6, 10, and 14 mm for a comparable follow-up period in contrast to the values of 14, 12, 17, and 13 mm in the contralateral toe pulp. Clearly, sensory re-education has a role to play in these new procedures.

Cross-Finger Flaps

The results of cross-finger flaps in terms of recovered functional sensation have been reported in general to be two to three times

the normal classic two-point discrimination of the contralateral fingertip[27,86,87] (These papers cannot be put into the %S3 or %S4 terminology). Others have commented upon the poor sensory recovery in these flaps.[88-91] Kleinert et al.[74] reported on a series of 20 children (less than 12 years of age) and 36 adults (greater than 12 years of age). These patients received postoperative sensory re-education. Ten percent of the children and 33% of the adults recovered to a S3+ sensory level. Ninety percent of the children and 42% of the adults recovered to a S4 (normal) sensory level.[74] These are the best reported results of cross-finger flaps of which I am aware.

How can sensory re-education benefit cross-finger flaps? As discussed in Chapter 2 and demonstrated at the end of Chapter 5, distal dorsal skin has rudimentary Meissner corpuscles as well as hair follicles. The dorsal skin from the dorsal cross-finger flap is reinnervated and connections, of one form or another, are made. Certainly, the total number of normal functional fiber/receptor systems maturing is greatly reduced. But, the potential is there for mechanoreceptor function. This provides the basis and potential for re-education of sensation.

SPASTIC, HEMI- AND TETRAPLEGICS

The extent of sensory recovery possible in these patients has been studied very little.

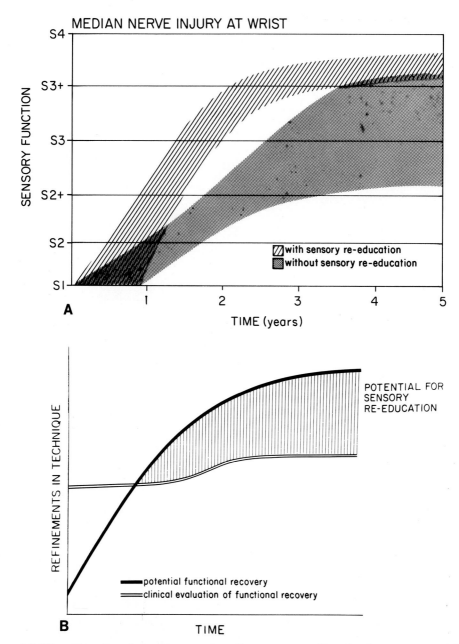

Figure 12.23.   Results of sensory re-education program. Graphs demonstrate ability of sensory re-education to help more patients achieve the highest level of sensory recovery (S4) in the shortest amount of time.

The pioneering work in retraining sensation in hemiplegics following cerebrovascular accidents was reviewed above under the "Roots of Re-education" section.

My experience with one patient has convinced me of the potential for functional sensation that may be present in these patients.

E. W., a seventeen-year-old, had sustained head trauma from a bike fall at age six. Cerebral hem-

Table 12.6
Results of Replants

Reference, Date	Type of Trauma	Repair Timing	No. of Cases	Age	% Children	Follow-up (yr)	Sensory Recovery (%)				
							S2	S2+	S3	S3+	S4
80, 1977	Civilian	All	70	1–70		¾–6	2		8	90	
81, 1978	Civilian	All	35	4–47	14	1–5	0	28	20	26	26
82, 1980	Civilian	All	25	2–72	13	1–3	0	26	13	9	52

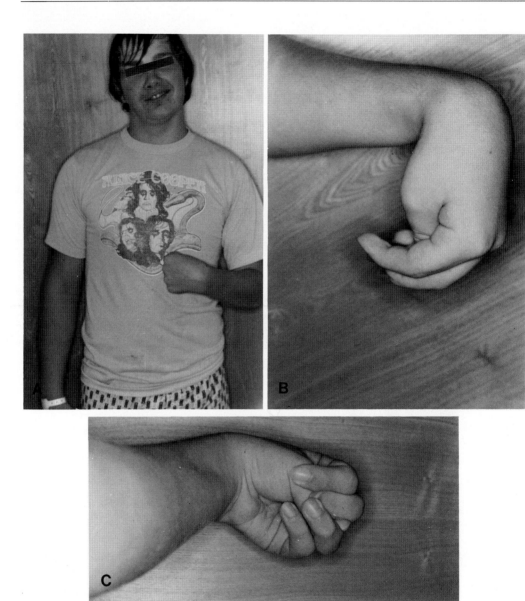

Figure 12.24. Spastic hemiplegic. *A*, Age 17 with posttraumatic left spastic hemiplegia. *B* and *C*, Note complete loss of use of fingertips, representing total sensory deprivation. Evaluation of sensibility demonstrated no constant-touch perception or classic two-point discrimination. There was moving-touch and 30-cps and 256-cps perception, but no moving two-point discrimination. Tactile gnosis was absent.

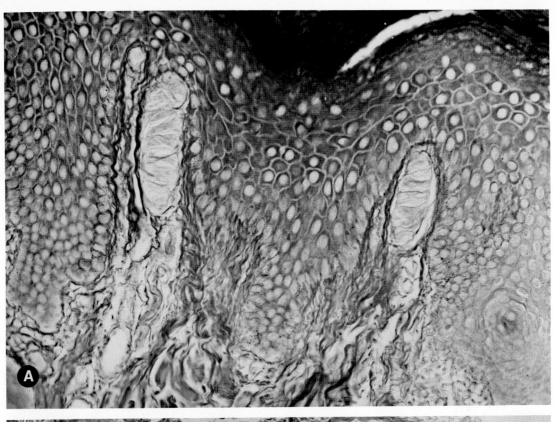

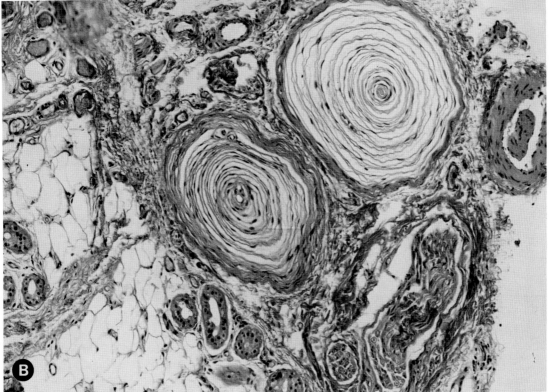

Figure 12.25. Spastic hemiplegia. At time of release of the thumb-in-palm deformity and tendon transfers, the middle fingertip was biopsied. Light microscopy demonstrated abundant innervated Meissner corpuscles (*A*, Silver stain; ×64), two innervated Pacinian corpuscles (*B*, hematoxylin and eosin stain; ×64), but few if any Merkel cell-neurite complexes (*arrow*) (*C*, Silver stain; ×125).

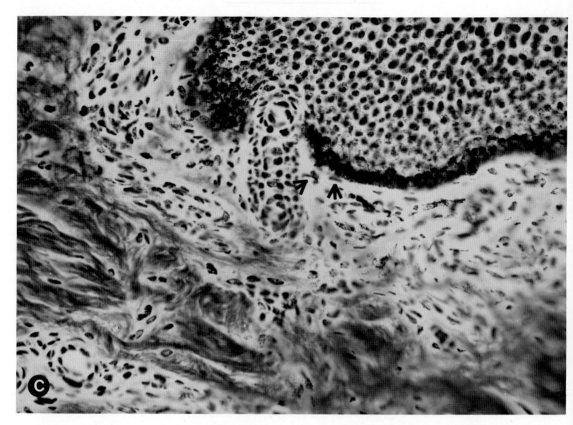

Figure 12.25. *C*, Possible Merkel cell-neurite complex (see legend on page 235).

orrhage resulted in left spastic hemiplegia (Fig. 12.24) and a severe thumb-in-palm deformity that had prevented any use of the hand for 11 years. If the fingers were forcefully pried apart and an object placed within, there was no ability to recognize the object. Preoperative evaluation of sensibility revealed just perception of moving-touch and the 30- and 256-cps tuning fork stimuli. At surgery, the thumb-in-palm deformity was released and appropriate tendon transfers carried out. A biopsy was done intraoperatively of his middle finger, which demonstrated normal quantity of innervated Meissner corpuscles and Pacinian corpuscles, but few innervated Merkel cell-neurite complexes (Fig. 12.25). Postoperatively he demonstrated increased use of his hand (Fig. 12.26), being able to pick-up and grasp objects voluntarily, and gradually coming to use the hand for activities of daily living. Evaluation of sensibility at 1 year after surgery demonstrated perception now of constant-touch, though there still was no classic two-point discrimination. Moving two-point discrimination was 6 mm and tactile gnosis was recovering.

This demonstrated unequivocally to me that the sensory deprivation *per se* which accompanied spastic hemiplegia can result in a severe loss of functional sensation beyond the true neurophysiologic loss resulting from loss of neural structures. This again represents a potential that may be regained through energetic sensory re-education. This is an entire area awaiting further investigation.

Fingertip Resurfacing

The reconstructed fingertip needs sensory re-education in all cases except local innervated flap reconstruction and healing by secondary intention. In each of these cases, normally innervated distal glabrous skin is the resurfacing agent. However, dorsal cross-finger flaps, palmar flaps, thenar flaps, more distal flaps, and skin grafts of all thickness and from all sources all share in common the

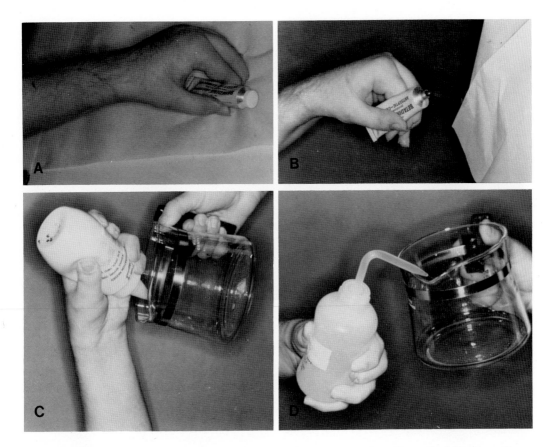

Figure 12.26. Spastic hemiplegia. After 1 year of postoperative rehabilitation, there now was (*A* and *B*) good pinch and (*C* and *D*) some grasp. He used this hand for the activities of daily living. There was now perception of constant-touch, but still no classic two-point discrimination. Moving two-point discrimination was 6 mm and tactile gnosis was recovering.

resurfacing of the fingertip with noninnervated skin. This skin is reinnervated by the digital nerves. Their regenerating axons enter or fail to enter whatever types of sensory receptors are present in the resurfacing material (including hair follicles). Thus, the fingertip reconstructed with noninnervated grafts or flaps should be viewed as a nerve repair from the standpoint of requiring sensory re-education.

When resurfacing with a graft is the method to be chosen, favor a full thickness graft from the hypothenar area because this contains the same type of sensory end organs as the fingertip. Resurfacing with nonglabrous skin never permits recovery of tactile gnosis.[92] With a glabrous skin graft, the regenerating end organs have the best chance to reinnervate appropriately. Skin from the plantar aspect of the foot has the same potential.[93] Many have described the use of hypothenar grafts for fingertip resurfacing,[94–96] but only recently has Thompson[97] provided us with a series in which two-point discrimination is reported. Five of his 10 patients had values between 4 and 6 mm, normal, while the other five ranged from 8 to 12 mm.

The ideal resurfacing material for a fingertip is, of course, another fingertip. Sometimes, in trauma with multiple finger injuries, the volar skin from one finger may be grafted to another fingertip. As my preliminary data

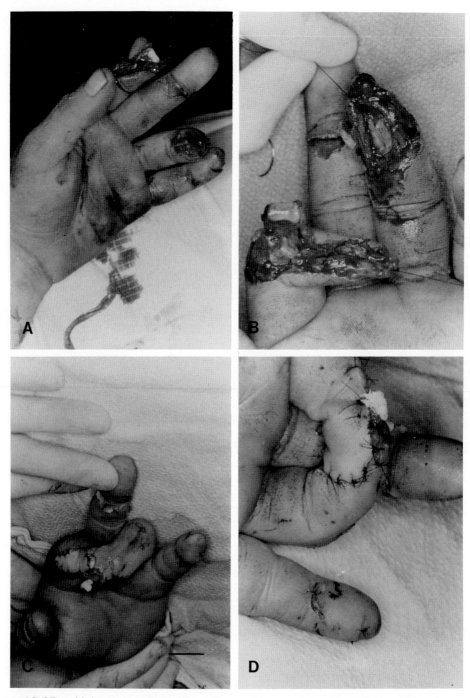

Figure 12.27.   Volar cross-finger flap. The trauma setting provided the opportunity (*A*) to use the volar surface of one finger (the index) to resurface and thereby conserve length with normal sensibility in a neighboring digit, the ring (*B*). After removing middle phalanx from index, the cross-finger flap was inset, and skin from the avulsed index distal phalanx was used as a graft to cover the underside of the flap (*C* and *D*).

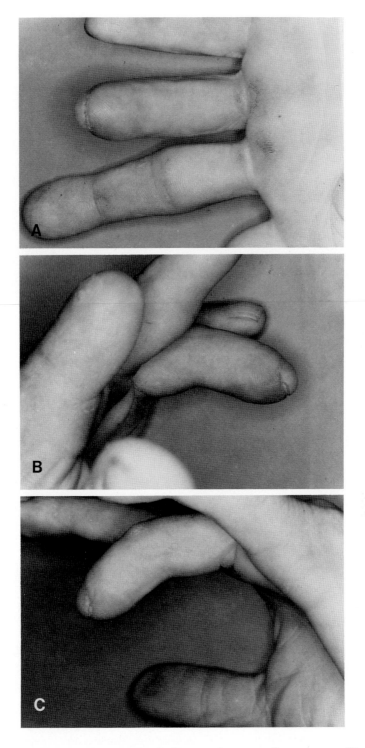

Figure 12.28.   Volar cross-finger flap: Follow-up 2 years after surgery. There is now 2 mm of moving two-point discrimination and 3 mm of constant two-point discrimination.

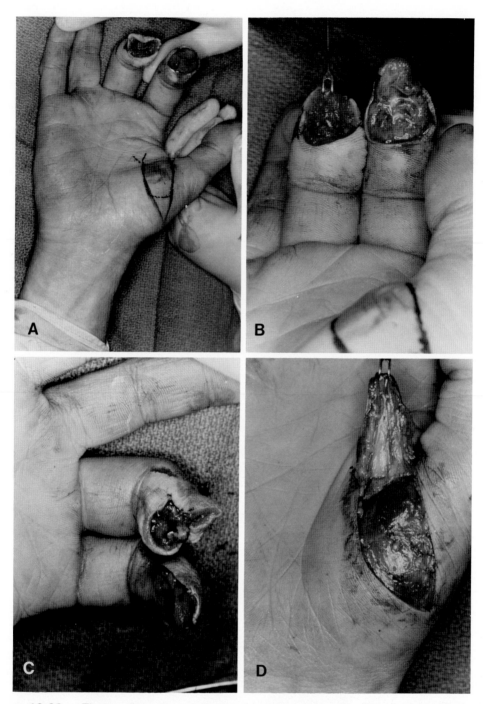

Figure 12.29.   Thenar flap: *A* and *B*, Injuries as shown with flap outlined for index fingertip. Note: Triangle marked at end of flap is saved as a graft to cover underside of flap and donor site (see below). *C* and *D*, Middle fingertip will be closed by subcutaneous pedicle flap technique.[117] Index is missing entire volar pulp, with phalanx and nail preserved.

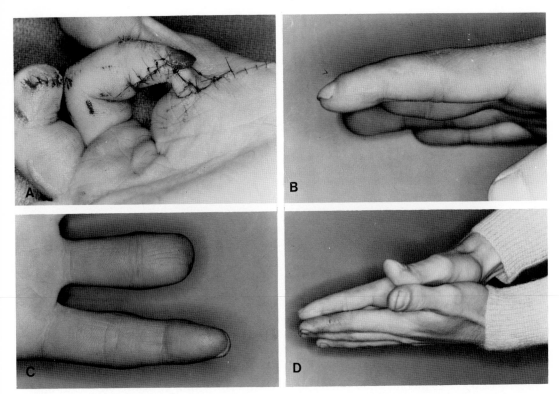

Figure 12.30. Thenar flap. *A*, I prefer to insert the distal tip of the thenar flap, which is, however, the more proximal and radial portion of thenar skin, into the proximal end of the defect. Blood supply is better here also. This approach permits, at inset, retention of a subcutaneous pedicle flap for a modest lengthening of tip or nail support (*B*). End result (*C* and *D*), at 6 months after inset, employing skin and full complement of sensory end-organs, there is 3 mm moving and 4 mm constant two-point discrimination after sensory re-education.

at the end of Chapter 5 demonstrated, there is the greatest conservation of sensory end organs with a flap, and so the ideal flap is a *volar* cross-finger flap. Again, the trauma setting can provide occasion to use a volar cross finger flap to salvage a neighboring digit (Figs. 12.27 and 12.28). The one flap of this type I have done did recover 2 mm of moving and 3 mm of constant two-point discrimination.

For loss of fingertip pulp where local flaps are insufficient, I favor the thenar flap, again because this region has the sensory end organ composition most similar to the distal phalanx. The technique I use places the proximal thenar skin into the proximal finger loss, the distal thenar skin (which has a slightly greater end-organ density) into the fingertip (see Figs. 12.29 and 12.30). Sensory re-education has resulted in recovery of 4-mm classic two-point discrimination and 3-mm moving two-point discrimination in the two cases done with this technique.

For loss of thumb pulp, I favor the volar advancement flap[9,97–100] which can be "extended" to provide up to 3 cm of distal coverage (Figs. 12.31 and 12.32) with excellent functional sensation.[101]

Innervated Flap Transfers

When a flap is transferred to the fingertip and the flap's nerve is sutured to the volar digital nerve of the recipient finger,[28,102–104] the need for sensory re-education is similar

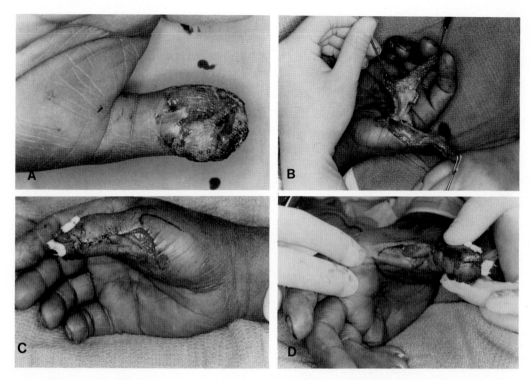

Figure 12.31. Extended volar advancement flap. To resurface extensive thumb pulp losses greater than 1.5 cm (*A*), an innervated extended volar advancement flap is created. By extending the flap proximally, the relative excess of skin over the thenar eminence can be utilized (*B*). The donor site defects on the radial and ulnar side of the flap are covered with two adjacent rotation flaps, respecting normal skin creases and dorsal versus palmar skin (*C* and *D*). (Reproduced with permission from A. L. Dellon, in press 1981.[101])

to that following nerve repair. But when an innervated flap is transferred and its nerve supply remains centrally unchanged, then the need for re-education is different. There has been no nerve repair.

One group of these transfers is the radial-innervated index dorsum to thumb pulp.[105–111] Sensory re-education in this group has two goals: (1) improve the tactile discrimination, as discussed above for the cross-finger flap and (2) correct "false localization." The normal classic two-point discrimination of the skin over the dorsum of the index finger's proximal phalanx is 12 to 15 mm.[112] Among the 34 reported cases,[105–111] there were five[106–107] with classic two-point discrimination of 6 mm or less and eight patients with 8 to 14 mm.[107,111] Two authors

believed that the flap was not good for restoring sensation other than protective.[105–110] Many of these patients had not learned to localize the stimulus to the thumb, but still referred it to the index finger.[105,109,110] One patient made the central adjustment by 10 months and one patient not for 10 years![107] Thus, the potential for central reorganization by sensory re-education exists and has been accomplished. Certainly this is an area for improved re-education efforts.

I have used this technique twice. At follow-up evaluation 3 years after surgery, both patients, who had received sensory re-education, had made the central adjustment. One had 5-mm moving two-point discrimination and 10-mm classic two-point discrimination. The other had no two-point discrimination.

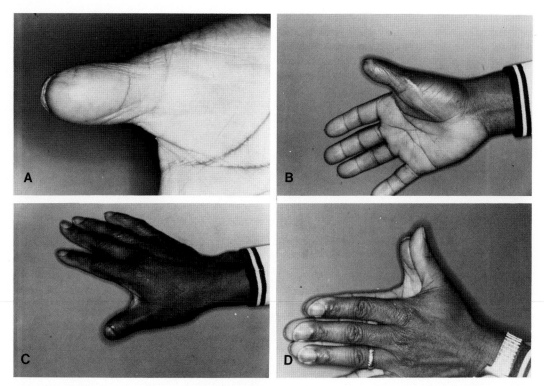

Figure 12.32.   Extended volar advancement flap. *A)* At 6 months postoperatively, there is a thumb with length conserved, tactile gnosis, and a (*C* and *D*) full thumb index web space preserved.

Both patients were dissatisfied with the scars. At present, this is a flap of last resort for me, and I prefer the extended volar advancement flap[101] (Figs. 12.31 and 12.32).

Neurovascular Island Flap

Four reports of long-term results in patients who have had a neurovascular island flap transferred have made the same general comments.[113–116] Initially, the skin island with digital artery and nerve intact lives and has normal tactile discrimination. Over time, the tested classic two-point discrimination greatly diminishes. Hand function related to this restored sensibility, however, consistently improves. Much theorizing goes on as to why two-point discrimination is lost, but the observed fact is that function has improved. Sensory re-education most certainly must take the credit for this, since the patient's use of the flap allows him to re-educate

himself despite the measurable loss in sensation.

Similar to the innervated cross-finger flap, there remains a significant problem with localization of the stimulus. Under slow, consciously directed activity, the ring finger island now on the thumb has its stimuli referred to the thumb. But if the thumb is surprisingly stuck by a pin, the patient believes his ring finger has been hurt! It remains unknown whether further sensory re-education can improve this.

I have had success with re-educating localization in two patients with these flaps, one followed for 3 years and one followed just 1 year. Two-point discrimination has fallen from normal to 5-mm moving and 15-mm classic in the first case, while remaining normal at 2-mm moving and 3-mm classic so far in the latter case. The first patient, in whom discrimination was clearly lost, is a poorly motivated person with a history of multiple self-inflicted wrist injuries, while the second patient is a higly motivated auto mechanic who has since returned to work. The role of sensory re-education in preventing the observed decline in tactile gnosis in neurovascular island flaps remains to be defined.

References

1. Bunnell S: Surgery of the nerves of the hand. Surg Gynecol Obstet 44:145–152, 1927.
2. Mountcastle VB: *Medical Physiology,* ed 12. Saint Louis: CV Mosby, 1968, Ch 61–62.
3. Dellon AL, Curtis RM, Edgerton MT: Re-education of sensation in the hand following nerve injury. (abstr). J Bone Joint Surg 53A:813, 1971.
4. Dellon AL, Curtis RM, Edgerton MT: Evaluating recovery of sensation in the hand following nerve injury. Johns Hopkins Med J 130:235–243, 1972.
5. Dellon AL, Curtis RM, Edgerton MT: Re-education of sensation in the hand following nerve injury. Plast Reconstr Surg 53:297–305, 1974.
6. Newton I, 1675. Cited by Boyes J: *On the Shoulders of Giants. Notable Names in Hand Surgery.* Philadelphia: JB Lippincott, 1976.
7. Hakstian RW: Funicular orientation by direct stimulation: An aid to peripheral nerve repair. J Bone Joint Surg 50A:1178–1186, 1968.
8. Nicholson OR, Seddon HJ: Nerve repairs in civil practice: Results of therapy of median and ulnar nerve lesions. Br Med J 2:1065–1071, 1957.
9. Moberg E: Aspects of sensation in reconstructive surgery of the upper extremity. J Bone Joint Surg 46A:817–825, 1964.
10. Seddon HJ, Medawar PB, Smith H: Rate of regeneration of peripheral nerves in man. J Physiol 102:191–215, 1943.
11. Sunderland S: Rate of regeneration in human peripheral nerves: Arch Neurol Psychiatry 58:251–295, 1947.
12. Davis RD: Some factors affecting the results of treatment of peripheral nerve injuries. Lancet 1:877–880, 1949.
13. Honner R, Fragiadakis EG, Lamb DW: An investigation of the factors affecting the results of digital nerve division. Hand 2:21–31, 1970.
14. Onne L: Recovery of sensibility and sudomotor function in the hand after nerve suture. Acta Chir Scand [Suppl] 300:1–70, 1962.
15. Heinrichs RW, Moorehouse JA: Touch perception in blind diabetic subjects in relation to the reading of Braille type. N Engl J Med 280:72–75, 1969.
16. Almquist EE: The effect of training on sensory function, in Mickon J, Moberg E (eds): *Traumatic Nerve Lesions of the Upper Limb.* Edinburgh: Churchill Livingstone, 1975, pp 53–54.
17. McEwan LE: Median and ulnar nerve injuries. Austr NZ J Surg 32:89–104, 1962.
18. Collins CC, Bach-y-Rita P: Transmission of pictorial information through the skin. Adv Biol Med Phys 14:285–315, 1973.
19. Bach-y-Rita P: Visual information through the skin—a tactile vision substitution system. Trans Am Acad Ophthalmol Otolaryngol 78:OP729–740, 1974.
20. Bach-y-Rita P: Plastic brain mechanisms in sensory substitution, in Zulch KJ, Creutzfeldt O, Galbraith GC (eds): *Cerebral Localization.* Berlin: Springer-Verlag, 1975, pp 203–216.
21. Bach-y-Rita P: Plasticity of the nervous system, in Zulch KJ, Creuzfeldt O, Galbraith GC (eds): *Cerebral Localization.* Berlin: Springer-Verlag, 1975, pp 314–327.
22. Mountcastle VB: The view from within: Pathways to the study of perception. Johns Hopkins Med J 136:109–131, 1975.
23. Bolton CF, Winkelmann RK, Dyk PJ: A quantitative study of Meissner's corpuscles in man. Neurology 16:1–9, 1966.
24. Rosenberg G: Effect of age on peripheral vibratory perception. J Am Geriatr Soc 6:471–481, 1958.
25. Dellon AL: The moving two-point discrimination test: Clinical evaluation of the quickly-adapting fiber/receptor system. J Hand Surg 3:474–481, 1978.
26. Hutchinson J, Tough JS, Wynburn GM: Regeneration of sensation in grafted skin. Br J Plast Surg 2:82–94, 1949.
27. Sturman MJ, Duran RJ: Late results of fingertip injuries. J Bone Joint Surg 45A:289–298, 1963.
28. May JW Jr, Chait LA, Cohen BE, et al: Free neurovascular flap from the first web of the foot in hand reconstruction. J Hand Surg 2:387–393, 1977.
29. Maquieric NO: An innervated full-thickness skin graft to restore sensibility to fingertips and heels. Plast Reconstr Surg 53:568–575, 1974.
30. May JW Jr, Daniel RK: Great toe to hand free tissue transfer. Clin Orthop 133:140–153, 1978.
31. O'Brien B, MacLeod AM, Sykes PJ, et al: Microvascular second toe transfer for digital reconstruction. J Hand Surg 3:123–133, 1978.
32. Norris TR, Poppen NK, Buncke HJ: Restoration of sensibility and function with microvascular transplants from the toe to the hand. Presented at Am. Soc Surg Hand Meeting, Feb 5, 1980.
33. Strauch B, Tsur H: Restoration of sensation to the hand by a free neurovascular flap from the first web space of the foot. Plast Reconstr Surg 62:361–367, 1978.
34. Buncke HJ, Rose EH: Free toe-to-fingertip neurovascular island flaps. Plast Reconstr Surg 63:607–612, 1979.
35. Parry CBW: *Rehabilitation of the Hand.* London: Butterworths, pp 92, 107–109, 112–113, 1966.
36. VanBuskirk C, Webster C: Prognostic value of sensory defect in rehabilitation of hemiplegics. Neurology 5:407–411, 1955.
37. Forster FM, Shields CD: Cortical sensory defects causing disability. Arch Phys Med Rehabil 40:56–61, 1959.
38. Vinograd A, Taylor E, Grossman S: Sensory retraining of the hemiplegic hand. Am J Occup Ther 5:246–250, 1962.
39. Bowden REM: Factors influencing functional recovery, in Seddon HJ (ed): *Peripheral Nerve Injuries.* London: Her Majesties Printing Office, 1954 Ch 7, pp 298–352.

40. Ruch TC, Fulton JF, German WJ: Sensory discrimination in monkey, chimpanzee and man after lesions of parietal lobe. Arch Neurol Psychiatry 39: 919–938, 1938.

41. Stopford JSB: An explanation of the two-stage recovery of sensation during regeneration of a peripheral nerve. Brain 49:372–386, 1926.

42. Horch K: Guidance of regrowing sensory axons after cutaneous nerve lesions in the cat. J Neurophysiol 42:1437–1449, 1979.

43. Parry CBW: Diagnosis and after-care of peripheral nerve lesions in the upper extremity (The Third Founder's Lecture, abstr). J Bone Joint Surg 48A: 607, 1966.

44. Dellon AL, Curtis RM, Edgerton MT: Program for sensory re-education in the hand following nerve injury, in Marshall E (ed): Hand Rehabilitation. Brookfield, Illinois: Fred Sammon, 1977, pp 110–112.

45. Maynard J: Sensory re-education after peripheral nerve injury, in Hunter J, Mackin E, Schneider L, et al (eds): Rehabilitation of the Hand. Baltimore: Williams & Wilkins, 1977.

46. Paul RL, Goodman H, Merzenick M: Alterations in mechanoreceptor input to Brodmann's area 1 and 3 of the post-central hand area of Macaco mulatto after nerve section and regeneration. Brain Res 39: 1–19, 1972.

47. Brushart TM, Terzis JK: Dorsal horn projections of normal and repaired sensory nerves. Presented at the Plastic Surgery Research Council Meeting, Hershey, Pa, April 21, 1980.

48. Dykes RW, Terzis JK: Reinnervation of glabrous skin in baboons: Properties of cutaneous mechanoreceptors subsequent to nerve crush. J Neurophysiol 42:1461–1478, 1979.

49. Dellon AL, Munger B: Correlation of sensibility evaluation, hand function and histology, in press 1981.

50. Mansat M, Delprat J: Reeducation de la sensibilité de la main. Ann Med Physique 18:527–538, 1975.

51. Millesi H, Rinderes D: A method for training and testing sensibility of the fingertips. Proc World Fed Occup Ther 7:122–125, 1979.

52. Carter MS: Re-education of Sensation. Presented at the Hand Rehabilitation Symposium, Philadelphia, March 23, 1980.

53. Reid RL, Werner J, Sunstrum C: Preliminary results of sensibility re-education following repair of the median nerve. Am Soc Surg Hand, Newsletter 15, 1977.

54. Narakas A: Surgical treatment of traction injuries of the brachial plexus. Clin Orthop 133:71–90, 1978.

55. Seddon HJ: Surgical Disorders of the Peripheral Nerves. Baltimore: Williams & Wilkins, 1972.

56. Moberg E: Future hopes for the surgical management of peripheral nerve lesions, in Michon J, Moberg E (eds): Traumatic Nerve Lesions. Edinburgh: Churchill Livingstone, 1975, pp 1–2.

57. Freshwater MF: The principles and purpose of plastic surgery—past and present, in Krizek TJ, Hoopes JE (eds): Symposium on Basic Science in Plastic Surgery. Saint Louis: CV Mosby, 1976, pp. 3–13.

58. Owen R: On the Archetype and Homologies of the Vertebrate Skeleton. London: J. Van Roost, 1848. Cited by Freshwater MF: The principles and purpose of plastic surgery—past and present, in Kruzik TJ, Hoopes JE (eds): Symposium on Basic Science in Plastic Surgery. Saint Louis: CV Mosby, 1976, p 3.

59. Curtis RM: Sensory re-education after peripheral nerve injury, in Frederick S, Brody GS (eds): Symposium on the Neurological Aspects of Plastic Surgery. Saint Louis: CV Mosby, 1978, pp 47–51.

60. Curtis RM, Dellon AL: Sensory re-education after peripheral nerve injury, in Omer G, Spinner M (eds): Management of Peripheral Nerve Injuries. New York: WB Saunders, 1980, pp 769–778.

61. Dellon AL, Jabaley ME: Re-education of sensation. Clin Orthop, in press 1981.

62. Dellon AL: Evaluation of sensibility and re-education of sensation, in Mansat M (ed): Proceedings: Symposium on Upper Extremity Sensory Problems, June, 1980.

63. Seddon HJ: Surgical Disorders of the Peripheral Nerves. Baltimore: Williams & Wilkins, 1972, p 239.

64. Weeks PM, Wray RC: Management of Acute Hand Injuries. St. Louis: CV Mosby, 1973, pp 302–303.

65. Ito T: Surgery of the Peripheral Nerve. Tokyo: Igaku Shoin, 1977, pp 110–111.

66. Daniel RK, Terzis JK: Reconstructive Microsurgery. Boston: Little, Brown, 1977, p 324.

67. Fess EE, Harmon KS, Strickland JW, et al: Evaluation of the hand by objective measurement, in Hunter JM, Schneider LH, Mackin EJ, et al (eds): Rehabilitation of the Hand. St. Louis: CV Mosby, 1978, Ch 5.

68. Bell JA: Sensibility evaluation, in Hunter JM, Schneider LH, Mackin EJ, et al (eds): Rehabilitation of the Hand. St Louis: CV Mosby, 1978, Ch 25.

69. Lister G: The Hand: Diagnosis and Indications. Edinburgh: Churchill Livingstone, 1977, p 73.

70. Sunderland S: Nerves and Nerve Injuries, Edinburgh: Churchill Livingstone, 1978, p 373.

71. Edshage S: Experience with clinical methods of testing sensation after peripheral nerve surgery, in Jewett DL, McCarroll HR Jr (eds): Nerve Repair and Regeneration. St. Louis: CV Mosby, 1980, pp 244–249.

72. Omer GE: Sensibility of the hand as opposed to sensation in the hand. Ann Chir 27:479–483, 1973.

73. Omer GE: Sensation and sensibility in the upper extremity. Clin Orthop 104:30–36, 1974.

74. Kleinert HE, McAlister CG, MacDonald CJ, et al: A critical evaluation of cross finger flaps. J Trauma 14:756–763, 1974.

75. Parry CBW, Salter M: Sensory re-education after median nerve lesions. Hand 8:250–257, 1976.

76. Tallis R, Staniforth P, Fisher TR: Neurophysiologic studies of autogenous sural nerve grafts. J Neurol Neurosurg Psychiatry 41:677–683, 1978.

77. Wilgis EFS, Maxwell GP: Distal digital nerve grafts: Clinical and anatomic studies. J Hand Surg 4:439–443, 1979.

78. Foucher G, Merle M, Maneaud M, et al: Microsurgical free partial toe transfer in hand construction:

A report of 12 cases. Plast Reconstr Surg 65:616–626, 1980.

79. Terzis J: Personal communication, May 20, 1980.
80. Morrison WA, O'Brien B, MacLeod AM: Evaluation of digital replantation—a review of 100 cases. Orthop Clin North Am 8:295–308, 1977.
81. Gelberman RH, Urbaniak JR, Bright DS, et al: Digital sensibility following replantation. J Hand Surg 3:313–319, 1978.
82. Schlenker JD, Kleinert HE, Tsai T: Methods and results of replantation following traumatic amputation of the thumb in sixty-four patients. J Hand Surg 5:63–70, 1980.
83. Kleinert HE, Juhalo CA, Tsai T, et al: Digital replantation—selection, techniques, and results. Orthop Clin North Am 8:309–318, 1977.
84. O'Brien B: Personal communication, 1979.
85. Urbaniak JR: Personal communication, 1979.
86. Smith JR, Bom AF: An evaluation of fingertip reconstruction by cross finger and palmar pedicle flaps. Plast Reconstr Surg 35:409–418, 1965.
87. Johnson RK, Inverson RE: Cross finger pedicle flaps in the hand. J Bone Joint Surg 53A:913–919, 1971.
88. Barclay TL: The late results of fingertip injuries. Br J Plast Surg 8:38–43, 1955.
89. Reid DAC: Experience of a hand surgery service. Br J Plast Surg 9:11–24, 1956.
90. Brady GS, Cloutier AM, Woolhouse FM: The fingertip injury: An assessment of management. Plast Reconstr Surg 26:80–90, 1960.
91. Holm A, Zacharial L: Fingertip lesions: An evaluation of conservative treatment versus free skin grafting. Acta Orthop Scand 45:382–392, 1974.
92. Mannerfelt L: Evaluation of functional sensation of skin grafts in the hand area. Br J Plast Surg 15:136–154, 1962.
93. Micks JE, Wilson JN: Full thickness sole-skin grafts for resurfacing the hand. J Bone Joint Surg 49A:1128–1134, 1967.
94. Patton H: Split-skin grafts from hypothenar area for fingertip avulsions. Plast Reconstr Surg 43:426–429, 1969.
95. Badim J, Lessa SF, Vieiro RC, et al: Regiao hipotenar coma area doadora para as lesoes de palpa digital. Rev Bras Chir 62:163–166, 1972.
96. Naso SJ: Full-thickness skin grafts from thenar eminence to cover volar avulsions of fingers. Orthop Rev 7:127–129, 1978.
97. Thompson JS: Free hypothenar full-thickness grafts for distal digital defects. Johns Hopkins Med J 145:126–130, 1979.
98. Snow JW: The use of a volar flap for repair of fingertip amputations: A preliminary report. Plast Reconstr Surg 40:163–168, 1967.
99. Keim HA, Grantham SA: Volar flap advancement for thumb and fingertip injuries. Clin Orthop 66:109–112, 1969.
100. Posner MA, Smith RJ: The advancement pedicle flap for thumb injuries. J Bone Joint Surg 53A:1618–1621, 1971.
101. Dellon AL: The extended volar advancement flap for thumb reconstruction, in press 1981.
102. Berger A, Meisse G: Innervated skin grafts and flaps for restoration of sensation to anesthetic areas. Chir Plast (Berl) 3:33–37, 1975.
103. Joshi BB: A sensory cross-finger flap for use on the index finger. Plast Reconstr Surg 58:210–213, 1976.
104. Joshi BB: Neural repair for sensory restoration in a groin flap. Hand 9:221–225, 1977.
105. Holevich J: A new method of restoring sensibility to the thumb. J Bone Joint Surg 45B:496–502, 1963.
106. Adamson JE, Horton CE, Crawford HH: Sensory rehabilitation of the injured thumb. Plast Reconstr Surg 40:52–57, 1967.
107. Gaul JS Jr: Radial-innervated cross-finger flaps from index to provide sensory pulp to injured thumb. J Bone Joint Surg 51A:1257–1263, 1969.
108. Braillar F, Horner RL: Sensory cross-finger pedicle graft. J Bone Joint Surg 51A:1264–1268, 1969.
109. Kim KL, Pasch JL: Island flap innervated by radial nerve for restoration of sensation in an index stump. Plast Reconstr Surg 47:386–388, 1971.
110. Foucher G, Braun JB: A new island flap transfer from the dorsum of the index to the thumb. Plast Reconstr Surg 63:344–349, 1979.
111. Lesavoy MA: The dorsal index finger neurovascular island flap. Orthop Rev 9:91–95, 1980.
112. Gellis M, Pool R: Two-point discrimination distances in the normal hand and forearm. Plant Reconstr Surg 59:57–62, 1977.
113. Reid DAC: The neurovascular island flap in thumb reconstruction. Br J Plast Surg 19:234–244, 1966.
114. Murray JF, Ord JVR, Gavelin GE: The neurovascular island flap pedicle flap. J Bone Joint Surg 49A:1285–1297, 1967.
115. Omer GE Jr, Day DJ, Ratliff H, et al: Neurovascular cutaneous island pedicles for deficient median nerve sensibility. J Bone Joint Surg 52A:1181–1192, 1970.
116. Krag C, Rasmussen KB: The neurovascular island pedicle flap for defective sensibility in the thumb. J Bone Joint Surg [Br] 57B:495–499, 1975.
117. Dellon AL: Subcutaneous pedicle flap technique for fingertip reconstruction, in press 1981.
118. Curtis RM, Engalitcheff J Jr: The work simulator, in press 1981.

COMBINED REFERENCES

1. Adamson JE, Horton CE, Crawford HH: Sensory rehabilation of the injured thumb. Plast Reconstr Surg 40:52–57, 1967.
2. Adeymo O, Wybrun GM: Inneration of skin grafts. Transplant Bull 4:152–153, 1957.
3. Adrian ED, Umrath K: The impulse discharge from the Pacinian corpuscle. J Physiol 78:139–154, 1929.
4. Adrian ED, Zotterman Y: The impulses produced by sensory nerve endings. Part 3. Impulses set up by touch and pressure. J Neurophysiol 61:464–483, 1926.
5. Adrian ED, Zotterman Y: The impulses produced by sensory nerve endings: The responses of a single nerve organ. J Physiol (Lond) 61:151–171, 1926.
6. Aitkens JT, Sharman M, Young JZ: Maturation of regenerating nerve fibres with various peripheral connections. J Anat 81:1–22, 1947.
7. Almquist E, Eeg-Olofsson O: Sensory nerve-conduction velocity and two-point discrimination in sutured nerves. J Bone Joint Surg 52A:791–796, 1970.
8. Almquist EE: The effect of training on sensory function, in Mickon J, Moberg E (eds): Traumatic Nerve Lesions of the Upper Limb. Edinburgh: Churchill Livingstone, 1975, pp 53–54.
9. Anderson S, Jones JK: Recent Mammals of the World: A Synopsis of Families. New York: Ronald Press, 1967.
10. Andres KH: The Peripheral Nervous System, Hubbard JI (ed). New York: Plenum Press, 1974, Ch 12.
11. Bach-y-Rita P: Plastic brain mechanisms in sensory substitution, in Zulch KJ, Creutzfeldt O, Galbraith GC (eds): Cerebral Localization, Berlin: Springer Verlag, 1975, pp 203–216.
12. Bach-y-Rita P: Plasticity of the nervous system, in Zulch KJ, Creutzfeldt O, Galbraith GC (eds): Cerebral Localization. Berlin: Springer-Verlag, 1975, pp 203–216, 314–327.
13. Bach-y-Rita P: Visual information through the skin—a tactile vision substitution system. Trans Am Acad Ophthalmol Otolaryngol 78:OP729–740, 1974.
14. Bach-y-Rita P, Collins CC, Saunders FA, et al: Vision substitution by tactile image projection. Nature 221:643–644, 1969.
15. Badim J, Lessa SF, Vieiro RC, et al: Regiao hipotenar como area doadora para as lesoes de palpa digital. Rev Bras Chir 62:163–166, 1972.
16. Barclay TL: The late results of fingertip injuries. Br J Plast Surg 8:38–43, 1955.
17. Bell JA: Sensibility evaluation, in Hunter JM, Schneider LH, Mackin EJ, et al (eds): Rehabilitation of the Hand. St. Louis: CV Mosby, 1978, Ch 25.
18. Bennett MR, Pettigrew AG, Taylor RS: The formation of synapsis in reinnervated and cross-reinnervated adult avian muscle. J Physiol 230:331–357, 1973.
19. Berger A, Meisse G: Innervated skin grafts and flaps for restoration of sensation to anesthetic areas. Chir Plast (Berl) 3:33–37, 1975.
20. Biedler LM, Nejad MS, Smallman RL, et al: Rat taste cell proliferation. Fed Proc 19:302, 1960.
21. Biemesderfer D, Munger BL, Binck J, et al: The Pilo-Ruffini complex: A non-sinus hair and associated slowly-adapting mechanoreceptor in primate facial skin. Brain Res 142:197–222, 1978.
22. Blackwelder RD: Classification of the Animal Kingdom. Carbondale, Ill: Southern Illinois Univ Press, 1963.
23. Blix M: Experimenteia bidrag till lösning of fragan om hudnervernas specifiko energi. Ups Lakarefor Forhandlingar 43:427–441, 1882.
24. Boeke J: On the regeneration of sensitive end-corpuscles after section of the nerve. K Acad van Wetenschoppen (Amsterdam) 25:319–323, 1922.
25. Boeke J: The Problems of Nervous Anatomy, London: Oxford University Press, 1940, pp 12–44.
26. Boeke J, Dijkstra C: De- and regeneration of sensible end-corpuscles in the duck's bill (corpuscles of Gandry and Herbst) after the cutting of the nerve, the removing of the entire skin or the transplantation of the skin in another region. K Acad van Wetenschoppen (Amsterdam) 35:1114–1119, 1932.
27. Bolton, CF, Winkelmann RK, Dyk PJ: A quantitative study of Meissner's corpuscles in man. Neurology 16:1–9, 1966.
28. Bora FW Jr: Peripheral nerve repair in cats: The fasicular Stitch. J Bone Joint Surg 49A:659–666, 1967.
29. Bora FW Jr, Pleasure DE, Didizan NA: A study of nerve regeneration and neuroma formation after nerve suture by various techniques. J Hand Surg 1:138–143, 1976.
30. Boring EG: Cutaneous sensation after nerve divisions. J Exp Physiol 10:1–95, 1916.
31. Boswick JA, Schneewind J, Stromberg W: Evaluation of peripheral nerve repairs below the elbow. Arch Surg 90:50–51, 1965.
32. Botezat E: Die Apparate des Gefühlssinnes der nackten und behaarten Saügetieshaut, mit Berucksechtegung des Menschen. Anat Anz 42:278–318, 1912.
33. Bowden REM: Factors influencing functional recovery, in Seddon HJ (ed): Peripheral Nerve Injuries. London: Her Majesty's Stationery Office, 1954, Ch 7, pp 298–354.
34. Brady GS, Cloutier AM, Woolhouse FM: The fingertip injury: An assessment of management. Plast Reconstr Surg 26:80–90, 1960.
35. Braillar F, Horner RL: Sensory cross-finger pedicle graft. J Bone Joint Surg 51A:1264–1268, 1969.
36. Breathnach AS: An Atlas of the Ultrastructure of Human Skin. London: JA Churchill, 1971.

37. Breathnach AS: Electron microscopy of cutaneous nerves and receptors. J Invest Dermatol 69:8–26, 1977.

38. Brooks D: The place of nerve grafting in orthopedic surgery. J Bone Joint Surg 37A:299–326, 1955.

39. Brown AG, Iggo A: The structure and function of cutaneous "touch corpuscles" after nerve crush. J Physiol 165:28P–29P, 1963.

40. Brown AG, Iggo A: A quantitative study of cutaneous receptor and afferent fibers in the cat and rabbit. J Physiol 193:707–733, 1967.

41. Brushart TM, Terzis JK: Dorsal horn projections of normal and repaired sensory nerves. Presented Plastic Surgery Research Council Meeting, Hershey, Pa, April 21, 1980.

42. Buncke HJ: Digital nerve repairs. Surg Clin North Am 52:1267–1285, 1972.

43. Buncke HJ, Rose EH: Free toe-to-fingertip neurovascular island flaps. Plast Reconstr Surg 63:607–612, 1979.

44. Bunnell S: Surgery of the nerves of the hand. Surg Gynecol Obstet 44:145–152, 1927.

45. Bunnell S, Boyes JH: Nerve grafts. Am J Surg 44:64–75, 1939.

46. Burgess PR, English KB, Horch KW, et al: Patterning in the regeneration of type I cutaneous receptors. J Physiol 236:57–86, 1974.

47. Burgess PR, Horch KW: Specific regeneration of cutaneous fibers in the cat. J Neurophysiol 36:101–114, 1973.

48. Cabaud HE, Rodkey WG, McCarroll HR Jr, et al: Epineural and perineural fascicular nerve repair: A critical comparison. J Hand Surg 1:131–137, 1976.

49. Campbell JN, Meyer RA, La Motte RH: Sensitization of myelinated nociceptive afferents that innervate monkey hand. J Neurophysiol 42:1669–1679, 1979.

50. Carter MS: Re-education of Sensation. Presented at the Hand Rehabilitation Symposium, Philadelphia, March 23, 1980.

51. Cauna N: Nature and functions of the papillary ridges of the digital skin. Anat Rec 119:449–468, 1954.

52. Cauna N: Nerve supply and nerve endings in Meissner's corpuscles. Am J Anat 99:315–350, 1956.

53. Cauna N: Structure of digital touch corpuscles. Acta Anat (Basel) 32:1–23, 1958.

54. Cauna N, Mannan G: Development and postnatal changes of digital Pacinian corpuscles (corpuscular lamellosa) in the human hand. J Anat 93:271–286, 1956.

55. Cauna N, Ross LL: The fine structure of Meissner's touch corpuscles of human fingers. J Cell Biol 8:467–482, 1960.

56. Celli L, Caroli A: La ripresa della sensibilita nei trapianti, ed. innesti cutanei della mano. Riv Chir Mano 8:23–62, 1970.

57. Chacha PB, Krishnamurti A, Soin K: Experimental sensory reinnervation of the median nerve by nerve transfers in monkeys. J Bone Joint Surg 59A:386–390, 1977.

58. Chambers MR, Andres KH, von Duering M, et al: The structure and function of the slowly-adapting type II mechanoreceptors in hairy skin. Q J Exp Physiol 57:417–445, 1972.

59. Clark FJ, Burgess PR: Slowly-adapting receptors in cat knee joint: Can they signal joint angle? J Neurophysiol 38:1448–1463, 1975.

60. Clark FJ, Horch KW, Bach SM, et al: Contributions of cutaneous and joint receptors to static knee-position sense in man. J Neurophysiol 42:877–888, 1979.

61. Cohen LH, Lindley SR: Studies in vibratory sensibility. Am J Psychol 51:44–51, 1938.

62. Collins CC, Bach-y-Rita P: Transmission of pictorial information through the skin. Adv Biol Med Phys 14:285–315, 1973.

63. Conomy JP, Barnes KL, Cruse RP: Quantitative cutaneous sensory testing in children and adolescents. Cleve Clin Q 45:197–206, 1978.

64. Corkin S, Milner B, Rasmussen T: Somatosensory threshold: Contrasting effects of post-central gyrus and posterior parietal lobe excision. Arch Neurol 23:41–58, 1970.

65. Cosh JA: Studies on the nature of vibation sense. Clin Sci 12:131–151, 1953.

66. Cramer LM, Chase RA: Symposium on the Hand. St. Louis: CV Mosby, 1971.

67. Currier RD: Nervous system, in Judge RD, Zuidema GD (eds): Physical Diagnosis: A Physiologic Approach to the Clinical Examination, ed 2. Boston: Little, Brown, 1968, Ch 20, pp 408–410, 424–425.

68. Curtis RM: Sensory re-education after peripheral nerve injury, in Frederick S, Brody GS (eds): Symposium on the Neurological Aspects of Plastic Surgery. St. Louis: CV Mosby, 1978, pp 47–51.

69. Curtis RM, Dellon AL: Sensory re-education after peripheral nerve injury, in Omer G, Spinner M (eds): Management of Peripheral Nerve Injuries. New York: WB Saunders, 1980, pp 769–778.

70. Curtis RM, Eversmann WW Jr: Internal neurolysis as an adjunct to the treatment of the carpal tunnel syndrome. J Bone Joint Surg 55A:733–740, 1973.

71. Daniel CR, Bower JD, Pearson JE, et al: Vibrometry and neuropathy. J Miss State Med Assoc 18:30–34, 1977.

72. Daniel RK: Microsurgery: Through the looking glass. N Engl J Med 300:1251–1257, 1979.

73. Daniel RK, Terzis JK: Reconstructive Microsurgery. Boston: Little, Brown, 1977, p 324.

74. David WB: The life of John Staige Davis, M.D. Plast Reconstr Surg 62:368–378, 1978.

75. Davis JS: Plastic Surgery, Principles and Practice. Philadelphia: Blakiston, 1919.

76. Davis JS, Kitlowski EA: Regeneration of nerves in skin grafts and skin flaps. Am J Surg 24:501–545, 1934.

77. Davis L: The return of sensation to the transplanted skin. Surg Gynecol Obstet 59:533–543, 1934.

78. Davis RD: Some factors affecting the results of treatment of peripheral nerve injuries. Lancet 1:877–880, 1949.

79. Dawson GD: The relative excitability and conduction velocity of sensory and motor nerve fibres in man. J Physiol 131:436–451, 1956.

80. Dellon AL: Changes in primate Pacinian corpuscles

after volar pad excision and skin grafting (Letter to the Editor). Plast Reconstr Surg 58:614–615, 1976.

81. Dellon AL: Clinical use of vibratory stimuli to evaluate peripheral nerve injury and compression neuropathy. Plast Reconstr Surg 65:466–476, 1980.

82. Dellon AL: Evaluation of sensibility and re-education of sensation, in Mansat M (ed): *Proceedings: Symposium on Upper Extremity Sensory Problems*, June, 1980.

83. Dellon AL: Reinnervation of denervated Meissner corpuscles: A sequential histological study in the monkey following fascicular nerve repair. J Hand Surg 1:98–109, 1976.

84. Dellon AL: Results of internal neurolysis in peripheral nerve compression, in press 1981.

85. Dellon AL: Subcutaneous pedicle flap technique for fingertip reconstruction, in press 1981.

86. Dellon AL: The extended volar advancement flap for thumb reconstruction, in press 1981.

87. Dellon AL: The moving two-point discrimination test: Clinical evaluation of the quickly-adapting fiber receptor system. J Hand Surg 3:474–481, 1978.

88. Dellon AL: The paper clip: Light hardware for evaluation of sensibility in the hand. Contemp Orthop 1:39–42, 1979.

89. Dellon AL: The plastic ridge device and moving two-point discrimination (Letter to the Editor). J Hand Surg 5:92–93, 1980.

90. Dellon AL: The vibrometer, in press 1981.

91. Dellon AL: Two-point discrimination and the Meissner corpuscle (Letter to the Editor). Plast Reconstr Surg 60:270–271, 1977.

92. Dellon AL, Curtis RM, Edgerton, MT: Evaluating recovery of sensation in the hand following nerve injury. Johns Hopkins Med J 130:235–243, 1972.

93. Dellon AL, Curtis RM, Edgerton MT: Program for sensory re-education in the hand following nerve injury, in Marshall E (ed): *Hand Rehabilitation*. Brookfield, Illinois: Fred Sammon, 1977, pp 110–112.

94. Dellon AL, Curtis RM, Edgerton MT: Re-education of sensation in the hand following nerve injury (abstr). J Bone Joint Surg 53A:813, 1971.

95. Dellon AL, Curtis RM, Edgerton MT: Re-education of sensation in the hand following nerve injury. Plast Reconstr Surg 53:297–305, 1974.

96. Dellon AL, Jabaley ME: Re-education of sensation. Clin Orthop in press 1981.

97. Dellon AL, Munger B: Correlation of sensibility evaluation, hand function and histology, in press 1981.

98. Dellon AL, Terrill RE: A protective acrylic cast for use in experimental hand surgery. Hand 8:165–166, 1975.

99. Dellon AL, Witebsky FG, Terrill RE: The denervated Meissner corpuscle: A sequential histologic study after nerve division in the Rhesus monkey. Plast Reconstr Surg 56:182–193, 1975.

100. Denny-Brown O, Brenner C: paralysis of nerve induced by direct pressure and by tourniquet. Arch Neurol Psychiatry 51:1–26, 1944.

101. Dickens WN, Winkelmann RK, Mulder DW: Cholinsterase demonstration of dermal nerve endings in patients with impaired sensation. Neurology (Minneap) 13:91–100, 1963.

102. Drachman DB (ed): *Tropic Functions of the Neuron*. New York: New York Academy of Sciences, 1974.

103. Dreyer DA, Schneider RJ, Metz CB, et al: Differential contributions of spinal pathways to body representation in post-central gyrus. J Neurophysiol 37:119–145, 1945.

104. Dykes RW, Terzis JK: Reinnervation of glabrous skin in baboons: Properties of cutaneous mechanoreceptors subsequent to nerve crush. J Neurophysiol 42:1461–1478, 1979.

105. Edshage S: Experience with clinical methods of testing sensation after peripheral nerve surgery, in Jewett DL, McCarroll HR Jr (eds): *Nerve Repair and Regeneration*. St Louis: CV Mosby, 1980, pp 244–249.

106. Edshage S: Peripheral nerve suture. Acta Chir Scand [Suppl] 331:1–101, (99 references), 1964.

107. Egger M: De la sensibilité osseuse. J Physiol (Paris) 1:511–520, 1899.

108. Elliott FA: *Clinical Neurology*. Philadelphia: WB Saunders, 1964, pp 419–420.

109. Engel AG, Stonnington HH: Morphologic effects of denervation of muscle: A qualitative ultrastructural study, in Drachman DB (ed): *Trophic Functions of the Neuron*. New York: New York Academy of Sciences, 1974, pp 68–88.

110. English KB: Cell types in cutaneous type I mechanoreceptors (Haarscheiben) and their alterations with injury. Am J Anat 1:105–126, 1974.

111. English KB: Morphogenesis of Haarscheiben in rats. J Invest Dermatol 69:58–67, 1977.

112. Erlanger J, Gasser HS: *Electrical Signs of Nervous Activity*. Philadelphia: Univ Penn Press, 1937.

113. Eskilden P, Morris A, Collins CC, et al: Simultaneous and successive cutaneous two-point threshold for vibration. Psychon Sci 14:146–147, 1969.

114. Farbman AI: Electron microscopic study of the developing taste bud in rat fungiform papillae. Dev Biol 11:110–135, 1965.

115. Farbman AI: Fine structure of degenerating taste buds after denervation. J Embryol Exp Morphol 22:55–68, 1969.

116. Fess EE, Harmon KS, Strickland JW, et al.: Evaluation of the hand by objective measurement, in Hunter JM, Schneider LH, Mackin EJ, et al (eds): *Rehabilitation of the Hand*. St Louis: CV Mosby, 1978, Ch 5.

117. Fitzgerald MJT, Martin F, Paletta FX: Innervation of skin grafts. Surg Gynecol Obstet 124:808–812, 1967.

118. Flynn JE, Flynn WF: Median and ulnar nerve injuries. Ann Surg 156:1002–1009, 1962.

119. Forster FM, Shields CD: Cortical sensory defects causing disability. Arch Phys Med Rehabil 40:56–61, 1959.

120. Foucher G, Braun JB: A new island flap transfer from the dorsum of the index to the thumb. Plast Reconstr Surg 63:344–349, 1979.

121. Foucher G, Merle M, Maneaud M, et al: Microsurgical free partial toe transfer in hand construction: A report of 12 cases. Plast Reconstr Surg 65:616–626, 1980.

122. Fox JC, Klemperer WW: Vibratory sensibility. Arch. Neurol Psychiatry 48:622–645, 1942.

123. Fredricks S, Brody GS: *Symposium on the Neurologic Aspects of Plastic Surgery.* St Louis: CV Mosby, 1978.

124. Freshwater MF: The principles and purpose of plastic surgery—past and present, in Krizek TJ, Hoopes JE (eds): *Symposium on Basic Science in Plastic Surgery.* St Louis: CV Mosby, 1976, pp 3–13.

125. Fujimoto S, Murray RG: Fine structure of degeneration and regeneration in denervated rabbit vallate taste buds. Anat Rec 168:393–414, 1970.

126. Gammon GS, Bronk DW: The discharge of impulses from Pacinian corpuscles in the mesentery and its relation to vascular change. Am J Physiol 114:77–84, 1935.

127. Gaul JS Jr: Radial-innervated cross-finger flaps from index to provide sensory pulp to injured thumb. J Bone Joint Surg 51A:1257–1263, 1969.

128. Gelberman RH, Blasingame JP, Fronek A, et al: Forearm arterial injuries. J Hand Surg 4:401–408, 1979.

129. Gelberman RH, Urbaniak JR, Bright DS, et al: Digital sensibility following replantation. J Hand Surg 3:313–319, 1978.

130. Geldard FA: The perception of mechanical vibration: IV. Is there a separate "Vibratory Sense"? J Gen Psychol 22:29–308, 1940.

131. Gelfan S, Carter S: Muscle sense in man. Exp Neurol 18:469–473, 1967.

132. Gillis M, Pool R: Two-point discrimination distances in the normal hand and forearm. Plast Reconstr Surg 59:57–62, 1977.

133. Gilmer B von H: A study of the regeneration of vibratory sensitivity. J Gen Psychol 14:461–462, 1936.

134. Gilray J, Meyer JS: *Medical Neurology.* Toronto: MacMillan, 1969, pp 2, 4, 59, 60.

135. Glees P, Mohiuddin A, Smith AG: Transplantation of Pacinian bodies in the brain and thigh of the cat. Acta Anat (Basel) 7:213–224, 1949.

136. Gordon I: The sensation of vibration with special reference to its clinical significance. J Neurol Psychopathol 17:107–134, 1936.

137. Gottschaldt KM, Lausmann S: Mechanoreceptors and their properties in the beak skin of geese (Anser anser). Brain Res 65:510–515, 1974.

138. Grabb WC, Bement SC, Koepke G: Comparison of methods of peripheral nerve suturing in monkeys. Plast Reconstr Surg 46:31–38, 1970.

139. Gradenigo G: A new optical method of acoumetrie. J Laryngol Rhin Otol 14:583–585, 1899.

140. Grandis V: Sur la mesure de l'acuite auditive au moyen de valeurs physiques entre elles. Arch Ital Biol 37:358–376, 1902.

141. Gray JAB, Malcolm JL: The initiation of a nerve impulse by mesenteric Pacinian corpuscles. Proc. R Aoc Lond [Biol] 137:96, 1950.

142. Gray JAB, Mathews PBR: A comparison of the adaptation of the Pacinian corpuscle with the accomodation of its own axon. J Physiol 114:454–464, 1951.

143. Gray RC: Quantitative study of vibration sense in normal and pernicious anemia. Minn Med 15:674–680, 1932.

144. Green D (ed): *Operative Treatment of Nerve Problems.* Edinburgh: Churchill Livingstone, in press 1980.

145. Grigg P, Finerman GA, Riley LH: Joint-position sense after total hip replacement. J Bone Joint Surg 55A:1061–1025, 1973.

146. Grigg P, Greenspan BJ: Response of primate joint afferent neurons to mechanical stimulation of knee joint. J Neurophysiol 40:1–8, 1977.

147. Gruber H, Zenker V: Acetylcholinesterase: Histological differentiation between motor and sensory nerve fibers. Brain Res 51:207–214.

148. Guth L: Degeneration and regeneration of taste buds, in Beidler LM (ed): *Handbook of Sensory Physiology.* Vol VI. Berlin: Springer-Verlag, 1971, pp 63–74.

149. Guth L: Taste buds in the rat's circumvallate papillae after reinnervation for the glossopharyngeal, vagus, and hypoglossal nerve. Anat Rec 130:25–37, 1958.

150. Guth L: The effects of glossopharyngeal nerve transection on the circumvallate papilla of the rat. Anat Rec 128:715–731, 1957.

151. Hakistian RW: Funicular orientation by direct stimulation: An aid to peripheral nerve repair. J Bone Joint Surg 50A:1178–1186, 1968.

152. Halata Z: Spezifische innervation, in Orfanos CE (ed): *Haar und Haarkrankheiten.* Stuttgart: Gustav Fischer Verlag, Ch 6, 1979.

153. Halata Z: The ultrastructure of the sensory nerve endings in the articular capsule of the knee joint of the domestic cat (Ruffini corpuscles and Pacinian corpuscles). J Anat 124:717–729, 1977.

154. Hamlin E, Watkins AL: Regeneration in the ulnar, median and radial nerves. Surg Clin North Am 27:1052–1061, 1947.

155. Harrington T, Merzenich MM: Neural coding in the sense of touch: Human sensations of skin indentation compared with responses of slowly-adapting mechanoreceptive afferents innervating the hairy skin of monkeys. Exp Brain Res 10:251–264, 1970.

156. Harris AJ: Inductive function of the nervous system. Annu Rev Physiol 36:251–305, 1974 (403 references).

157. Hashimoto K: Fine structure of the Meissner corpuscle of human palmar skin. J Invest Dermatol 60:20–28, 1973.

158. Head H: *Studies in Neurology.* Cited by Fox JC, Klemperer WW: Vibratory sensibility. Arch Neurol Psychiatry 48:623–645, 1942.

159. Head H: The afferent nervous system from a new aspect. Brain 28:99–115, 1905.

160. Head H, Sherren J: The consequences of injury to the peripheral nerves in man. Brain 28:116–337, 1905.

161. Heinrichs RW, Moorehouse JA: Touch perception

in blind diabetic subjects in relation to the reading of Braille type. N Engl Med 280:72–75, 1969.

162. Henderson WR: Clinical assessment of peripheral nerve injuries: Tinel's test. Lancet 2:801–805, 1948.

163. Hensel H, Boman KA: Afferent impulses in cutaneous sensory nerves in human subjects. J Neurophysiol 23:564–578, 1960.

164. Hoffman H: Local re-innervation in partially denervated muscle: A histo-physiological study. Aust J Exp Biol Med Sci 28:384–398, 1950.

165. Holevich J: A new method of restoring sensibility to the thumb. J Bone Joint Surg 45B:496–502, 1963.

166. Holm A, Zacharias L: Fingertip lesions: An evaluation of conservative treatment versus free skin grafting. Acta Orthop Scand 45:382–392, 1974.

167. Holmes W: Histologic observations on the repair of nerves by autografts. Br J Surg 35:167–173, 1947.

168. Honner R, Fragiadahis FG, Lamb DW: An investigation of the factors affecting the results of digital nerve division. Hand 2:21–31, 1970.

169. Horch K: Guidance of regrowing sensory axons after cutaneous nerve lesions in the cat. J Neurophysiol 42:1437–1449, 1979.

170. Horch KWM, Burgess PR: Responses to threshold and suprathreshold stimuli by slowly-adapting cutaneous mechanoreceptors in the cat. J Comp Physiol 110:307–315, 1976.

171. Horch KWM, Burgess PR, Whitedorn D: Ascending collaterals of cutaneous neurons in the fasciculus gracilis of the cat. Brain Res 117:1–17, 1976.

172. Horch KWM, Tuckett RP, Burgess PR: A key to the classification of cutaneous mechanoreceptors. J Invest Dermatol 69:75–82, 1977.

173. Horch KWM, Whitehorn D, Burgess PR: Impulse generation in type I cutaneous mechanoreceptors. J Neurophysiol 37:267–281, 1974.

174. Hulliger M, Nordh E, Thelin AE, et al: The response of afferent fibers from the glabrous skin of the hand during voluntary finger movements in man. J Physiol 291:233–249, 1979.

175. Hunter JM, Schneider LH, Mackin EJ, et al: Rehabilitation of the Hand. St. Louis: CV Mosby, 1978.

176. Hurley HG, Koelle GB: The effect of inhibition of nonspecific cholinesterase in perception of tactile sensation in human volar skin. J Invest Dermatol 31:243–245, 1958.

177. Hutchinson J, Tough JS, Wynburn GM: Regeneration of sensation in grafted skin. Br J Plast Surg 2: 82–94, 1949.

178. Ide C: The fine structure of the digital corpuscle of the mouse toe pad, with special reference to nerve fibers. Am J Anat 147:329–356, 1977.

179. Iggo A: Cutaneous and subcutaneous sense organs. Br Med Bull 33:97–102, 1977.

180. Iggo A: Cutaneous receptors, in Hubbard JI (ed): The Peripheral Nervous System. New York: Plenum Press, 1974, Ch 12, pp 347–404 (101 references).

181. Iggo A: New specific sensory structures in hairy skin. Acta Neuroveg 24:175–180, 1963.

182. Iggo A, Muir AR: A cutaneous sense organ in the hairy skin of cats. J Anat 97:151, 1963.

183. Iggo A, Muir AR: The structure and function of a slowly-adapting touch corpuscle in hairy skin. J Physiol 200:763–796, 1969.

184. Ito T: Surgery of the Peripheral Nerve. Tokyo: Igaku Shoin, 1977.

185. Jabaley ME: Recovery of sensation in flaps and skin, in Tubiana R (ed): The Hand. Philadelphia: WB Saunders, 1981.

186. Jabaley ME, Burns JE, Ortt BS, et al: Comparison of histologic and functional recovery after peripheral nerve repair J. Hand Surg. 1:119–130, 1976.

187. Jabaley ME, Dellon AL: Evaluation of sensibility through microhistological studies, in Omer GE, Spinner M (eds): Management of Peripheral Nerve Problems. Philadelphia: WB Saunders, 1980, Ch 23, 62.

188. Jabaley ME, Wallace WH, Heckler FR: Internal topography of major nerves of the forearm and hand: A current review. J Hand Surg 5:1–18, 1980.

189. Jewett DL, McCarroll HR Jr: Nerve Repair and Regeneration. St Louis: CV Mosby, 1980.

190. Johnson KO: Reconstruction of population response to a vibratory stimulus in quickly-adapting mechanoreceptive afferent fiber population innervating glabrous skin of the monkey. J Neurophysiol 37:48–71, 1974.

191. Johnson RK, Inverson RE: Cross finger pedicle flaps in the hand. J Bone Joint Surg 53A:913–919, 1971.

192. Joshi BB: A sensory cross-finger flap for use on the index finger. Plast Reconstr Surg 58:210–213, 1976.

193. Joshi BB: Neural repair for sensory restoration in a groin flap. Hand 9:221–225, 1977.

194. Kaas JH, Nelson RJ, Sur M, et al: Multiple representations of the body within the somatosensory cortex of primates. Science 204:521–523, 1979.

195. Kappers CVA, Huber GC, Crosby EC: The Comparative Anatomy of the Nervous System of Vertebrates, including Man. New York: Hafner, 1960.

196. Karthals JK, Wisniewski HM, Ghetti B, et al: The fate of the axon and its terminal in the Pacinian corpuscle following sciatic nerve section. J Neurophysiol 3:385–403, 1974.

197. Kasprzak H, Tapper DN, Craig PH: Functional development of the tactile pad receptor system. Exp Neurol 26:439–446, 1970.

198. Kawamura T: Fine structure of the dendritic cells and Merkel cells in the epidermis of various mammals. Jpn J Dermatol 81:343–351, 1971.

199. Kawamura T, Nishiyama S, Ikeda S, et al: The human haarscheibe, its structure and function. J Invest Dermatol 42:87–90, 1966.

200. Keim HA, Granthan SA: Volar flap advancement for thumb and fingertip injuries. Clin Orthop 66: 109–112, 1969.

201. Kim KL, Pasch JL: Island flap innervated by radial nerve for restoration of sensation in an index stump. Plast Reconstr Surg 47:386–388, 1971.

202. Kingsley NW, Stein JM, Levenson SM: Measuring tissue pressure to assess the severity of burn induced ischemia. Plast Reconstr Surg 63:404–408, 1979.

203. Kirklin JW, Murphy F, Berkson J: Suture of peripheral nerves: Factors affecting prognosis. Surg. Gynecol Obstet 88:719–730, 1959.

204. Kleinert HE, Juhalo CA, Tsai T, et al: Digital replantation—selection, techniques, and results. Orthop Clin North Am 8:309–318, 1977.
205. Kleinert HE, McAllister CG, MacDonald CJ, et al: A critical evaluation of cross finger flaps. J Trauma 14:756–763, 1974.
206. Knibestol M, Vallbo AB: Single unit analysis of mechanoreceptor activity from the human glabrous skin. Acta Physiol Scand 80:178–195, 1970.
207. Konietzny F, Hensel H: Response of rapidly and slowly-adapting mechanoreceptors and vibratory sensitivity in human hairy skin. Pfluegers Arch 368:39–44, 1977.
208. Krag K, Rasmussen KB: The neurovascular island flap for defective sensibility of the thumb. J Bone Joint Surg [BR] 57B:495–499, 1975.
209. Kredel FE, Evans JP: Recovery of sensation in denervated pedicle and free skin grafts. Arch Neurol Psychiatry 29:1203–1221, 1933.
210. Krishnamurti A, Kanagasuntheram R, Vÿ S: Failure of reinnervation of Pacinian corpuscle after nerve crush: An electron microscopic study. Acta Neuropathol (Berl) 23:338–341, 1973.
211. LaMotte RH: psychophysical and neurophysical studies of tactile sensibility, in Hollies N, Goldman R (eds): Clothing Comfort: Interaction of Thermal, Ventilation, Construction and Assessment Factors. Amer Arbr Sci, Amer Arbor, 1977, by report to the international union, LaMotte R, Mountcastle B: Symposium on "Active Touch," Beaune, France, 1977.
212. LaMotte RH, Campbell JN: Comparison of response of warm and nociceptive C-fiber afferents in monkey with human judgments of thermal pain. J Neurophysiol 41:509–528, 1978.
213. LaMotte RH, Mountcastle VB: Capacities of humans and monkeys to discriminate between vibratory stimuli of different frequency and amplitude: A correlation between neural events and psychophysical measurements. J Neurophysiol 38:539–559, 1975.
214. LaMotte RH, Mountcastle VB: Disorders in somesthesia following lesions of parietal lobe. J Neurophysiol 42:400–419, 1979.
215. Landau W, Bishop GH: Pain from dermal, periosteal and fascial endings and from inflammations. Arch Neurol Psychiatry 51:1–26, 1944.
216. Lansen RD, Posch JL: Nerve injuries in the upper extremity. Arch Surg 77:469–482, 1958.
217. Lee FC: A study of the Pacinian corpuscle. J Comp Neurol 64:497–522, 1936.
218. Lefkowitz M: A Model of the Glabrous Skin of the Fingertip, Master's thesis. Johns Hopkins University, Baltimore, 1979.
219. Lesavoy MA: The dorsal index finger neurovascular island flap. Orthop Rev 9:91–95, 1980.
220. Levin S, Pearsall G, Ruderman RJ: von Frey's method of measuring pressure sensibility in the hand: An engineering analysis of the Weinstein-Semmes pressure aesthisiometer. J Hand Surg 3:211–216, 1978.
221. Lewis T, Pickering GW, Rothschild P: Centripetal parapysis arising out of arrested bloodflow to the limbs. Heart 61:1, 1931.

222. Lin C, Merzenich MM, Sur M, et al: Connections of areas 3b and 1 of the parietal somatosensory strip with the ventroposterior nucleus in the Owl Monkey (Aotus trivirgatus). J Comp Neurol 185:355–372, 1979.
223. Lindblom U: Properties of touch receptors in distal glabrous skin of the monkey. J Neurophysiol 28:966–985, 1965.
224. Lindblom V, Meyerson BA: Influence on touch, vibration and cutaneous pain of dorsal column stimulation in man. Pain 1:257–270, 1975.
225. Lindsay WK: Hand injuries in children. Clin Plast Surg 3:65–75, 1976.
226. Lister G: The Hand: Diagnosis and Indications. Edinburgh: Churchill Livingstone, 1977, p 73.
227. Livingstone WK: Evidence of active invasion of denervated areas by sensory fibers from neighboring nerves in man. J Neurosurg 4:140–145, 1947.
228. Lofgren L: Recovery of nervous function in skin transplants with special reference to the sympathetic functions. Acta Chir Scand 102:229–239, 1952.
229. Lowenstein WR: Biological transducers. Sci Am 203:99–108, 1960.
230. Lowenstein WR: Development of a receptor on a foreign nerve fiber n a Pacinian corpuscle. Science 177:712–715, 1972.
231. Lowenstein WR: On the "specificity" of a sensory receptor. J Neurophysiol 24:150–158, 1961.
232. Lowenstein WR, Mendelson M: Components of receptor adaptation in a Pacinian corpuscle. J Physiol 177:377–397, 1965.
233. Lowenstein WR, Rothkamp R: The sites for mechanoelectric conversion in a Pacinian corpuscle. J Gen Physiol 41:1245–1265, 1958.
234. Lunborg G: Structure and function of the intraneural microvessels as related to trauma, edema formation and nerve function. J Bone Joint Surg 57A:938–948, 1975.
235. Lyons WR, Woodhall B: Atlas of Peripheral Nerve Injury. Philadelphia: WB Saunders, 1949, p 215.
236. Major RH, Delp MH: Physical Diagnosis, ed 6. Philadelphia: WB Saunders, 1962, pp 300, 320–323.
237. Mann SJ, Straille WE: Tylotrich (hair) follicle: Association with a slowly-adapting tactile receptor in the cat. Science 147:1043–1045, 1965.
238. Mannerfelt L: Evaluation of functional sensation of skin grafts in the hand area. Br J Plast Surg 15:136–154, 1962.
239. Mansat M, Delprat J: Reeducation de la sensibilite de la main. Ann Med Physique 18:527–538, 1975.
240. Maquieric NO: An innervated full-thickness skin graft to restore sensibility to fingertips and heels. Plast Reconstr Surg 53:568–575, 1974.
241. Marshall AJ (ed): Biology & Comparative Physiology of Birds. New York: Academic Press, 1960.
242. Matsen FA, Mayo KA, Kriegmire RB Jr, et al: A model compartmental syndrome in man with particular reference to the quantification of nerve function. J Bone Joint Surg 59A:648–653, 1977.
243. Matsen FA, Weinquist RA, Kriegmire RB: Diagnosis and management of compartment syndromes. J Bone Joint Surg 62A:286–291, 1980.
244. May JW Jr, Chait LA, Cohen BE, et al: Free neu-

rovascular flap from the first web of the foot in hand reconstruction. J Hand Surg 2:387–393, 1977.

245. May JW Jr, Daniel RK: Great toe to hand free tissue transfer. Clin Orthop 133:140–153, 1978.

246. Mayamoto Y: Experimental study of results of nerve suture under tension vs. nerve grafting. Plast Reconstr Surg 64:540–549, 1979.

247. Maynard J: Sensory re-education after peripheral nerve injury, in Hunter J, Mackin E, Schneider L, et al (eds): Rehabilitation of the Hand. Baltimore: Williams & Wilkins, 1977.

248. McCarroll HR: The regeneration of sensation in transplanted skin. Ann Surg 108:309–320, 1938.

249. McEwan LE: Median and ulnar nerve injuries. Aust NZ J Jurg 32:89–104, 1962.

250. McFarlane RM, Moyer JR: Digital nerve grafts with the lateral antebrachial cutaneous nerve. J Hand Surg 1:169–173, 1976.

251. McLachlean EM, Taylor RS, Bennett MR: The site of synapsis formation in reinnervation and cross-reinnervation mammalian muscle. Proc. Aust Physiol Pharmacol Soc 3:62–69, 1972.

252. McQuillan WM: Sensory recovery after nerve repair. Hand 2:7–9, 1970.

253. McQuillan WM, Neilson JMM, Boardman AK, et al: Sensory evaluation after median nerve repair. Hand 3:101–111, 1971.

254. Meissner G: Beiträge sur Kenntnis der Anatomie and Physiologie der Haut. Leipzig, Leopold Voss, 1853, p 47, and Untersuchungen uber den Tostsuin, Z Rat Med 7:92–119, 1859. Cited by Winkelman RK: Nerve Endings in Normal and Pathologic Skin. Springfield: Charles C Thomas, 1960.

255. Melvin JL, Harris DH, Johnson EW: Sensory and motor conduction velocities in the ulnar and median nerves. Arch Phys Med Rehabil 47:511–519, 1966.

256. Merkel F: Tastzellen und Tastkorperchen bei den Hausthieren und beim Menschen. Arch Mikrosk Anat 11:636–652, 1875.

257. Merzenich MM, Harrington T: The sense of flutter-vibration evoked by stimulation of the hairy skin of primates: Comparison of human sensory capacity with the responses of mechanoreceptive afferents innervating the hairy skin of monkeys. Exp Brain Res 9:236–260, 1969.

258. Merzenich MM, Kaas JH, Sur M, et al: Double representation of the body surface within cytoarchitecture areas 3b and 1 in "S1" in the Owl Monkey (Aotus trivirgatus). J Comp Neurol 181: 41–74, 1978.

259. Michon J, Moberg E: Traumatic Nerve Lesions of the Upper Extremity. London: Churchill Livingstone, 1975.

260. Micks JE, Wilson JN: Full thickness sole-skin grafts for resurfacing the hand. J Bone Joint Surg 49A: 1128–1134, 1967.

261. Miller MR, Ralston HJ, Kasahara M: The pattern of cutaneous innervation of the human hand. Am J Anat 102:183–201, 1958.

262. Miller SH, Rusennas I: Changes in primate Pacinian corpuscles following volar pad excision and skin grafting: A preliminary report. Plast Reconstr Surg 57:627–636, 1976.

263. Millesi H, Meisse G, Berger A: Further experience with interfascicular grafting of the median, ulnar and radial nerves. J Bone Joint Surg 58A:209–218, 1976.

264. Millesi H, Meisse G, Berger A: The interfascicular nerve grafting of the median and ulnar nerves. J Bone Joint Surg 54A:727–750, 1972.

265. Millesi H, Rinderes D: A method for training and testing sensibility of the fingertips. Proc World Fed Occup Ther 7:122–125, 1979.

266. Minor L: Uber die Localisation used klinische Bedeutung der sog. "Knochensensibilitat" oder das "Vibrationsgefuhls." Neurol Centralbl 23:146–199, 1904.

267. Mirsky IA, Futterman P, Brohkahn RH: The quantitative measurement of vibratory perception in subjects with and without diabetes mellitus. J Lab Clin Med 41:221–235, 1953.

268. Mitchell SW: Injuries of Nerves and Their Consequences, 1872. American Academy of Neurology Reprint Series. New York: Dover, 1965, pp 19, 84, 179, 183, 184.

269. Moberg E: Aspects of sensation in reconstructive surgery of the upper extremity. J Bone Joint Surg 46A:817–825, 1964.

270. Moberg E: The Upper Limb in Tetraplegia. New York: Grune & Stratton, 1978.

271. Moberg E: Criticism and study of methods for examining sensibility in the hand. Neurology (Minnlap) 12:8–19, 1962.

272. Moberg E: Emergency Surgery of the Hand. New York: Churchill Livingstoner, 1968.

273. Moberg E: Fingers were made before forks. Hand 4:201–206, 1972.

274. Moberg, E: Future hopes for the surgical management of peripheral nerve lesions, in Michon J, Moberg E (eds): Traumatic Nerve Lesions. New York: Churchill Livingstone, 1975.

275. Moberg E: Methods for examining sensibility in the hand, in Flynn JE (ed): Hand Surgery, ed 1. Baltimore: Williams & Wilkins, 1966, pp 435–439.

276. Moberg E: Objective methods for determining the functional value of sensibility in the skin. J Bne Joint Surg [Br] 40:454–466, 1958.

277. Moberg E: Reconstructive hand surgery in tetraplegia, stroke and cerebral palsy: Some basic concepts of physiology and neurology. J Hand Surg 1:29–34, 1976.

278. Montagna W: Comparative anatomy and physiology of the skin. Arch Dermatol 96:357–363, 1967.

279. Morrison WA, O'Brien B, MacLeod AM: Evaluation of digital replantation—a review of 100 cases. Orthop Clin North Am 8:295–308, 1977.

280. Mountcastle VB: Discussion section of Abo Foundation Symposium on Touch, Heat and Pain. London: JA Churchill, 1966.

281. Mountcastle VB: Medical Physiology, ed 12. St Louis: CV Mosby, 1968, Ch 61–63.

282. Mountcastle VB: Modality and topographic properties of single neurons of cat's somatic sensory cortex. J Neurophysiol 20:408–434, 1957.

283. Mountcastle VB: The view from within: Pathways to the study of perception. Johns Hopkins Med J 136:109–131, 1975.

284. Mountcastle, VB, Darian-Smith I: Neural mecha-

nisms in somesthesic, in Mountcastle VB (ed): *Medical Physiology*, ed 12. St. Louis: CV Mosby, 1968, Ch 62.

285. Mountcastle VB, Henneman E: The representation of tactile sensibility in the thalamus of the monkey. J Comp Neurol 97:409–440, 1952.

286. Mountcastle VB, Poggio GF, Werner G: The relation of thalamic cell response to peripheral stimuli varied over an intensive continuum. J Neurophysiol 26:807–834, 1963.

287. Mountcastle VB, Powell TPS: Neural mechanisms subserving cutaneous sensibility, with special reference to the role of afferent inhibition in sensory perception and discrimination. Bull Johns Hopkins Hosp 105:201–232, 1959.

288. Mountcastle VB, Talbot WH, Darian-Smith I, et al: A neural base for the sense of flutter-vibration. Science 155:597–600, 1967.

289. Mountcastle VB, Talbot WH, Kornhuber HH: *The Neural Transformation of Mechanical Stimuli Delivered to the Monkey's Hand*. Ciba Foundation Symposium on Touch, Heat and Pain, de Rueck AVS, Knight J (eds). London: JA Churchill, 1966.

290. Muller J: *Uber die phantastischen Gesichtserscheinungen*. Koblenz: J Holscher, 1826.

291. Munger BL: The intraepidermal innervation of the snout skin of the opossum: A light and electron microscopic study, with observations on the nature of the Merkel's Tastzellen. J Cell Biol. 26:79–96, 1965.

292. Munger BL: Neural-epithelial interactions in sensory receptors. J Invest Dermatol 69:27–40, 1977.

293. Munger BL: Patterns of organization of peripheral sensory receptors, in Lowenstein WR (ed): *Handbook of Sensory Physiology*. Berlin: Springer-Verlag, 1971, Ch. 17.

294. Munger BL: The comparative ultrastructure of slowly and rapidly adapting mechanoreceptors, in Dubner R, Kawamuro Y (eds): *Oral-Facial Sensory and Motor Mechanisms*. New York: Appleton-Century-Crofts, 1971, Ch 6.

295. Munger BL, Page RB, Pubols BH Jr: Identification of specific mechanosensory receptors in glabrous skin of dorsal root ganglionectomized primates. Anat Rec 93:630–631, 1979.

296. Munger BL, Pubols LM: The sensorineural organization of the digital skin of the raccoon. Brain Behav Evol 5:367–393, 1972.

297. Munger BL, Pubols LM, Pubols BH Jr: The Merkel rete papilla—a slowly-adapting sensory receptor in mammalian glabrous skin. Brain Res 29:47–61, 1971.

298. Murabeck, SJ, Owen CA, Hargen AR, et al: Acute compartment syndromes: Diagnosis and treatment with the aid of a wick catheter. J Bone Joint Surg 60A:1091–1095, 1978.

299. Murray JR, Ord JVR, Gavelin GE: The neurovascular island flap pedicle flap. J Bone Joint Surg 49A:1285–1297, 1967.

300. Napier, JR: The significance of Tinel's sign in peripheral nerve injuries. Brain 72:63–82, 1949.

301. Narakas A: Surgical treatment of traction injuries of the brachial plexus. Clin Orthop 133:71–90, 1978.

302. Naso SJ: Full-thickness skin grafts from thenar eminence to cover volar avulsions of fingers. Orthop Rev 7:127–129, 1978.

303. Newman HW, Corbin KB: Quantitative determination of vibratory sensibility. Proc. Soc Exp Biol 35:273–276, 1936.

304. Newton I, 1675. Cited by Boyes J: *On the Shoulders of Giants. Notable Names in Hand Surgery*. Philadelphia: JB Lippincott, 1976.

305. Nicholson OR, Seddon HJ: Nerve repair in civilian practice: Results of treatment of median and ulnar lesions. Br Med J 2:1065–1071, 1957.

306. Nielsen JB, Torup D: Nerve injuries in the upper extremities. Dan Med Bull 11:92–95, 1964.

307. Nishi K, Oura C, Paillie W: Fine structure of Pacinian corpuscles in the mesentery of the cat. J Cell Biol 43:539–552, 1969.

308. Norris TR, Poppen NK, Buncke HJ: Restoration of sensibility and function with microvascular transplants from the toe to the hand. Presented Am Soc Surg Hand Meeting, Feb 5, 1980.

309. O'Brien B, MacLeod AM, Sykes PJ, et al: Microvascular second toe transfer for digital reconstruction. J Hand Surg 3:123–133, 1978.

310. Oester YT, Davis L: Recovery of sensory function, in Woodhall B, Beebee GW (eds): *Peripheral Nerve Regeneration*. Washington DC: US Gov Printing Office, 1956, Ch 5, pp 241–310.

311. Omer G: Injuries to nerves of the upper extremities. J Bone Joint Surg 56A:1615–1624, 1974.

312. Omer GE: Sensation and sensibility in the upper extremity. Clin Orthop 104:30–36, 1974.

313. Omer GE: Sensibility of the hand as opposed to sensation in the hand. Ann Chir 27:479–483, 1973.

314. Omer, GE: Sensibility testing, in Omer GE, Spinner M (eds): *Management of Peripheral Nerve Problems*. Philadelphia: WB Saunders, 1980, Ch 1.

315. Omer GE, Day DJ, Ratliff H, et al: Neurovascular cutaneous island pedicles for deficient median nerve sensibility. J Bone Joint Surg 52A:1181–1192, 1970.

316. Omer GE, Spinner M: *Management of Peripheral Nerve Problems*. Philadelphia: WB Saunders, 1980.

317. Onne L: Recovery of sensibility and sudomotor activity in the hand after nerve suture. Acta Chir Scand [Suppl] 300:1–70, 1962 (135 references).

318. O'Rain S: New and simple test of nerve function in the hand. Br Med J 3:615–616, 1973.

319. Orgel MG, Aguayo, A, Wiliams HB: Sensory nerve regeneration: An experimental study of skin grafts in the rabbit. J Anat 111:121–135, 1972.

320. Orgel MG, Terzis JK: Epineurial vs perineurial repair: An ultrastructural and electrophysiologic study of nerve regeneration. Plast Reconstr Surg 60:80–91, 1977.

321. Orphanos CE, Mahrle G: Ultrastructural and cytochemistry of human cutaneous nerves. J Invest Dermatol 61:108–120, 1973.

322. Osborne G: The surgical treatment of tardy ulnar neuritis (abstr). J Bone Joint Surg 39B:782, 1957.

323. Osler W: The student life, in Franklin AW (ed): *A Way of Life and Selected Writings of Sir William Osler*. New York: Dover, 1958, pp 172–173.

324. Owen R: *On the Archetype and Homologies of the*

Vertebrate Skeleton, London: J Van Roost, 1848. Cited by Freshwater MF: The principles and purpose of plastic surgery—past and present, in Kruzik TJ, Hoopes JE (eds): *Symposium on Basic Science in Plastic Surgery*. St. Louis: CV Mosby, 1976, p 3.

325. Pacini F: *Nuovo Giornalle Letherali*, 1836, p 109. Cited by Winkelmann RK: *Nerve Endings in Normal and Pathologic Skin*. Springfield: Charles C Thomas, 1960.

326. Palmer P: Ultrastructural alterations of Merkel cells following denervation. Anat Rec 151:396-397, 1965.

327. Parry CBW: *Rehabilitation of the Hand*, ed 2. London: Butterworths, 1966, pp 19, 107-108.

328. Parry CBW, Salter M: Sensory re-education after median nerve lesion. Hand 8:250-257, 1976.

329. Patton H: Split-skin grafts from hypothenar area for fingertip avulsions. Plast Reconstr. Surg 43:426-429, 1969.

330. Paul RL, Goodman H, Merzenick M: Alterations in mechanoreceptor input to Brodmann's area 1 and 3 of the post-central hand area of Macaco mulatto after nerve section and regeneration. Brain Res 39:1-19, 1972.

331. Paul RL, Merzenich M, Goodman H: Representation of slowly- and rapidly-adapting cutaneous mechanoreceptors of the hand on Brodmann's area 3 and 1 of Macaca mulatta. Brain Res 36:229-249, 1972.

332. Pearson, GHJ: Effect of age in vibratory sensibility. Arch Neurol Psychiatry 20:482-496, 1928.

333. Pease DC, Quilliam TA: Electron microscopy of the Pacinian corpuscle. J Biophys Biochem Cytol 3:331-342, 1957.

334. Penfield W, Rasmussen AT: *The Cerebral Cortex of Man: A Clinical Study of Localization of Function*. New York: MacMillan, 1950.

335. Perry JR, Hamilton GF, Lachenbuch PA, et al: Protective sensation in the hand and its correlation to the ninhydrin sweat test following nerve laceration. Am J PHys Med 53:113-118, 1974.

336. Phelps PE, Walker E: Comparison of the finger wrinkling test results to established sensory tests in peripheral nerve injury. Am J Occup Ther 31:565-572, 1977.

337. *Physical Diagnosis: A Physiologic Approach to the Clinical Examination*. Boston: Little Brown, 1968, Ch 20, pp 408-410.

338. Pinkus F: Uber Hautsinnesorgane neben den menshlichen Haar (Haarscheiben) und ihre vergleichenden anatomische Bedeutung. Arch Mikrosk Anat Entu Mech 65:124-179, 1904.

339. Ponten B: Grafted skin: Observation on innervation and other qualities. Act Chir Scand [Suppl] 257:1-78, 1960.

340. Poppen NK, McCarroll HR Jr: Reply. J Hand Surg 5:92-93, 1980.

341. Poppen NK, McCarroll HR Jr, Doyle JR, et al: Recovery of sensibility after suture of digital nerves. J Hand Surg 4:212-226, 1979.

342. Porter RW: Functional assessment of transplanted skin in volar defects of digits: A comparison between free grafts and flaps. J Bone Joint Surg 50A:955-963, 1968.

343. Porter RW: New test for fingertip sensation. Br Med J 2:927-928, 1966.

344. Posch JL, dela Cruz-Saddul F: Nerve repair in trauma surgery: A ten year study of 231 peripheral injuries. Orthop Rev 9:35-45, 1980.

345. Posch JL, Marcotte DR: Carpal tunnel syndrome: An analysis of 1,201 cases. Orthop Rev 5:25-35, 1976.

346. Posner MA, Smith RJ: The advancement pedicle flap for thumb injuries J Bone Joint Surg 53A:1618-1621, 1971.

347. Powell TPS, Mountcastle VB: Some aspects of the functional organization of the cortex of the post-central gyrus of the monkey: A correlation of findings obtained in a single unit analysis with cytoarchitecture. Bull Johns Hopkins Hosp 105:133-162, 1959.

348. Powell TPS, Mountcastle VB: The cytoarchitecture of the post-central gyrus of the monkey Macaca mulatta. Bull Johns Hopkins Hosp 105:108-131, 1959.

349. Pubols LM, Pubols BH Jr, Munger BL: Functional properties of mechanoreceptors in glabrous skin of the raccoon's forepaw. Exp Neurol 31:165-182, 1971.

350. Ranson SW: Degeneration and regeneration of nerve fibers. J Comp Neurol 22:487-546, 1912.

351. Reid DAC: Experience of a hand surgery service. Br J Plast Surg 9:11-16, 1956.

352. Reid DAC: The neurovascular island flap in thumb reconstruction. Br J Plast Surg 19:234-244, 1966.

353. Reid RL, Werner J, Sunstrum C: Preliminary results of sensibility re-education following repair of the median nerve. Am Soc Surg Hand, Newsletter 15, 1977.

354. Remensnyder JP: Physiology of nerve healing and nerve grafts, in Krizek TJ, Hoopes JE (eds): *Symposium on Basic Science in Plastic Surgery*. St. Louis: CV Mosby, 1976, Ch 24.

355. Renfrew S: Fingertip sensation: A routine neurological test. Lancet 1:396-370, 1969.

356. Renfrew S, Melville ID: The somatic sense of space (choraesthesia) and its threshold. Brain 83:93-112, 1960.

357. Ridley A: A biopsy study of the innervation of forearm skin grafted to the fingertip. Brain 93:547-554, 1970.

358. Ridley A: Silver staining of nerve endings in human digital glabrous skin. J Anat 104:41-48, 1969.

359. Ridley A: Silver staining of the innervation of Meissner corpuscles in peripheral neuropathy. Brain 91:539-552, 1968.

360. Rivers WHR, Head H: A human experiment in nerve division. Brain 31:323-450, 1908.

361. Roland PE: Asterognosis: Tactile discrimination after localized hemisphere lesions in man. Arch Neurol 33:543-550, 1976.

362. Rorabeck CH, Clarke KM: The pathophysiology of the anterior tibial compartment syndrome: An experimental investigation. J Trauma 18:229-304, 1978.

363. Rosen JM, Kaplan EN, Jewett DL, et al: Fascicular sutureless and suture repair of the peripheral

nerves: A comparison study in laboratory animals. Orthop Rev 8:85–92, 1979.

364. Rosenberg G: Effect of age on peripheral vibratory perception. J Am Geriatr Soc 6:471–481, 1958.

365. Rothschild NMV: *A Classification of Living Animals*. New York: John Wiley & Sons, 1961.

366. Ruch TC, Fulton, JF, German WJ: Sensory discrimination in monkey, chimpanzee and man after lesions of parietal lobe. Arch Neurol Psychiatry 39:919–938, 1938.

367. Rumpf J: Ueber exinem Fall von Syringomjlie nebst Beitragen zur Untersuchung der Sensibilitat. Neurol Centralbl 8:183–190, 222–230, 1890.

368. Rydel A, Seifer W. Untersuchungen ueber das Vibrationsgefuhl oder die sogenannte Knochensensibilitat (Pallasthesie). Arch Psychiatr Nervenkr 37:488–536, 1903.

369. Sakellarides H: A follow-up study of 173 peripheral nerve injuries in the upper extremity of civilians. J Bone Joint Surg 44A:140–148, 1962.

370. Salisbury RE, Taylor JW, Levine NS: Evaluation of digital escarotomy in burned hands. Plast Reconstr Surg 58:440–443, 1976.

371. Sanders FK: Histopathology of nerve grafts, in Seddon HJ (ed): *Peripheral Nerve Injuries*. London: Her Majesty's Printing Office, 1954, pp 134–155.

372. Sanders FK, Young JZ: The influence of peripheral connections on the diameter of regenerating nerve fibers. J Exp Biol 22:203–212, 1947.

373. Sanders FK, Young JZ: The role of the peripheral stump in the control of fibre diameter in generating nerves. J Physiol 103:119–136, 1944.

374. Satinsky, D, Pepe FA, Liu CN: The neurilemma cell in peripheral nerve degeneration and regeneration. Exp Neurol 9:441–451, 1964.

375. Santoni-Rugiu P: Experimental study on reinnervation of free grafts and pedicle flaps. Plast Reconstr Surg 38:98–104, 1966.

376. Saxod R: Developmental origin of the Herbst cutaneous sensory corpuscle: Experimental analysis using cellular markers. Dev Biol 32:167–178, 1973.

377. Schlenker JD, Kleinert HE, Tsai T: Methods and results of replantation following traumatic amputation of the thumb in sixty-four patients. J Hand Surg 5:63–70, 1980.

378. Schneider RJ, Kulis AT, Ducker TB: Proprioceptive pathways in the spinal cord. J Neurol Neurosurg Psychiatry 40:417–433, 1977.

379. Seddon HJ: Methods of investigating nerve injuries, in Seddon HJ (ed): *Peripheral Nerve Injuries*. London: Her Majesty's Stationery Office, 1954, pp 1–15.

380. Seddon HJ: Nerve grafting and other unusual forms of nerve repair, in Seddon HJ (ed): *Peripheral Nerve Injuries*. London: Her Majesty's Printing Office, 1954, pp 389–417.

381. Seddon HJ: *Surgical Disorders of the Peripheral Nerves*. Baltimore: Williams & Wilkins, 1972.

382. Seddon HJ: The use of autogenous grafts for repair of large gaps in peripheral nerves. Br J Surg 35:151–167, 1947.

383. Seddon HJ, Medawar PB, Smith H: Rate of regeneration of peripheral nerves in man. J Physiol 102:191–215, 1943.

384. Shaffer JM, Cleveland F: Delayed suture of sensory nerves of the hand. Ann Surg 131:556–563, 1950.

385. Silver A, Montagna W, Versaci A: The effect of denervation on sweat glands and Meissner Corpuscles of human hands. J Invest Dermatol 42:307–324, 1964.

386. Silver A, Versaci A, Montagna W: Studies of sweating and sensory function in cases of peripheral nerve injuries of the hand. J Invest Dermatol 40:243–258, 1963.

387. Siminoff R: Quantitative properties of slowly-adapting mechanoreceptors in alligator skin. Exp Neurol 21:290–306, 1968.

388. Simpson SA, Young JZ: Regeneration of fiber diameter after cross-unions of visceral and somatic nerves. J Anat 79:48–64, 1944.

389. Smith HR: The ultrastructure of the human haarscheibe and Merkel cell. J Invest Dermatol 54:150–159, 1970.

390. Smith J: Microsurgery of peripheral nerves. Plast Reconstr Surg 33:317–329, 1964.

391. Smith JR, Bom AF: An evaluation of fingertip reconstruction by cross-finger and palmar pedicle flaps. Plast Reconstr Surg 35:409–418, 1965.

392. Smith KR: The structure and function of the Haarscheibe. J Comp Neurol 131:459–474, 1967.

393. Snow JW: The use of a volar flap for repair of fingertip amputations: A preliminary report. Plast Reconstr Surg 40:163–168, 1967.

394. Spencer PS, Schaumberg HH: An ultrastructural study of the inner core of the Pacinian corpuscle. J Neurocytol 2:217–235, 1973.

395. Spindler H, Dellon AL: Results of electrodiagnostic studies in a well-defined population of peripheral compression neuropathies, in press 1981.

396. Spinner M: *Injuries to the Major Branches of the Peripheral Nerves of the Forearm*, ed 2. Philadelphia: WB Saunders, 1978.

397. Stopford JSB: An explanation of the two-stage recovery of sensation during regeneration of a peripheral nerve. Brain 49:372–386, 1926.

398. Stopford JSB: *Sensation and the Sensory Pathway*. London: Longsmans, Green, 1930, Ch XI.

399. Straille WE: Sensory hair follicles in mammalian skin: The tylotrich follicle. Am J Anat 106:133–148, 1960.

400. Strauch B, Tsur H: Restoration of sensation to the hand by a free neurovascular flap from the first web space of the foot. Plast Reconstr Surg 62:361–367, 1978.

401. Stromberg WB, McFarlane RM, Bell LL, et al: Injury of the median and ulnar nerves. J Bone Joint Surg 43A:717–730, 1961.

402. Sturman MJ, Duran RJ: Late results of fingertip injuries. J Bone Joint Surg 45A:289–298, 1963.

403. Sunderland S: Capacity of reinnervated muscles to function efficiently after prolonged denervation. Arch Neurol Psychiatry 64:755–771, 1950.

404. Sunderland S: Funicular suture and funicular exclusion in repair of several nerves. Br J Surg 40:580–587, 1953.

405. Sunderland S: *Nerves and Nerve Injuries*, ed 2. Edinburgh: Churchill-Livingstone, 1978.

406. Sunderland S: Rate of regeneration in human pe-

ripheral nerves. Arch Neurol Psychiatry 58:251–295, 1947.

407. Sunderland S: The pros and cons of funicular nerve repair. J Hand Surg 4:201–211, 1979.

408. Swanson AB, Goran-Hagert C, Swanson GD: Evaluations of impairment of hand functions, in Hunter JM, Schneider LH, Mackin EJ, et al (eds): *Rehabilitation of the Hand*. St Louis: CV Mosby, 1978, Ch 4.

409. Symns JLM: A method of estimating the vibratory sensation, with some notes on its application in diseases of the central and peripheral nervous system. Lancet 1:217–218, 1918.

410. Talbot WH, Darian-Smith I, Kornhuber HH, et al: The sense of flutter-vibration: Comparison of the human capacity with response patterns of mechanoreceptive afferents from the monkey hand. J Neurophysiol 31:301–334, 1968.

411. Tallas R, Staniforth P, Fisher TR: Neurophysiological studies of autogenous nerve grafts. J Neurol Neurosurg Psychiatry 41:677–683, 1978.

412. Terui A: Reinnervation in the free skin graft. Jpn J Plast Reconstr Surg 18:392–399, 1975.

413. Terzis JK: Functional aspects of reinnervation of free skin grafts. Plast Reconstr Surg 58:142–156, 1976.

414. Thompson JS: Free hypothenar full-thickness grafts for distal digital defects. Johns Hopkins Med J 145:126–130, 1979.

415. Thomson JL, Ritchie WP, French LO: A plan for care of peripheral nerve injuries overseas. Arch Surg 52:557–570, 1946.

416. Tilney F: A comparative sensory analysis of Helen Keller and Laura Bridgman: Mechanisms underlying sensorium. Arch Neurol Psychiatry 21:1227–1269, 1929.

417. Tomson WB: The general appreciation of vibration as a sense extraordinare. Lancet 2:1299, 1890.

418. Torebjork HE, Hallin RG: Perceptual changes accompanying controlled preferential blocking of A and C fiber responses in intact human skin nerves. Exp Brain Res 16:321–332, 1973.

419. Treitel L: Arch Psychol Bd, 29:633, 1897. Cited by Merzenich MM: Some observations on the encoding of somesthetic stimuli by receptor populations in the hairy skin of primates, doctoral dissertation. Baltimore: Johns Hopkins Univ (Physiol), 1968, pp 145–179.

420. Trotter WM, Davies HM: Experimental studies in the innervation of the skin. J Physiol 38:134–246, 1909.

421. Trotter WB, Davies HM: The peculiarities of sensibility found in cutaneous areas supplied by regenerating nerves. J Psychol Neurol 20:102–131, 1913.

422. Truex RC, Carpenter MB: *Human Neuroanatomy*, ed 5. Baltimore: Williams & Wilkins, 1964, pp 149, 203–212.

423. Tsatsos C: Address by His Excellency, President of the Hellenic Republic, to the Institute of Management Science, Athens, Greece, July 1977, quoted by Conomy JP, Barnes KL, Cruse RP: Quantitative cutaneous sensory testing in children and adolescents. Cleve Clin Q 45:197–206, 1978.

424. Turnbull F: Radial-medial anastamosis. J Neurosurg 5:562–566, 1948.

425. Valentin G: Ueber die Dauer der Tasteindrucke. Arch Physiol Heilk 11:438–478, 587–621, 1852.

426. Vallbo AB, Hagbarth KE: Activity from the skin mechanoreceptors recorded percutaneously in awake human subjects. Exp Neurol 21:270–289, 1968.

427. VanBuskirk C, Webster C: Prognostic value of sensory defect in rehabilitation of hemiplegics. Neurology 5:407–411, 1955.

428. Vierck CJ Jr, Jones MB: Size discrimination on the skin. Science 163:488–489, 1969.

429. Vinograd A, Taylor E, Grossman S: Sensory retraining of the hemiplegic hand. Am J Occup Ther 5:246–250, 1962.

430. von Frey M: Beitrage zur Physiologie des Schmerzsinns, Ber Sachs Ges Wiss 46:283–296, 1894.

431. von Frey M: Beitrage zur Physokogie zur Sinnesphysiologie der Haut, III. Ber Sachs Ges Wiss 47:166–184, 1895.

432. von Frey M: Physiologische Versuche uber das Vibrationsgefuhl. Biol 65:417–427, 1915.

433. von Frey M: The distribution of afferent nerves in the skin. JAMA 47:645–648, 1906.

434. von Frey M: Untersuchungen über die Sinnesfunktionen der menschlichen Haut. Abh Sächs Ges (Akad) Wiss 40:175–266, 1896.

435. von Prince K, Butler B Jr: Measuring sensory function of the hand in peripheral nerve injuries. Am J Occup Ther 21:385–395, 1976.

436. Wall P, Dubner R: Somatosensory pathways. Annu Rev Physiol 34:315–336, 1972.

437. Wallace AA: The damaged digital nerve. Hand 7:139–144, 1975.

438. Wallace WA, Coupland RE: Variations in the nerves of the thumb and index finger. J Bone Joint Surg 57B:491–494, 1975.

439. Waller A: Experiments on the section of the glossopharyngeal and hypoglossal nerves of the frog, and observations of the alterations produced thereby in the structure of their primitive fibers. Philos Trans R Soc Lond 140:423–429, 1850.

440. Walsche FMR: The anatomy and physiology of cutaneous sensibility: A critical review. Brain 65:45–112, 1942.

441. Walton R, Finseth F: Nerve grafting in the repair of complicated peripheral nerve trauma. J Trauma 17:793–796, 1977.

442. Weber E: Ueber den Tastsinn. Arch Anat Physiol, Wissen Med Muller's Archives 1:152–159, 1835.

443. Webster HF: The relationship between Schmidt-Lantermann incisures and myelin segmentation during Wallerian degeneration. Ann NY Acad Sci 122:29–38, 1965.

444. Webster N: *The Living Webster Encyclopedic Dictionary*. Chicago: English Language Inst of America, 1975.

445. Weckesser EC: The repair of nerves in the palm and the fingers. Clin Orthop 19:200–207, 1961.

446. Weckesser EC: *Treatment of Hand Injuries*. Chicago: Western Reserve Press, 1974.

447. Weddell G: Multiple innervation of sensory spots in skin. J Anat 75:441–446, 1941.

448. Weddell G: Nerve endings in mammalian skin. Biol Rev 30:159-195, 1955.

449. Weddell G, Guttmann L, Guttmann E: The local extension of nerve fibres into denervated areas of skin. J Neurol Neurosurg Psychiatry 4:206-225, 1941.

450. Weddell G, Palmer E, Palli W: Nerve endings in mammalian skin. Biol Rev 30:159-195, 1955.

451. Weddell G, Sinclare DC: "Pins and Needles": Observation on some of the sensations aroused on a limb by the application of pressure. J Neurol Neurosurg Psychiatry 10:26-46, 1947.

452. Weddell G, Sinclair DC, Feindel WH: Anatomical basis for alterations in quality of pain sensibility. J Neurophysiol 11:99-109, 1948.

453. Weeks PM, Wray RD: Management of Acute Hand Injuries. St Louis: CV Mosby, 1973, pp 302-303.

454. Weeks PM, Wray RC: Management of Acute Hand Injuries: A Biological Approach, ed 2. St. Louis: CV Mosby, 1978.

455. Weiland AJ, Villarreal-Rios A, Kleinert HE, et al: Replantation of digits and hands: Analysis of surgical techniques and functional results in 71 patients with 86 replantations. J Hand Surg 2:1-12, 1977.

456. Weinstein S: Tactile sensitivity in the phalanges. Percept Mot Skills 14:351-354, 1962.

457. Werner G, Mountcastle VB: Neural activity in mechanoreceptive afferents: Stimulus-response relations, Weber functions, and information transmission. J Neurophysiol 28:359-397, 1965.

458. Werner JK: Tropic influence of nerves in the development and maintenance of sensory receptors. Am J Phys Med 53:127-142, 1974 (68 references).

459. Werner JK, Omer GE Jr: Evaluating cutaneous pressure sensation of the hand. Am J Occup Ther 24:347-356, 1970.

460. Whitesides TE, Haney TC, Harado H, et al: A simple method for tissue pressure determination. Arch Surg 110:1311-1313, 1975.

461. Whitsel BL, Petrucelli LM, Ha H, et al: The resorting of spinal afferents as antecedent to the body representation in the post-central gyrus. Brain Behav Evol 5:303-341, 1972.

462. Whitsel BL, Petrucelli LM, Sapiro G, et al: Modality representation in the lumbar and cervical fasciculus gracilis of squirrel monkeys. Brain Res 15:67-78, 1969.

463. Wilgis EFS, Maxwell GP: Distal digital nerve grafts: Clinical and anatomic studies. J Hand Surg 4:439-443, 1979.

464. Williamson RT: The vibratory sensation in diseases of the nervous system. Am J Med Sci 164:715-727, 1922.

465. Winkelmann RK: Effect of sciatic nerve section on enzymatic reactions of sensory end-organs. J Neuropathol Exp Neurol 21:655-657, 1962.

466. Winkelmann RK: Nerve Endings in Normal and Pathologic Skin. Springfield: Charles C Thomas, 1960.

467. Winkelmann RK, Breathnach AS: The Merkel cell. J Invest Dermatol 60:2-15, 1973.

468. Woltman HW: Neuritis associated with acromegaly. Arch Neurol Psychiatry 45:680-682, 1941.

469. Woltman HW, Wilder RM: Diabetes mellitus: Pathologic changes in the spinal cord and peripheral nerves. Arch Intern Med 44:576-603, 1929.

470. Wong WC, Kanagastuntheram R: Early and late effects of median nerve injury on Meissner's and Pacinian corpuscles in the hand of the macaque (M. fascicularis). J Anat 109:135-142, 1971.

471. Woodhall B, Beebe GW: Peripheral Nerve Regeneration—A Follow-Up Study of 3635 World War II Injuries. Washington, DC: US Govt Print Office, 1956, p 309.

472. Woolard HH, Weddell G, Harpman JA: Observations on the neurohistologic basis of cutaneous pain. J Anat 74:413-419, 1940.

473. Woolsey CN: Organization of somatic sensory and motor areas of cerebral cortex, in Harlow HF, Woolsey CN (eds): Biological and Biochemical Basis of Behavior. Madison: Univ Wisc Press, 1958.

474. Yahr MD, Beebe GW: Recovery of motor function, in Seddon HJ (ed): Peripheral Nerve Regeneration. Washington DC: US Govt Printing Office, 1956, Ch III, pp 71-202.

475. Young VL, Wray CR, Weeks PM: The results of nerve grafting in the wrist and hand. Ann Plast Surg 5:212-215, 1980.

476. Zachary RB: Results of nerve suture, in Seddon HJ (Ed): Peripheral Nerve Injuries. London: Her Majesty's Stationary Office, 1954, Ch VIII, pp 354-388.

477. Zachary RB, Holmes W: Primary suture of nerves. Surg Gynecol Obstet 83:632-651, 1946.

478. Zaleski AA: Regeneration of taste buds after transplantation of tongue and ganglia grafts to the anterior chamber of the eye. Exp Neurol 35:519-528, 1972.

479. Zalewski AA: Combined effects of testosterone motor, sensory or gustatory nerves on reinnervation of taste buds. Exp Neurol 24:285-297, 25:29-37, 1969.

480. Zollman PE, Winkelmann RK: The sensory innervation of the common North American raccoon (Procyon lotor). J Comp Neurol 119:149-157, 1962.

INDEX